American Medical Association
Physicians dedicated to the health of America

The
Continuing
Professional
Development
of
Physicians

From Research
to Practice

Edited by
Dave Davis, MD
Barbara E. Barnes, MD
Robert Fox, EdD

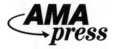

The Continuing Professional Development of Physicians: From Research to Practice

AMA Press
Vice President, Business Products: Anthony J. Frankos
Publisher: Michael Desposito
Director, Production and Manufacturing: Jean Roberts
Senior Acquisitions Editor: Suzanne Fraker
Project/Developmental Editor: Anne Serrano
Director, Marketing: John Kinney
Marketing Manager: John Kinney
Senior Production Coordinator: Rosalyn Carlton
Senior Print Coordinator: Ronnie Summers

Internet address: www.amapress.com

This book is for informational purposes only. It is not intended to constitute legal or financial advice. If legal, financial, or other professional advice is required, the services of a competent professional should be sought.

Additional copies of this book may be ordered by calling 800-621-8335 or visiting www.amapress.com. Mention product number OP230503

ISBN 1-57947-403-9
BP17:02-P-064:5/03

Library of Congress Cataloging-in-Publication Data

The continuing professional development of physicians : from research to practice / Dave
  Davis, Barbara E. Barnes, Robert Fox, editors.
    p. cm.
  Includes bibliographical references and index.
  ISBN 1-57947-403-9
  1. Medicine--Study and teaching (Continuing education) 2. Physicians--In-service
training. 3. Medical personnel--In-service training. I. Davis, David A., M.D. II. Barnes,
Barbara E., M.D. III. Fox, Robert D.

R845.C66 2003
610'.71'5—dc21
                                                                          2003045239

ACKNOWLEDGMENTS

The editors express our thanks to our patient family, hard-working staff members, and the many thought leaders and colleagues in the discipline of physician continuing professional development who have supported the creation of this book.

Thanks also go to the AMA Press staff members who worked on the book: Suzanne Fraker, Fred Donini-Lenhoff, John Kinney, Anne Serrano, Rosalyn Carlton, and Ronnie Summers.

CONTENTS

FOREWORD

The editors, Dave Davis, MD, Barbara E. Barnes, MD, and Robert Fox, EdD, are leaders in the field of what was formerly called continuing medical education, now expanded to the continuing professional development (CPD) of physicians They have assembled a virtual who's who of CPD researchers and practitioners to discuss the elements directors of CPD programs need to understand.

The book takes a forward look at the field, discarding the term *continuing medical education*, which all too frequently connotes only lecture presentations. The concept of CPD, which has been adopted by the American Medical Association, greatly expands what physicians can do with the help of educational experts to provide optimal patient care. To clarify the linkages between the world of the educator and the world of the medical practitioner, the book uses case studies or clinical thematics. To my knowledge, this book represents the first attempt to discuss and assess most of the activities that medical education directors should consider as they enter the expanding field that strives for better physician performance.

There is an excellent discussion of the forces that are changing the practice of medicine and how these affect directors of CPD. Such forces as the aging population, managed care, advances in medical science, and evolving changes in the physician workforce are definitely affecting the approach to lifelong learning. The authors strongly encourage directors to consider the needs of the patient population in addition to the specific needs of the practicing physician.

Elements that can affect a physician's performance, such as feedback from chart audits, HMO data, and state and federal databases, are also discussed. Providing physicians with performance feedback by comparing their results with those of others is a powerful tool for improving physician behavior. The importance of physicians reflecting on their clinical experience to direct their study is emphasized, and specific examples of ways to help the self-directed learner are useful.

The value of self-assessment programs, learning contracts, and portfolios of learning will be of special interest to directors. How to gain the most from large- and small-group teaching activities is carefully described, with attention to faculty development by improved lecture presentations, integration of case examples in courses, application of the most effective educational technology, and inclusion of small-group discussions in large-group programs.

Many methods of improving health care and physicians' performance have little or nothing to do with formal education, but improvements are often best accomplished by implementation of organizational changes within a hospital or office practice. The remarkable advances in information technology have created many new models to help the physician use the best scientific approaches in patient care. Reminder systems that can be built into an electronic medical record should prevent many errors of omission. Directors of CPD must always evaluate not only the performance of physicians they serve but their own as well. This type of evaluation ranges from satisfaction to actual assessment of how a teaching activity has changed the health status of patients or the health of the population at large. The methods of evaluation described in this book should be valuable to directors of physician education.

I enjoyed reading the manuscripts that led to the final version of this all-inclusive book and I was pleased that the authors took the broad view of lifelong learning for physicians. I approve their recommendation that we no longer think of continuing medical education as limited to a lecture-room activity and that we broaden the approaches to helping physicians improve the care they deliver. All who are dedicated to assisting physicians in lifelong learning and improving health care are indebted to the editors and the contributors for their forward look in describing the expanding techniques that will help physicians offer their patients optimal health care.

Phil R. Manning, MD
Paul Ingalls Hoagland-Hastings Foundation
Professor of Continuing Medical Education
Keck School of Medicine
University of Southern California, Los Angeles

Barbara E. Barnes, MD, MS, received her BS degree in psychology from the University of Maryland and her MD degree from the Pennsylvania State University. She is Assistant Vice Chancellor for Continuing Education in the Health Sciences and Associate Dean for Continuing Medical Education at the University of Pittsburgh.

Dave Davis, MD, is Associate Dean for Continuing Education and leader of the knowledge translation program for the Faculty of Medicine, University of Toronto. A family physician and health services researcher, he has had a 25-year career devoted to understanding physician learning and the effectiveness of continuing medical education.

Robert Fox, EdD, is currently Professor of Adult and Higher Education at the University of Oklahoma in Norman. He teaches masters and doctorate students in theory and research related to continuing professional development and instructional strategies in adult and higher education.

ABOUT THE CONTRIBUTORS

Geoffrey M. Anderson, MD, PhD, is a Professor in the Department of Health Policy, Management and Evaluation, Faculty of Medicine, University of Toronto where he is the Liberty Health Chair of Health Management Strategies and a senior adjunct scientist at the Institute for Clinical Evaluative Sciences. His research is focused on developing and testing ways to understand and improve health care performance.

Mary Carol Badat, MAd Ed, received her BS degree in psychology from the University of Illinois at Champaign and her MEd in adult education from the National Louis University. Since 1999, she has been manager of Online CME at the American Academy of Pediatrics, engaged in developing and implementing an online learning system for pediatricians.

Nancy L. Bennett, PhD, is the Assistant Dean for Continuing Education at Harvard Medical School. Her primary interests center on the professional development of those in health care.

Adalsteinn (Steini) D. Brown, DPhil, is Assistant Professor in the Department of Health Policy, Management, and Evaluation, Faculty of Medicine, at the University of Toronto, and principal investigator for the Hospital Report 2001 Series. He is an adjunct scientist at the Institute for Clinical Evaluative Sciences in Ontario and an honorary lecturer in the Department of Epidemiology and Biostatistics and an instructor in the Department of Family Medicine at the University of Western Ontario.

Craig Campbell, MD, is a specialist in internal medicine and an Associate Professor of medicine in the Faculty of Medicine at the University of Ottawa, Ontario, Canada. Dr Campbell serves as the Deputy Chair, Education, in the Department of Medicine at the University of Ottawa and is Director Professional Development of the Maintenance of Certification Program of the Royal College of Physicians and Surgeons of Canada.

Linda Casebeer, PhD, is Associate Professor and Associate Director of Continuing Medical Education at the University of Alabama School of Medicine, Birmingham. Her work focuses on translating biomedical research into practice.

Robert M. Centor, MD, is Professor of Medicine and Associate Dean of Primary Care and of Continuing Medical Education of the University of Alabama School of Medicine, Birmingham. He is a general internist and chief of the Division of General and Internal Medicine, with special research interests in medical decision-making and effective teaching methodologies.

Karen Costie, RN, a registered nurse with more than 15 years of clinical experience, is president of Professional Development Associates. Her professional work has focused on health care education research and continuing professional development of physicians.

Charles P. Friedman, MD, is Professor of Medicine, Associate Vice Chancellor for Biomedical Informatics, and Director of the Medical Informatics Training Program at the University of Pittsburgh. He has a longstanding research interest in the uses of information technology to improve education across the health professions and the continuum of professional practice.

Mark H. Gelula, PhD, is Director of Faculty Development and Research Assistant Professor of Medical Education and Adjunct Assistant Professor of Psychiatry at the University of Illinois at Chicago College of Medicine. As Director of Faculty Development for the College of Medicine, he is responsible for organizing college-wide faculty development strategies and subsequent programs; he also directs and teaches the Faculty Development Fellowship.

S. Tunde Gondocz, MSc, received her BA degree in psychology from Chatham College, Pittsburgh, and her MSc degree in health administration and planning from the University of British

Columbia, Vancouver. She has been instrumental in developing and evaluating the Maintenance of Competence (MOCOMP®) Program, and since 1998, has been manager of the Office of Professional Development at the Royal College of Physicians and Surgeons of Canada.

Joseph S. Green, PhD, is Associate Dean for Continuing Medical Education at the Duke University School of Medicine and Clinical Associate Professor in the Department of Community and Family Medicine. Dr Green has been involved in continuing medical education and continuing professional development for nearly 30 years in positions within the Veterans Administration Health Care System, the Association of American Medical Colleges, the University of Southern California School of Medicine, and Sharp HealthCare in San Diego, California.

R. Van Harrison, PhD, is an Associate Professor in the Department of Medical Education and Director of the Office of Continuing Medical Education at the University of Michigan Medical School. He is currently on the editorial board of the *Journal of Continuing Education in the Health Professions*, a reviewer for the journals *Medical Care* and *Academic Medicine*, a reviewer for the annual Research in Medical Education Conference of the Association of American Medical Colleges, and an accreditation reviewer for the Accreditation Council for Continuing Medical Education.

Marcia J. Jackson, PhD, Education Division Vice President at the American College of Cardiology, oversees administration of and assists with the strategic leadership of the the American College of Cardiology. She is President of the Alliance for Continuing Medical Education, a member of the Task Force on CME Provider/Industry Collaboration, as well as a member and former chair of the Monitoring Committee of the Accreditation Council for Continuing Medical Education.

Penny A. Jennett, PhD, is head of the Health Telematics Unit, professor of community health sciences, and previous director of the Office of Medical Education in the Faculty of Medicine, University of Calgary. Recognized internationally for her expertise in continuing medical education, telehealth, health telematics, health informatics, health education, and program evaluation, she serves as Vice-Chair of the Board of Netera; is President-Elect, Treasurer, and a founding member of the Canadian Society of Telehealth; and is a member of the Board of CANARIE Inc.

Robert E. Kristofco, MSW, is Associate Professor and Director of Continuing Medical Education at the University of Alabama School of Medicine, Birmingham. He has been involved in academic continuing medical education for the past 20 years.

James C. Leist, EdD, recently retired from the faculty and administration at Wake Forest University School of Medicine (formerly Bowman Gray School of Medicine), where he served as an Associate Professor of Community Medicine in the Department of Family and Community Medicine and Associate in Medical Education. Dr Leist is the part-time Co-Director of Faculty Development in the Department of Community and Family Medicine at Duke University School of Medicine and a part-time staff member for the Alliance for Continuing Medical Education.

Jocelyn Lockyer, PhD, is Director of Continuing Medical Education and Professional Development and an Associate Professor of Community Health Sciences, Faculty of Medicine, University of Calgary. Dr Lockyer has served on the Alliance for Continuing Medical Education Board and assumed leadership roles for many Alliance for CME, Society of Academic CME, and Association of Canadian Medical Colleges committees.

Karen V. Mann, PhD, is Professor and Director of the Division of Medical Education at Dalhousie University. She serves on the editorial boards of *Medical Education* and the *Journal of Continuing Education in the Health Professions* and is involved in faculty and curriculum development and education research.

Phil R. Manning, MD, a career-long advocate for individualized learning based on practice analysis to determine educational deficits of physicians, has been active in continuing medical education for 47 years. He is the Paul Ingalls Hoagland-Hastings Foundation Professor of Continuing Medical Education at the Keck School of Medicine, University of Southern California, Los Angeles.

Paul E. Mazmanian, PhD, serves as Associate Dean for Continuing Medical Education. He is a professor in the Department of Preventive Medicine and Community Health, Virginia Commonwealth University.

Donald E. Moore, Jr, PhD, is currently Director, Division of Continuing Medical Education, and Associate Professor in the Department of Medical Administration at Vanderbilt University School of Medicine in Nashville, Tennessee. Dr Moore received his PhD in education from the University of Illinois at Urbana-Champaign.

John Parboosingh MB, is Professor Emeritus of Obsterics and Gynecology and former Associate Dean of Continuing Medical Education at the University of Calgary. In 1993 he established the Maintenance of Competence (MOCOMP®) Program at the Royal College of Physicians and Surgeons of Canada where he served as Director of Professional Development from 1998 to 2001. Dr Parboosingh is a consultant to PediaLink™, the American Academy of Pediatrics' recently developed knowledge management program.

Linda Raichle, PhD, is Associate Director of Academic Affairs at Merck & Company, Inc, where she directs the development and implementation of strategies for continuing medical education initiatives for multiple therapeutic areas. She is Chair of the Pharmaceutical Alliance for Continuing Medical Education, a special interest section of the Alliance for CME, and serves as a member of the AMA's Task Force on Continuing Medical Education.

Lynne Sinclair, BSc (PT), MA (Ad Ed), is the Associate Chair of the University of Toronto, Department of Physical Therapy, where she is also the Academic Coordinator of Clinical Education and the Graduate Coordinator for the MScPT Program.

Dennis K. Wentz, MD, joined the American Medical Association in 1988 as director of the Division of Continuing Medical Education (now the Division of Continuing Physician Professional Development). He now serves as the AMA staff representative to the ACCME.

Douglas L. Wooster, MD, is Chief of Vascular Surgery at St Joseph's Health Centre and an Associate Professor of Surgery at the University of Toronto. He is Chair of the Standards Committee of the Royal College of Physicians and Surgeons of Canada; serves on the boards various surgical societies in Canada and the United States; and is the coordinator of the Vascular Self-Evaluation Program and section editor for CME on the VascularWeb site of the joint societies.

A Clinical Thematic

Dave Davis, MD; Robert Fox, EdD;
Barbara E. Barnes, MD; Karen Costie, RN

John Premi, one of the contributors to *The Physician as Learner: Linking Research to Practice*[1] and a participant in the consensus processes that led to this book, once said, "It all begins in the clinical encounter," meaning, of course, that continuing professional development (CPD) is grounded in medical practice. The true beneficiaries of this book therefore are our clients' clients—physicians' patients and communities. To keep us mindful that the purpose of CPD is to improve individual and population health, we have created a clinical thematic that is threaded throughout the book. Although individual chapters employ vignettes and cases that exemplify specific issues, the clinical thematic weaves together the core concepts of the book and, perhaps more clearly than in any other way, demonstrates the true purpose of the CPD professional's task.

For the purposes of this book, we take the word *thematic* to mean a central motif or framework in which the topics of each chapter can be applied. We have chosen a clinical thematic as the chief way by which we can ground the theory and practice of CPD in order to achieve at least two purposes. First, for our readers who are physicians or other health professionals, the thematic will prompt reflection on the connection between patient care and education. The use of a clinical scenario will help them to understand the relevance of the research and practice of CPD to day-to-day clinical care. Second, for educators, the clinical theme provides a window into the clinical realities that physicians face on a regular basis. Educators, like health care professionals, may use the issue-generation component of the case to prompt internal reflection, either alone or in a group learning setting.

The case may also serve as a basis for bringing CPD professionals and clinicians together to develop common ground relative to vocabulary and shared understanding of how physicians learn and change. In some ways, the thematic can be seen as a bridge between the world of the educator and the world of the clinician. That is our purpose in constructing it.

We have written the clinical thematic as though it were an unfolding case, a technique called *progressive disclosure*, which attempts to simulate the way in which clinical issues present, develop, and unfold in clinical practice. Like all such simulation, this one may appear artificial at first. However, it is our hope that as the reader progresses through the book, the scenario becomes progressively more realistic. Further, there are many elements to this case. By introducing the reader to them sequentially, we will attempt to weave them together in a coherent manner—dealing with the context in which the CPD professional practices, his or her ability to determine where and how to start the CPD process, the development of educational and other interventions, and, finally, the determination of success. The case, that of a diabetic patient, appears at the beginning of each major section, reinforcing previous material and introducing the material that follows.

You might ask, "Why this case? Why diabetes?"

Diabetes met several disease-based criteria: it is commonplace (the American Diabetic Association indicates 4% of the adult population suffer from diabetes); it affects many organ systems and is therefore rich in its clinical context; it has both acute and chronic components that may be managed in a variety of settings—primary, secondary, and tertiary care; and it demonstrates both individual and population health issues. These characteristics are prototypical of the major causes of morbidity and mortality in North America such as atherosclerosis, cancer, arthritis, and Alzheimer's disease.

We also had several educational criteria in constructing the clinical case. First, it had to be broad enough to cover knowledge, skills, and attitudes as exemplified in prevention and management. Second, like most diseases and medical conditions, it had to exist in both the biomedical and the psychosocial realm, with implications for learning from the molecular/cellular level, through the personal and psychological, and finally to the family and community. Third, it had to be sufficiently commonplace to allow readers and learners in all professions to be familiar with the disease. Finally, it had to represent a field with advancing medical knowledge, requiring that physicians remain abreast of current recommendations for management. We felt that diabetes met all of these criteria.

Let us begin with an introduction to the case.

The Clinical Scenario

Ms Marjory Hall is a 58-year-old self-employed accountant who has noticed increasing fatigue, weight loss, and thirst for several weeks. An independent woman, she has ignored most of these symptoms (she has even been happy with the weight loss) and has not taken time off work to visit her physician. She realizes that she must now seek medical care, since she has started to note some worrisome deterioration in her vision, an important consideration for her job. She is motivated to take care of herself because she is the sole support to her grand-daughter, age 9. However, she is concerned about how she will pay the medical bills if she does have a serious condition because her health insurance does not cover most outpatient services or prescriptions.

Dr Ted Brucken, age 42, is a graduate of a large central US medical school with a traditional undergraduate curriculum and teaching methods. He subsequently trained in family medicine in San Francisco before settling back home in a suburban community in the Pacific Northwest. He is a relatively senior member of the Mountainside Medical Group, a primary care association of family physicians, internists, pediatricians, and obstetricians. Ted has a busy practice, seeing mostly adult women and men, with a few children and teenagers thrown in for good measure. He no longer does obstetrics, having found that the increased workload afforded him little time for family or other hobbies and pursuits.

The Mountainside Medical Group is affiliated with the Central-North HealthCare System, an integrated delivery network composed of a tertiary medical center and several community hospitals. Although Dr Brucken and his colleagues are generally happy with their practice arrangements, the mix of the patients, and the community in which they practice, they are increasingly frustrated by requirements promulgated by insurers, governmental agencies, and the quality assurance committee at the local hospital. Declining reimbursement is causing them to extend office hours and decrease the time spent with each patient. Dr Brucken formerly had a volunteer faculty appointment with the University of the Northwest Medical School. Several medical students per year did clinical rotations in the office and the physicians routinely attended grand rounds and other CPD activities at the medical school's campus. However, the practice administrator no longer allows physicians to take time out of the office and they stopped taking students because the physicians see fewer patients per hour when they are teaching. Dr Brucken realizes that he has not attended a formal CPD activity in several months and is concerned about how he will prepare for his mandatory board recertification examination in two years. He also notices that the pile of unread journals on his desk is getting higher and higher. Ted knows that there have been many new recommendations for taking care of the common problems he sees in the office but is not sure if he is incorporating these into his practice. He even wonders if it is worth learning about these new developments; many insurance programs will not pay for some of the new, expensive medications or other interventions.

THIS CASE IN THE CONTEXT OF CPD

Even before the clinical encounter with Ms Hall has occurred, it is obvious that Dr Brucken will have to take into account a number of factors as he constructs a professional development plan that will help him care for her problem. Although the practice of medicine is centered in the patient–physician relationship, care is delivered in the context of societal needs and systems of delivery (Figure I-1). The core competencies established by the Accreditation Council for

FIGURE I-1

The Patient–Physician Relationship is developed in the Context of Societal Imperatives and Systems of Care

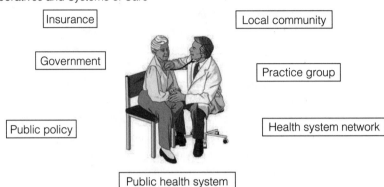

Graduate Medical Education (www.acgme.org/outcome) and adopted by the American Board of Medical Specialties address the skills required to function in this larger framework. In addition to possessing an appropriate body of medical knowledge, physicians must be able to effectively communicate with their patients, improve their practice through CPD activities and continuous quality improvement processes, understand the needs of not only each individual patient but also the community and society in which they practice, work with the organizations that deliver and regulate health care, and adhere to acknowledged professional standards. The needs that drive CPD, methods used to deliver education, and criteria on which learning is evaluated must therefore reflect these diverse dimensions. In order to conceptualize how these factors can be incorporated into the practice of CPD, it is helpful to look at a physician's professional development from four different perspectives: the patient, the physician, the system of care delivery, and community and societal interests.

The Patient

The first issue, and one we would argue is the most important to address, is the patient, in this case, an independent, self-directed professional who must manage her illness in the context of her family responsibilities. We recognize that—with some exceptions explored here and throughout the book—the patient is *not* the client of the CPD professional. Nonetheless, Dr Brucken must understand what information and skills are required by Ms Hall to manage her illness. Her insurance plan, for example, may not cover prescriptions, and so Ted may need to discuss various management options, reviewing the costs and benefits of different therapies.

Marjory's ethical values and her family situation and cultural beliefs will also determine the strategies employed to control her disease.

The Physician

The second issue revolves around the physician. Dr Brucken's learning activities will be shaped by his learning styles and preferences, the setting in which he practices, patient–physician communication strategies, and his motivation to change. Having trained in a medical school with a traditional curriculum, he may feel more comfortable learning in a didactic, large-group setting rather than a problem-based discussion group. However, given the pressure for clinical productivity in his office, Ted might be driven to consider self-study venues. He may notice that he is always the first one in his group to try a new therapy and wonder why his colleagues are not as willing to incorporate innovations into their practice.

The System of Care Delivery

The third issue relates to the clinical context in which these two elements come together. They refer to the characteristics of Dr Brucken's practice setting: its patient demographics, organizational and administrative structure, and fiscal incentives and disincentives. The increased complexity of health care delivery and financing demands that physicians make decisions not only in the context of their patients' needs and preferences but also according to the directives of their practice group, hospital, health network, and third-party payers. Dr Brucken must see more patients in order to assure that his group is profitable, providing a barrier to attending grand rounds and teaching students in his office. The increased focus on ambulatory care means that he has less opportunity to interact with consultants in the hospital. When prescribing diagnostic tests or medications for Marjory, he must consider not only what is medically indicated and what she might prefer but also the tests and pharmaceutical products covered by her insurance company. He also likely receives data on his performance compared to others in his group or hospital department that identifies areas of subpar performance, triggering the development of a learning plan.

Community and Societal Interests

Fourth and finally, the broader community or population in which the patient and physician exist requires consideration. Dr Brucken must be aware of the prevalence of disease in the population that he serves. If his community is experiencing a large influx of immigrants from Southeast Asia, he might have to learn more about

Hepatitis B or other infectious diseases. He is also subject to regional (eg, state), national, and specialty society requirements for maintenance of competency and reporting of medical errors. Ted may realize that his license may not be renewed if he lacks the required number of continuing medical education credits. Although he has little interest in dermatology and routinely refers these patients to a colleague in his office, he may need to attend a course in this area in order to prepare for a recertification exam.

SUMMARY

It is against this framework that the three major sections or elements of the book are projected, represented in diagrammatic form (Table I-1). We have chosen to leave the cells blank in order that, at each step, the reader may insert notations, questions, or points of learning about the issues to be studied or points to be applied.

The first section of the book addresses the questions: What is the first step in planning for CPD activities and programs? How can we determine what to do in the context of CPD? These questions are addressed against the framework presented by Ms Hall, Dr Brucken, the Mountainside Medical Group, and the community in which they exist—from the broadest, population perspective, down to the picture presented by the physician and his patient. The second section of the book presents an interventionist perspective, addressing issues of developing and implementing CPD activities. Although these CPD methods are described by the type of activity, eg, those targeted to groups of physicians or those that use educational technologies, each must be considered in the context of the patient, physician, clinical setting, and community in order to have relevance. Finally, the third section of the book presents a schema by which we can assess the impact of CPD interventions.

TABLE I-1

Schematic Overview of the Book in the Context of Clinical Practice

	Patient	Physician	Clinical Context	Community
Determining what to do				
Developing CPD activities				
Evaluating outcomes				

In this section, perhaps more than in any other, a consideration of the clinical context affecting the outcomes of CPD interventions is helpful. Each of these areas is represented in Table I-1.

These three sections are prefaced by two chapters attempting to "set the stage" on which the case for the continuing professional development of physicians is made. The first of these addresses the domain of CPD itself in its structure, issues, and evolution. The second chapter paints a broader picture, outlining external (and internal) forces affecting the shape and future of CPD.

REFERENCE—INTRODUCTION

1. Davis DA, Fox RD, eds. *The Physician as Learner: Linking Research to Practice.* Chicago, Ill: American Medical Association; 1994.

chapter 1

The Horizon of Continuing Professional Development: Five Questions in Knowledge Translation

Dave Davis, MD; Robert Fox, EdD; Barbara E. Barnes, MD

A news reporter's questions—who, what, when, where, why, and how—are familiar in the description of most events. And a book, despite its solid, three-dimensional nature, is an event in its own right. We will use these questions to our own purposes, introducing this book about continuing medical education (CME) and continuing professional development (CPD) and about the translation of knowledge into practice.

We have divided this chapter into five parts to answer the following questions:

- What do CME, CPD, and knowledge translation mean?
- Why a book on this subject?
- For whom is it written?
- How did it come to be? and
- Where and how does it apply?

WHAT DO CONTINUING MEDICAL EDUCATION AND CONTINUING PROFESSIONAL DEVELOPMENT MEAN?

About a dozen books, perhaps a hundred monographs, and thousands of articles touch on the subject of CME and CPD, and the issues related to physician or health professional learning and their outcomes. In contrast, relatively few publications relate specifically to the subject of turning the knowledge acquired by these processes into performance change.

Some Definitions

Continuing Medical Education

A recent American Association of Medical College's statement about CME provides us with a holistic definition, as follows:

> "Continuing medical education is a distinct and definable activity that supports the professional development of physicians and leads to improved patient outcomes. It encompasses all the learning experiences that physicians engage in with the conscious intent of regularly and continually improving their performance . . . . "[1]

Despite this holistic and comprehensive definition, it seems to us that, perhaps because of the commonplace nature in medicine of the acronym CME, it is the "gestalt" or the picture of the term *CME* that truly carries the day. Physicians most often see CME in quite narrow and constraining ways, usually as the lecture-based experience in a resort or hotel. As a result, most physicians still conjure up images of darkened meeting rooms with slides presented by a distant speaker, a picture eloquently described by George Miller in the 1960s.[2] Some individuals equate the term *CME* with the credit system itself, for example, by using the phrase, "don't forget to sign up to get your CMEs."

None of this picture, however, seems to capture the essence of the continuous learning of physicians in their quest to maintain competence and provide quality health care for their patients, perhaps calling for a new name.

Continuing Professional Development

In the context of attempting to change physician behavior, a further, and perhaps more holistic, term has come into common use in the United Kingdom, Australia, Canada, and in parts of the United States: *CPD* or *continuing professional development*. Derived from the fields of CME and continuing professional education, CPD, as outlined by Stanton and Grant,[3] includes educational methods beyond the didactic, embodies concepts of self-directed learning and personal development, and considers organizational and system factors.

Apart from the still-pervasive narrower picture of CME described earlier, we prefer the term *CPD* for three reasons. First, it establishes greater content depth, encompassing not only the narrower clinical dimensions of cardiology or infectious disease (what Miller calls a categorical content model[2]) but also the broader field of practice management, ethical decision-making, evidence-based care, managed care principles, and other, broader aspects of medical practice.

Second, the formats conjured by the phrase *CPD* appear to us to be more comprehensive than those that arise from considering CME. Perhaps because of the relative newness of the term, we see

CPD as being the umbrella for all sorts of interventions, not just the traditional conference or mailed material. In this area, CPD more easily encompasses other learning formats such as reminders, audit and feedback, academic detailing, and Web-based guidelines.

Third, the difference between CME and CPD for us resides in the venue of the learning or setting of the educational intervention. CME, still in its traditional mode, makes us think of the lecture hall or conference room, often miles, both physically and symbolically, from the real practice setting. On the other hand, CPD can be seen more readily to occur in practice settings, as well as other learning sites, the nearer to the practice setting as possible. Further and perhaps more importantly, CPD reflects the variety of independently developed and managed learning activities that make up the development of a competent practitioner. The phrase more accurately reflects this observation: the theme in adult learning that has emerged over the past 25 years, beginning with Knowles,[4] that adults learn independently of teachers and in a manner that is closely tied to their experience. The term *CPD* ties the study and practices of facilitating learning to the broader concepts of CPD and adult learning. In this sense, it situates the learning in the learner, perhaps the ultimate venue in which CPD may occur.

We can conceptualize the difference between CME and CPD in a three-dimensional matrix (Figure 1-1), using the three sets of issues we have just described. Although there are lots of ways to conceptualize this field, the following highlights the differences for us between the two definitions. In this diagram, the first axis deals with the educational content issue, a second with the formats of CME and CPD, and the third with setting of the educational development, learning, or change intervention. Using this matrix, it is easy to see that CME subsumes a smaller area, marked in dark gray, compared to its much larger and more holistic cousin, CPD.

Throughout this book, we will use the broader term *CPD* to describe the processes outlined above.

The Translation of Knowledge into Practice

Whatever we call it, the subject matter of CME and CPD is clearly important: it focuses, after all, on the longest and clearly the most complex phase of education related to physicians, and perhaps other health professionals, as they struggle with the issues of providing optimal health care. The subject is also clearly broad and rich.

The final piece in this puzzle derives from a consideration of the purpose of CPD. In this context we maintain that the term *knowledge translation* is a term more frequently used as the outcome of CPD.

With increasing regularity in health services research, this term has come to mean the transfer of knowledge to the practitioner or

F I G U R E   1-1

A Diagrammatic Comparison of CME and CPD

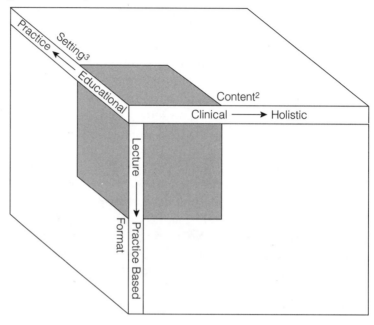

Notes:

1) CME is shown by the shaded area.

2) Content ranges from the purely clinical to more holistic topics such as ethics, practice management.

3) Setting refers to the venue of the learning—ranging from the traditionally educational (eg, the lecture hall or conference room) to practice settings.

the health system in such a way that it becomes imbedded in performance and therefore, ultimately, in health care outcomes. In this construct, knowledge is digested and set in order so that practice and its outcomes are changed or maintained. Knowledge translation in our context implies more than direct application and assumes a process of reformulation and interpretation—translating a scientific finding into a conclusion, into an interpretation, into an invention or principle, into a practice, into an interaction, or into an outcome. Each of these reflects the need by the clinician to adjust the information to fit the uniqueness and conflict endemic in the context of application.

We see two ways of understanding this phenomenon: the conceptual or theoretical and the practical, using an example from recent CME experience. We believe these examples will help the readers to translate CPD theory and principles into a more holistic and effective application of the concepts.

The first example comes from the area of guideline dissemination, an attempt to consolidate and disseminate clinical information

FIGURE 1-2

Knowledge Creation to Health Care Outcomes Process

Knowledge creation/ research ➡	Distillation, review of findings, publications, clinical application of research (eg, guidelines development) ➡	Dissemination of guidelines, other data ➡	Implementation of optimal practice ➡	Improved practitioner performance and health care outcomes

in such a way that practitioners can readily use it in clinical decision-making. Figure 1-2 outlines a simplistic and highly stylized view of the knowledge creation-to-application model, outlining several steps.

The first step, the creation of knowledge, resides with basic and applied health science researchers, whose task, once discoveries are made and validated, is to publish their findings, most often in peer-reviewed journals. The second step, made necessary for today's clinicians by the sheer volume of such publications, involves the review and distillation of these findings in ways that practitioners can use, generally referred to as clinical practice guidelines, or CPGs. Although not without their critics, CPGs are intended to be "systematically developed statements . . . used to aid practitioner and patient decisions."[5] This work resides in the clinical domain, driven by the efforts of clinical epidemiologists and others and often supported/encouraged by such groups as the Cochrane Collaborative,[6] national specialty societies, and the evidence-based medicine (EBM) movement itself.

The third phase, the dissemination of guidelines, has occupied national specialty societies, among other groups, using the print medium almost exclusively. To a lesser extent, CME providers have offered venues such as conferences, conventions, and rounds to disseminate these findings.

Studies of the fourth step have been widely neglected. Apart from a few systematic efforts to incorporate guideline-derived knowledge into practice undertaken by quality improvement initiatives, most outcomes-oriented educational interventions have derived from research-funded health services initiatives. Further, there exists no concerted, central repository of studies and activities aimed at this critical element of the implementation of critical knowledge into practice. This "macro process" in guideline dissemination and adoption is parallel, we hold, to the more "micro" process we refer to as *knowledge translation*. Further deficiencies in understanding the fourth step derive from our failure to apply models of the dissemination of knowledge to practice, as described by Rogers;[7] Bennis, Benne, and Chin;[8] or Fox.[9]

Understanding this expanding notion of the outcomes of education, the broadened role of CME and CPD, and their place in "translating" knowledge into practice, might also be helped by the example provided below.

CME and CPD and HIV-AIDS: A Case Study

The sudden rise of a new clinical entity—HIV and AIDS—in the 1980s provided instruction for the field of CME and CPD. Seen from its clearly biological and therapeutic perspectives, CME providers were quick to respond to the call for courses, rounds, and other methods to disseminate knowledge about this disease and its clinical diagnosis and management. We can be quite confident that hundreds of such events were held, virtually worldwide in the first decade of the disease, from basic sciences research symposia to primary care meetings and workshops. Although clearly necessary, and of impact to those physicians and researchers engaged in fighting this disease, it is apparent to us that the wide scope of HIV and AIDS could have been better served by applying the concepts of CPD.

Such a process would have considered nonclinical aspects of the disease (eg, ethical issues, communication about sexual behavior and risk factors, attitudes toward and relationships with disenfranchised or uninsured patents and populations), the formats of the educational interventions (addressing the issue that not all physicians attend conferences and, if they do attend, may not identify the need in this area), and the location of these interventions—the clinical practice setting, home, or community clinic—instead of, or in addition to, the conference hall.

WHY A BOOK ON CME, CPD, AND KNOWLEDGE TRANSLATION?

There are several clusters of reasons behind the writing of this book, apart from those that are expressed in Chapter 2. They may be—in parallel with our understanding of clinical knowledge translation—seen across a continuum ranging from the academic or theoretical to the practical needs of the CPD professional.

Earlier we alluded to the large number of publications, monographs, texts, and journal articles that have filled the educational and clinical literature about CME, CPD, health professional learning, and change. And there are, just as in CME itself, a wide variety of other methods, from traditional courses and conferences, such as those held by the Society for Academic CME or the Alliance for CME, to the many articles that address questions of importance to the field of CME. These are regularly found in key medical—educational journals, including the *Journal for Continuing Education in the Health Professions (JCEHP), Medical Education, Academic*

Medicine, and *Teaching and Learning in Medicine*. With somewhat more difficulty (given problems with keyword listing and subsequent searching or retrieval), editors of clinical journals have shown an increased willingness to publish articles of clinical relevance but that address the continuing education of clinicians. Largely fugitive until two decades ago, much of this literature now resides in a computerized database called the *Research and Development Resource Base in Continuing Education*. This database, described in detail elsewhere,[10] resides at the University of Toronto (www.cme.utoronto.ca/RDRB) and is supported by the University of Toronto Academic Development Fund in Continuing Education, the Society for Academic CME, the Alliance for CME, and the American Medical Association. However, storing information and distilling and synthesizing information are two entirely different processes, yet both are important to the field. It is clear to us that the fields of CPD and, earlier, CME have failed to do so.

And although failures and shortcomings are unpleasant to contemplate, they can provide effective ways to learn about and change how researchers and practitioners of CPD work, especially in terms of generating and using new knowledge. We see several areas for consideration and have attempted to address them in this book.

First, over the last decade, researchers in CME (the branch of CPD that applies to medicine) have been more effective at generating more knowledge but less effective at generating useful knowledge. The lessons to be learned and the changes that must be made to correct this imbalance are difficult but essential to the future of CPD. They require that we change the way we approach the research and practice of CPD if we are to be more effective at facilitating learning and change. This is the work of researchers and change agents who use knowledge to make a difference in the ways physicians practice and the ways patients live.

Second, the enterprise responsible for the CPD of physicians has a problem: there is a growing gap between the work of those who study the field and the work of those who use knowledge about CPD in practice. Research has not changed the practice of CPD very much, and the practice of CPD has not appeared to change research in the field. That is partly because practitioners and researchers have different perspectives on the needs of the field. Most of those who work in this field are engaged in the practice of educating and facilitating planned change. We believe that CPD professionals want studies that will guide them through everyday problems of practice rather than studies that address broad areas of interest or respond to conceptual curiosities. CPD professionals want useful guidance and tools that support their decisions. CPD professionals wish to simplify their work and increase their feelings of confidence in their actions. They also want direct and clear suggestions to come from research. These practitioners want information when they need it, not "just-in-time" learning but timely guidance, the purpose of this book.

Third, to a remarkable level, there has been a misperception of the role of CPD professionals. Because they are accountable for their actions and because their actions contribute to the health of the public, their priorities are these: more time, more fiscal support, and more recognition for providing high-quality learning experiences to physicians. Earlier theoreticians and scholars in CPD may have been misdirected in their belief that CPD professionals needed to become more "academic" and intellectual; time, practicality, and other pressures do not permit this phenomenon.

Fourth, translating theory into practice requires a process that incorporates planned, developmentally oriented systems and processes that foster the integration of interpretation and application based on the relationships among practice problems and research findings. The corporate world speaks about research and development, only rarely referring to research without considering its uses. The field of CPD suffers from separate discussions about research and practice, neglecting intelligent conversations about the development of research into practice. Innovations must be disseminated systematically through a process that assures applicability, quality, and ongoing evaluation. If we are to effectively translate theory to practice and improve the way we facilitate the teaching and development of physicians, we need a new and strong dissemination instrument—a further role for this book.

In addition, a system must be built around the research knowledge base that allows a place for the scholarly practitioner. We have failed to develop this concept as fully as we should. A more robust way of viewing CPD allows for the role of scholarship in every CPD activity. To the extent that the book's chapters are based on literature and encourage readings on the part of the CPD professional, this goal, too, can be attained.

Finally, and as a result of the earlier issues, the field of CPD suffers from the following phenomenon: few bridges span the huge gulf from theory to research on physician learning to practice. The product of most CME providers, however innovative and responsive to adult learner needs, remains inadequate. The field neither supports nor encourages better (let alone best) practices; and there is a lack of common conceptual and best practices framework and a strong need for understanding of physician learning and change. Thus, opportunities exist for change in the CPD model, perhaps even more than in older visions of CME: they are neither seized nor used.

This book attempts to bridge that gap.

FOR WHOM IS THIS BOOK DESIGNED?

In some ways, we hope that the previous introductory paragraphs make it apparent to the reader that the book was designed (or not!) for them. Adapting the principles articulated by Sackett and Haynes[11] and others, readers might well ask themselves:

- Is this book based on subject areas or topics of interest to me?
- Do the method, tools, and interventions described in the book apply to my setting?
- Are the theories and concepts applied here of intuitive sense to me?
- Are the sources of evidence used in this book clearly indicated?

We would hope that, based on these principles, most readers would extract, digest, and apply (translate) whatever they read in order to practice and improve outcomes. In fact, and to help this process, we do have specific audiences in mind for this book—one primary and several secondary.

The major target audience for this book is the provider of CME or CPD. These are individuals trained as physicians, other health professionals, and managers who have found themselves associate deans and directors of CME and CPD. They work in a variety of settings such as medical schools, hospitals, specialty organizations, managed care organizations, or commercial units with an interest in changing provider performance. Important but perhaps secondary audiences for this book include, though are clearly not limited to, the following:

- Policy-setters in government, insurance industry, licensing bodies, regulatory agencies
- Researchers in CME, CPD, faculty development, health services, continuing and higher education, adult education
- Managers in health care maintenance organizations, hospitals, and other integrated health systems
- Health professionals themselves. Among the many movements/trends in undergraduate education is the movement toward self-directed learning. This book may help you meet this increasingly important need.
- Educators in medical schools and other training centers.

An International Audience?

A final word in this section about a possible international audience for this book. Although many of the references here stem from a strong North American influence on (some would say bias toward) CME and CPD, we are aware of a clear and powerful movement elsewhere in the world—in the United Kingdom and the rest of Europe, Australia, South America, and elsewhere—to develop and evaluate models of continuing education and CPD delivery. It is our intention that this book be used with that basis and that readers in Australia, Switzerland, Brazil, California, and Ontario feel equally at home in its content.

HOW DID THIS BOOK COME TO BE? WHAT PROCESSES DROVE THE WRITING OF THIS BOOK—CONSENSUS VERSUS EVIDENCE?

In some ways, perhaps in most, the process of writing this book has paralleled the process of our clinical colleagues in their search for the development of practice guidelines. You will recall that there are two basic processes that distill the literature and lead to such statements of care.

The first of these is called *consensus,* a process of gathering together experts (and occasionally consumers and other practitioners) to discuss best practices and to distill what might be called an agreement regarding best methods of providing clinical care. The second of these is evidence-based and reflects the appropriate distillation and synthesis of the best available literature and information of a scientific nature regarding practice principles. Although the two are not mutually exclusive, the methodology and its underlying culture has shifted in medicine toward the use of evidence and away from the opinions of a few experts. The process of developing evidence-based recommendations differs substantially from those used by our clinical colleagues and is referred to elsewhere in this book in sections devoted to research.

And so, CPD has shifted, although with several differences. The field has also held consensus conferences, permitting and encouraging distillations of thought-leaders, based to an increasing extent on the literature.

A good example of this consensus-to-evidence process in CME and CPD comes from observing the Banff and Beaver Creek conferences evolve over a decade and a half. The first of these meetings (in Banff, Alberta, in 1989) produced a statement, shown in Figure 1-3,[12] reflective of the need to leave behind the term *CME* and to move forward in a way that was more holistic and encompassing, reflective of learning, change, and the practice environment. Not in common usage at that time, the phrase *CPD* could well have been applied to the statement in Figure 1-3.

A second consensus meeting held in Beaver Creek, Colorado, in 1992, displayed a more concerted effort to categorize the areas of study in CME and to utilize the literature of the field more widely. Both meetings were co-sponsored and supported by the American

The Banff Summary Statement

The Banff Summary Statement

To be effective, Continuing Medical Education . . . can no longer be seen as a unidirectional delivery system. It must be aware of and responsive to the needs of the practitioner/learner . . . understanding of the principles of adult education, education and cognitive psychology. It must understand, work with, and even begin to direct the realities of practice and health care delivery, including patient forces and the practice environment, and continue to develop the delivery systems of continue education in order that they may be practice-based, appropriate, effective and integrated within the practice and professional life of the physician.

In order to accomplish this goal, it may be that a new phrase is required to describe the vacuum which CME researchers and providers may fill—that between the learner, the practice environment and the educational delivery system.

---

and Canadian Medical Associations and were led by two of us (Robert Fox and Dave Davis). Finally, a third conference, Beaver Creek II, was held in May of 1999, supported solely by the American Medical Association (AMA) and led by this book's editors.

The migration from consensus-based statements to those that derive from evidence is apparent in the process and products of these three conferences, mimicking and in some ways differing from our clinical colleagues. As an example, the first (Banff) document was a much more consensus-based product, articulating the theoretical basis of understanding of CME at the time (the late 1980s). Although this conference did employ the literature to a certain extent, it used a nominal group process to develop a consensus statement about a future research agenda as the nature of CME itself. The outcome emerging from the Beaver Creek conference of 1989 was a book titled, *The Physician as Learner*,[13] published by the AMA in 1994. This book used the literature much more extensively, while employing the consensus-building process evident among its writers and colleagues at the meeting.

In contrast, and further along the continuum of evidence-based practice, this book has taken shape, with several differences from its earlier counterparts. First, the discussion, to which many published researchers and academics in CME were invited, established many useful understandings and constructs of the state of the art of CME. Many of them are included here, referenced and highlighted where possible. Interested in moving both the process and the outcome along so that as much of the field as possible could be represented, the editors chose chapter subjects as well as primary and secondary authors both beyond the Beaver Creek group and within it. This process also recognizes the complex and interdisciplinary world in which CPD exists. And so it is, in many ways, less the individuals (the consensus) and more the evidence (the literature) that drives this text beyond that of its earlier cognate cousins.

Evidence: A Word about the Word

We need to say a couple things at this juncture about the word *evidence*—how our clinician colleagues use it and how we see it being used in continuing professional education and development.

First, in clinical care, health disciplines are interested in such items as the evidence for the effectiveness of new medications or the pre-test probability of a specific investigation. These phenomena, more easily measured and observable than those in the educational realm, lend themselves to testing, often by means of the randomized controlled trial (RCT). In contrast, in CPD, although many RCTs test the complex interventions of continuing education, the degree to which they depend on hard or objective outcomes (eg, prescribing rates or patient length of stay data), limits the interpretability of this trial methodology. Here interpretation and understanding often require qualitative methods to "get inside the head" of the physician or other health professional-learner, or into the health care team or the practice setting, in order to determine what has happened (or not) during the trial and the context in which this has occurred.

Research in CPD is fundamentally different than its clinical counterpart.

Evidence in continuing education comes in a variety of forms, from the RCT to the descriptive study, from those trials using quantitative methods to those that employ qualitative methods, from surveys and interviews, from key informants, and from many other sources. This is not to say that all studies are good studies. Where we can, we will describe those that employ sound, reliable, and valid methods to reach conclusions and indicate means by which the reader can develop and apply his or her own critical appraisal skills.

The Literature: A Word about the Database

We have referred to "the literature" in this section as though it were a readily identifiable and easily searchable phenomenon. It is not. Highly fugitive, existing in many data categories (principally, education and medicine), the literature of CME, CPD, and knowledge translation is difficult to retrieve and in some ways even more difficult to categorize. Since the mid-1980s, much of the literature has been placed into the database called the Research and Development Resource Base in continuing medical education (RDRB/CME) referred to earlier.

WHERE AND IN WHAT WAYS CAN I USE THIS BOOK? HOW IS THIS BOOK DIFFERENT FROM OTHERS?

The Book's Format

The Text

There are several features we have employed in the formatting of this book, making (we think) it more readable and useful:

- *The book's sections:* Although highly nontraditional in scope and content, we have used a traditional educational model to organize and direct our thinking. First, the book opens with an introduction, which includes chapters on forces for change in the health care and educational environment, and this one. Second, a section on needs assessment focuses on the question, How do I determine what needs to be done or changed? Here, authors sequentially focus on the broadest population health perspective, through intermediate steps such as concentrating on the needs of groups of physicians, and finally concentrating on means by which individual learning needs may be determined. The third section outlines the tools for learning and change and describes educational or professional development tools that may be applied to a variety of "target organs." These include individuals, groups of learners, organizations, practices, and communities. Fourth, a subsequent section on evaluation describes in greater detail the question of determining whether interventions have made an impact on physician learning, performance, or health care outcomes. In this section, tools of the trade are described, a categorization of these methods provided, and a sketch of the purposes and roles of evaluation is outlined. Finally, the book includes references to next steps in the application of theory to practice in the field of CPD.

- *A clinical thematic:* In many ways, this book is about CPD and its environment and about the tools of education; however, it is, most importantly, about the patient and population that our clients serve. To facilitate the bridging between the clinical world and that of the educator or CME/CPD provider, each of the book's three sections begins with a patient-centered theme, a progressively disclosing case that outlines the issues that the clinician faces at individual, practice, and community levels. We know that clinicians will derive some educational understanding as a result of this thematic and that educators and health services researchers will derive some understanding of the clinical experience.

- *Cases, vignettes:* We have encouraged authors to include illustrative cases and vignettes in each of the book's chapters to highlight common educational-provider problems, solutions, and issues. Nonclinical, they are meant to provide examples of both common and best practice.

- *Annotated bibliographies:* We have asked each author to generate a short list of those articles, texts, and monographs that they thought were most instrumental to their writing—seminal pieces that helped them construct and understand their work. These pieces, annotated by the authors themselves, form the final section.

- *The chapters:* Finally, to help the reader and to provide a template for the book's contributors, we have attempted to formulate chapter outlines along this pattern:

  - An educational problem or case presentation, called a vignette
  - An exploration of the problem, providing the reader with some delineation of the issues and questions, leading to a synthesis of major themes
  - An attempt to present what evidence has been found to address the question(s) presented, using the literature to explore and expand the issues
  - An application of the evidence, including practical applications, theoretical questions, and, where possible, ethical considerations
  - A presentation of the challenges still faced: what we do not know and what the future might look like, especially concentrating on the role of the CPD professional as he or she faces (and helps shape) this future.

USING THE BOOK

By now, the reader may have thought of several ways in which this book could be used, beyond the temptation to employ it as a door stop or a booster for the CME office projector. Here are several that we envisage:

- To develop an evidence base regarding CME and CPD, enlarging the repertoires of the CME provider
- To create faculty or staff development activities in order that they may become familiar with the "science" of CME, CPD, and knowledge translation. There is a wide variety of these, from the formal to informal, from one-on-one consultation to group teaching sessions.

TABLE 1-1

Using this Book

Application	User			
	Clinician	**CME Provider**	**Manager**	**Researcher**
Understanding theoretical constructs of CPD				
Faculty/staff development				
Developing programs				
Generating research questions and studies				
Assessing the impact of CPD programs/ interventions				

■ To provide material by which health care managers can make intelligent and informed decisions regarding CE provision in order to create the context in which knowledge translation and improved health care outcomes can be realized.

In summary, the context and utility of this book may be portrayed in Table 1-1, a device to end this introduction and one to refer back to as a device to organize its reading.

REFERENCES

1. Bennett NL et al. Continuing medical education: a new vision of the professional development of physicians. *Acad Med.* 2000;75:1167–1172.

2. Miller GE. Continuing education for what? *J Med Ed.* 1967;42:320–326.

3. Stanton F, Grant J. The effectiveness of continuing professional development. In: *The Effectiveness of Continuing Professional Development.* London: Joint Centre for Medical Education, Open University; 1997.

4. Knowles MS, Holton EF, Swanson RA, Holton E. *The Adult Learner: The Definitive Classic in Adult Education and Human Resource Development.* Houston, TX: Gulf Publishing Company; 1998.

5. Institute of Medicine/Committee on Quality of Health Care in America. *Crossing the Quality Chasm: A New Health System for the 21st Century/Committee on Quality Health Care in America.* Washington, DC: National Academy Press, 2001.

6. Bero LA, Grilli R, Grimshaw JM, Harvey E, Oxman AD, Thomson MA. Closing the gap between research and practice: An overview of systematic reviews of interventions to promote the implementation of research findings. The Cochrane Effective Practice and Organization of Care Review Group. *BMJ.* 1998;317:465–468.

7. Rogers EM. *Diffusion of Innovations.* 4th ed. New York, NY: Free Press; 1995.

8. Bennis WG, Benne KD, Chin R, eds. *The Planning of Change.* London: Holt, Rinehart & Winston; 1985.

9. Fox RD. Using theory and research to shape the practice of continuing professional development. *J Contin Educ Health Prof.* 2000;20:238–246.

10. Taylor-Vaisey A. Information needs of CME providers: research and development resource base in continuing medical education. *JCEHP.* 1995;274:700–705.

11. Haynes RB, McKibbon KA, Fitzgerald D, Guyatt GH, Walker CJ, Sackett DL. How to keep up with the medical literature: 1.Why try to keep up and how to get started. *Ann Intern Med.* 1986;105:149–153.

12. McMaster University. *Banff Monograph.* Hamilton, Ont: McMaster University Faculty of Health Sciences Press, 1987.

13. Davis D, Fox R, eds. *The Physician as Learner: Linking Research to Practice.* Chicago, Ill: American Medical Association; 1994.

chapter 2

Forces for Change in the Landscape of CME, CPD, and Health Systems-Linked Education

Dennis K. Wentz, MD; Marcia J. Jackson, PhD; Linda Raichle, PhD; Dave Davis, MD

INTRODUCTION

Consider how rapidly the major scenarios and players have altered the delivery of care in the United States. Only 9 years ago, forces related to physician accountability, universal accessibility to care, and cost containment were pushing the United States toward a nationalized system of health and medical care, a system proposed by the Clinton Administration. Now, at the start of the twenty-first century, it is important to note that this proposed nationalized system never materialized and may never do so, arguing articulately and clearly for a separate, related, and potent force in health care—the political forces of society. In its place has arisen a pluralistic system of group practices, managed care organizations, independent practice organizations, preferred provider organizations, government programs such as Medicare and Medicaid, to name only a few—all driven by cost issues. These are some of the factors that impact on physicians' practices and relate to their subsequent learning, as well as the education and practice of the team members with whom they work.

What are these attending factors? How have they shaped the delivery of continuing medical education and the continuing professional development of physicians? What might the future hold in this arena?

In the United States, managed health care was embraced in the 1990s by business and government to an unprecedented degree as a solution to the soaring costs of medical care. This free-market approach penetrated every aspect of health care—from individual physician practice, to hospitals (especially the nation's teaching hospitals and academic medical centers), to the organization of practice, to patients, and to its impact on practitioner motivation, morale, and learning. An American Medical Association (AMA) survey in 1998 revealed that 92% of physicians had a contract or some sort of a relationship with a managed care organization.[1]

These economic and practice issues are not confined to the United States. Sizable forces of economic and political change regularly stir the health care delivery systems of Canada, the United Kingdom, the European Community, Australia, and elsewhere.[2] Although the many examples in this chapter focus on American experiences, we attempt to use other, worldwide experiences where they exist in the literature. The issues range from the costs of the health care system, to increasing societal concern about the quality of the physicians in practice, to the size of the physician workforce, to ensuring universal access to comprehensive health care, and to measurement of performance and medical outcomes. The end result has an impact on continuing medical education (CME).

During the last decade, on a worldwide basis, we have observed sizable changes in the health care environment and, at the same time, constancy in many aspects of the setting and delivery of health care and its educational system. Wentz and colleagues in *The Physician as Learner* published in 1994, addressed the powerful environmental forces for change at that time.[3] These forces continue to drive the health care environment in the United States, Canada, the United Kingdom and Australia, and elsewhere.[3] Because these forces have a major impact on physician behavior, they drive change in the environment facing CME and the continuing professional development (CPD) of physicians, as CME/CPD attempts to stay relevant to physicians' learning needs and practices.

FIGURE 2-1

A Conceptual View of Forces Affecting The Provision of CME and the Practice of CPD

	Personal/Social Forces	Health Care Forces
M A C R O	**Societal Forces**	**Professional Forces**
M I C R O	**Personal/Learner Forces**	**CME/CPD Provider Forces**

This chapter reviews some of these issues in order to provide an appropriate background for reading, interpreting, and incorporating the ideas and concepts outlined in this book. It looks at some of these forces for change in the CME and CPD environments from several perspectives, using the broad conceptual model for change outlined by Fox and colleagues in their study of physician learning and change.[4] By adapting these forces from the "micro" perspective of the physician-learner to the more "macro" forces affecting the provision of practice education and the translation of knowledge into practice, we believe that an understanding of these forces is an important attribute for physicians and health professionals, their CME providers, and managers in health care systems. These forces include:

I.   Societal forces that impact the health professions and the delivery of health care

II. Professional forces that operate within the practice of medicine and the allied disciplines

III. Forces that operate in the provision or delivery of CME and CPD

IV. Forces generated by the health professional as learner.

We recognize, however, that this is a highly artificial classification, and many forces slip readily from one category to another. We have conceptualized these forces as a two-by-two table (Figure 2-1): the macro forces (societal and professional) represent the top half of the square, the more micro forces (learner and CME provider) the lower half. In general, the macro forces are more powerful and provide considerably more influence than those we have characterized as micro. However, there are many exceptions, and a true working knowledge of these four areas, or forces, for change requires an understanding of their interplay. This diagram may help that process.

SOCIETAL FORCES

Physicians, other health care professionals, and the delivery of health and medical care do not exist in a vacuum. Rather, they are subject to a myriad of forces, both indirect and direct, that exert their influences on society as a whole.

Indirect Influences: The Changing Face of Society

Although many societal forces are at play, perhaps none has more significance for health care than this: The population of developed nations is aging rapidly and, simultaneously, the average life expectancy continues to rise.[5] Related to this is clear evidence that a large and probably increasing percentage of disease, morbidity, and mortality relates to personal behaviors that are therefore largely preventable.[6]

Thus, the US Department of Health and Human Services, in its year 2000 blueprint for health care titled "Healthy People 2010," highlights 10 areas to be measured as a "report card" on health status. These areas, intended to guide the nation toward better health, include physical activity, overweight status and obesity, tobacco use, substance abuse, mental health, injury and violence, immunization, responsible sexual behavior, environmental quality, and access to health care.

Koplan and Fleming, of the US Centers for Disease Control and Prevention, recently challenged physicians and health care professionals to think boldly and proactively about how today's actions and lack of actions, which will be regarded decades from now, in terms of what could have been changed for the better: "In the decades ahead—in our lifetimes—physicians and public health professionals have both a responsibility and an unprecedented opportunity to apply our current knowledge to improve the health of the nation."[7] The authors later added overpopulation and global environmental degradation to the list of public health challenges.

Other societal forces for change in the delivery of health care and continuing education exist. While the ethnic, socioeconomic, and cultural diversity of American, Canadian, British, and other populations changes rapidly, this change has received scant attention from physicians or health care organizations.[8] Another major issue is the health literacy of patients and the public. The migration of individuals from vastly different cultures, as well as the active out-migration of travelers of an expanding business or tourist nature, has caused a steady and marked increase in the prevalence of infectious diseases.[9,10] Only partly related to the rise and treatment, not only is HIV infection and the full-blown disease of AIDS of epidemic proportion in many parts of the world, Ebola virus, West Nile fever, polio and others have crossed oceans. With a growing threat and likelihood of bioterrorism (eg, the 2001 anthrax attack in the United States) and growing fears about smallpox, bubonic plaque, and other infectious diseases, these areas must become subject matter for CME providers.

Each issue translates into other contexts or subject matter for CME—geriatric care and the care of chronically ill individuals, preventive medicine, health education of the public, population health issues, and other multicultural health issues, among a myriad of others. These issues dictate that CME providers equip themselves to help physicians deal with lifelong CPD. Subjects for CME must include improving learners' communication skills; understanding and applying the principles of health promotion and prevention in busy practice settings; and increasing knowledge of health economics.

Fluency in statistics may be as important as the ability to provide clinical diagnoses and medical care.

Direct Influences: Society's Impact on the Health Care Professions

Societal or population forces have a direct impact on the shape, nature, and delivery of health care. The environment for medical care itself is caught directly in and reflective of turbulent change in many areas, most often the product of social forces.

There are many issues involved. Health economist, Ian Morrison, has pointed out several key driving forces in the reshaping of health care and CME.[11] Among the most important are the growing public discontent with current health care practices and the subsequent emergence of what he terms a "reluctantly empowered consumer." Clearly, this movement to consumerism in health care exists. It is fed by rising education levels, relentless media coverage of health issues, proliferation of direct-to-consumer advertising, systems of "tiering" of benefits, and increased rationing of access (either by denying the choice of health care provider or by a system of queuing to obtain desired care). It is made more complex by a strong interest by many patients in alternative and complementary health care practices and self-care.

These forces, of course, have a direct impact on health care provision and, as a result, on CME and CPD. Teaching physicians to deal with these issues calls upon the trio of components of competency: knowledge about patient concerns and issues; skills in dealing with patients fairly, openly, and in a shared manner; and, most importantly and with the most difficulty, attitudes.

PROFESSIONAL FORCES

We conceive of three separate but equal strands in the cord of professional forces affecting CME/CPD providers and their clients, ie, health practitioners. They are continuing new developments in science and technology; the integration of the Internet into practice and education; and changes in health systems and the workforce, including health care financing, systems for continuous performance measurement, and regulatory forces.

Developments in Science and Technology

Genetics
Developments in science and technology continue to advance medical practice dramatically and will certainly increase. A leading example comes with the completion of the Human Genome Project

in 2003. As a result, medicine will eventually be armed with better information to treat genetic disorders, knowledge with the real potential to lead to new treatments, genetic-mediated pharmaceuticals, and other interventions.[12]

The response to this genetic revolution is substantially split along two lines. On the one hand, many scientists and scholars argue that genetic manipulation to alter the course of, or possibly even eliminate, certain chronic diseases will be commonplace. It is possible that this type of innovation will not only lead to a higher quality of life but also provide tangible improvements to the general health and even economic status of populations. Exactly which institutions will disseminate this information to practicing physicians remains in doubt, as does the nature and scope of the educational exercise itself. The revolution could represent a new opportunity for academic medical centers that emphasize "translational" research, converting new knowledge into the knowledge base and skill sets of daily practice.

On the other hand, global public response to advances in genetics reflects fears about mishandling of the technology as well as the fundamental beliefs about such issues as the creation of life and the definition of *human and organ regeneration,* to name a few. Thus, it is clear that physicians will face ethical dilemmas as they advise patients, and that patient education and the securing of informed consent will be a major challenge. Further, these forces, like those of the consumerism movement outlined earlier, require not only the knowledge of this genetic revolution but also an understanding of patient beliefs and values and an attitude of shared decision-making. Peter Singer, in the edited series on bioethics in the *Canadian Medical Association,* indicates that "bioethics is not an esoteric pursuit removed from . . . everyday practice, but rather bioethics is in the background of every encounter between physicians and patents and families."[13]

Advances in Science and Information Distribution

Advances continue to occur in the science and technology of health care. Although not part of the purview of this book, advances as imaging technology, for example, enable physicians to examine the functionality of organs without surgery. Further, miniaturized devices have expanded the opportunities for replacing traditional open surgeries with minimally invasive surgical techniques.

The largest single force for change that we envisage, however, comes from the field of informatics, the Internet, and the World Wide Web. A National Academy of Science report concluded that medicine has been slower than other industries to adopt and use new information technology.[14] Many now see the promise of the Web but also note the lack of an information technology infrastructure.

Information and communication technology will, within this decade, have the capacity to transform medicine in several critical ways. We outline six of them here: 1) the automation of office logistics and procedures; 2) the adoption of electronic patient records; 3) the creation of platforms for online outcomes research; 4) improvements in the systems for telemedicine, telemetry, and distance education; 5) increased access to information and educational materials via the Internet; and 6) information delivered to the doctor at point of patient need, "just-in-time" information for informed patient management. So transformative is the potential of the Internet that a survey of government and the Internet called for "digital democracy," symbolic of the new environment engendered by this technology.[15]

Changes in Physician Workforce and Health Systems

There are changes in the once relatively constant physician workforce in every country, producing changes in the production of physicians on a worldwide basis. A comparison between Canada and the United States illustrates this powerful phenomenon.

In the American health care marketplace, the supply of physicians continues to grow, outpacing the growth of the US population.[16] While the enrollment at allopathic medical schools in the United States has actually stabilized or decreased, there are several new osteopathic medical schools. Additional physicians in the United States also come from the large number of international medical graduates who successfully complete accredited residency programs. Moreover, particularly in the United States, the demographic characteristics of the physician population are changing. Not only is the proportion of physicians approaching retirement age increasing, many are opting for early retirement. Societal moves to increase the number of primary care physicians and decrease the number of specialists also have had an effect. More recently, a serious concern is emerging about the wisdom of that strategy, as specialist shortages are felt around the country.[17]

In Canada, the federal government reduced the amount of money available to provinces for health care in the 1990s. Provinces, in turn, have set up a strict control process for the number of graduate medical education training slots, leading to country-wide physician shortages. Recognizing the problem, provinces like Ontario have recently increased enrollments, but the pipeline is long and new graduates will not enter the workforce until at least 2006–2007. In the European Union, large numbers of physicians are being trained in some countries; these physicians are unable to find specialist training or maintain their medical careers. Migration of these physicians to other EU countries, which is permitted under the treaties in place, is a source of anxiety. The entrance requirements, specific training, knowledge bases, and professional expectations still differ greatly from country to country.

In the United States, to the extent that government programs such as Medicare and Medicaid embrace managed care plans, it is likely that more health care services will be provided by nonphysician providers, specifically nurse practitioners and physician assistants. The number of nonphysician providers is rapidly growing, and their scope of practice is expanding, often by legislative mandate.[18] There is evidence that industry is now directing significant marketing dollars to these nonphysician providers in recognition of their role as influencers of therapy choices and their importance in patient compliance with treatment regimes.

Hospital consolidation and restructuring is a phenomenon occupying health care managers in virtually all developed nations. In the United States, the number of operational hospital beds has decreased markedly, from a high of slightly more than 1 million in 1983 to just above 850,000 in 1999. In another significant development with at least some impact for CME/CPD, the hospital occupancy rate has dropped to 62% while the ratio of employees to beds has increased.[19] In part, this reflects the fact that more patients are treated in outpatient settings and those entering or remaining in the hospital tend to be sicker and require more intensive care. There is also a move to identify "Centers of Excellence" because the growing literature shows that high-volume hospitals have lower mortality rates than low-volume hospitals for certain conditions.[20] Internationally, hospital restructuring has proceeded along similar lines, most frequently with a view to reduce labor expenses through the redesign of job descriptions, especially in nursing. This has translated into new job definitions, decrease in numbers of registered nurses, and changes in the skill mix of many nursing tasks, often leading to complete reorganization of care at the clinical care level, rarely if ever with any systematic study of outcomes.[21]

Finally, the move to push health care into the community by means of ambulatory care clinics, primary care offices, and home care has implications for undergraduate education. Most medical schools and even residency programs are scrambling to find new ways to teach basic clinical skills, because patients often enter the hospital only for select procedures and complicated care. This push also has implications for the provision of CME and the continuing professional development of physicians. A new specialty of "hospitalist" physician is emerging, while many doctors are increasingly ambulatory and community based. Again, changes in the delivery system of CME are needed.

Health Care Expenditures

In this section, we explore the effect of health care financing issues at four levels: the national level, local levels (including managed care), the level of academic health science centers, and the actual practice site for the patient-physician encounter.

First, despite increasing concern and attention, health care expenditures continue to grow as a percentage of the gross national domestic product; this is occurring most rapidly in the United States. It is certain that physicians will continue to face further pressure to reduce health care costs, creating ethical and financial dilemmas for physicians as they struggle to provide appropriate health care services to patients.

In most countries, there are at least two faces to the financial crunch in health care. On the one hand, futurist Leland Kaiser says that, with finite resources, society will need to limit its expenditures on health care by some kind of rationing, either implicit or explicit.[22] However, a free market approach to control costs that favored managed care and similar systems has clearly not worked. In 1999, the California Medical Association predicted bankruptcy for up to 90% of physician organizations in the state because of the financial collapse of two of the largest physician-practice management companies, in turn leaving more than $100 million in unpaid bills to these physicians.[23]

Second, at the level of the integrated care system, the question exists, at least in the United States: Can managed care exist without raising prices as the costs of care increase? This question raises the possibility of creating instability for patients and physicians and increasing the likelihood of new initiatives for some sort of universal coverage plan. Is it possible, as some have commented, that the managed care movement that led to most of these changes in the environment "will soon be rubble?" An article in the *Wall Street Journal* discusses the investor rebellion faced by major insurers now operating managed care plans, appropriately titled "In Boom Times, Managed Care is a Bust!"[24]

Coupled with this instability is the fact that under the current market-driven health care system, the number of Americans without health insurance continues to increase (to more than 41 million) while those who are still insured are paying a larger portion of insurance premiums.[25] As the health care safety net for patients disintegrates, what will legislators and politicians do? Will they turn to other models, none of which have been totally satisfactory, eg, the models of the United Kingdom, Canada, and elsewhere? And if so, what will the effect be on physicians, on other players in the health care system, on CME and CPD, and, most importantly, on the patient?

Third, at the front lines of practice, physician practice arrangements continue to evolve; the percentage of physicians who are employed is continuing to rise, seen especially in the increasing numbers of group practices. Increasingly, physicians provide their care through medical systems and groups organized in a variety of ways, emphasizing ambulatory care. And yet another concern: As patient care continues to shift from the inpatient to the outpatient ambulatory setting, is there potentially increased risk for both patients and physicians?

Fourth, medical schools and academic medical centers, particularly in the United States, are now heavily dependent on the income generated from clinical practice, not only to compensate faculty but also to cover operating expenses. At the same time, revenue from clinical practice in academic settings is threatened from competition with managed care organizations that do not see it as their role to support medical education or research. As a result, although public support for biomedical and clinical research is at an all-time high, academic physicians find themselves with less time, fewer patients, and constricted financial resources, which are needed to teach and conduct research. Their colleagues in clinical practice, no less constrained by fiscal and logistical barriers, suffer from lack of time and resources to spend in educational and professional development.

Continuous Quality Improvement

All health care systems, and especially the physicians within them, are pressed more than ever to demonstrate quality of care on a quantitative basis, a movement generally referred to as continuous quality improvement (CQI) or total quality management. This movement has been defined as "the disruption, measurement and constant improvement of key processes to better meet customer needs,"[26] and has been well articulated by Berwick, among others.[27] This global phenomenon, primarily characterized by small local tests of CQI processes, occurs despite the fact that the ability to measure quality is currently limited by the inadequacies of information systems, the complexity of health plans, and the overall availability of funding. A confounding variable arises from the probabilistic nature of measurement of health care outcomes, especially when the disease is rare or its management complicated, thus falling outside of standard evidence-based guidelines or "care maps." Patients worldwide are voicing their expectations directly and through regulatory agencies, demanding documentation and evidence of physician and hospital quality. For example, in the United States, the Joint Commission on Accreditation of Health Care Organizations (JCAHO) (www.jcaho.org) launched its new "ORYX" initiative in July 2002, with a requirement of a data-driven evaluation process that includes outcomes data to be in place in accredited institutions.

The very nature of the patient–physician relationship may be at stake. The increasing prominence of cost containment in medical practice and resulting pressures on physicians to see more patients per unit time in a day may fundamentally change this relationship. This relationship depends on trust, which requires time to develop, and is threatened when the time allotted for patient visits drops to 8 minutes a patient, as has been noted in some managed care plans. There is increasing evidence that physician satisfaction has plummeted in light of the interference with the traditional patient–physician relationship. Some see a major challenge to medical professionalism in society.[28]

As patient access to health care information continues to increase, physicians will be increasingly challenged by patients to justify their diagnoses and treatment decisions and to avoid medical errors. At the same time, the medical records of patients have too often become a vehicle to justify payment by a third party, perhaps serving this purpose even more than being the long-standing record of the patient's illness.

FORCES AFFECTING CME AND CPD PROVIDERS

Credit for CME: Recertification, Relicensure, and Mandatory Continuing Education

Roles of Professional Associations: The Credit System in CME
The forces that have created the CME credit systems in the United States and Canada continue to exert their influence. These forces are aided by increasing societal and professional pressures for accountability and are altered by the principles of adult education, research in CME, and a better understanding of longitudinal theoretical models of learning and change. The latter forces, more in the mainstream in the United Kingdom and Australia, often lead to merged quality assurance and CME activities, ensuring that CME activities are, on the one hand, converted into practice and performance changes and that practice data, on the other hand, are used as a more objective form of needs assessment. Examples of this shift are the reaccreditation (recertification) of general practitioners in the United Kingdom, modeled after that of the Royal Australasian College of General Practitioners,[29] the Royal College of Family Physicians of Canada, the Royal College of Physicians and Surgeons of Canada,[30] and the Royal New Zealand College of General Practitioners.[31] The latter program has documented changes in CME activities on the part of its members.

In the United States, the American Medical Association's Physician Recognition Award (AMA PRA) is moving to recognize many new activities that reflect physician-initiated and self-directed learning for category 1 credit. Included are activities as diverse as authorship of articles in indexed peer-reviewed journals, teaching in credit-certified CME courses, specialty board certification and re-certification, and the attainment of a medically related advanced academic degree.[32] Two AMA pilot projects currently underway will add to this list. The first examines CME provided on the Internet through which the physician learner begins an Internet journey by searching for instantaneous information to assist in patient management. This can then lead to a tailored CME program for the individual physician. Most CME credit activities on the Internet in 2002 were still predeveloped enduring materials that could be downloaded. A second AMA pilot project is examining how physicians participating in performance review and organized quality improvement/outcomes activities can earn CME credit. Finally, in a major move to embrace the concepts of evidence-based medicine in CME, the American Academy of Family Physicians (AAFP) began, in 2002, to require documentation that CME accredited as AAFP "Prescribed Credit" is either evidence-based (preferable) or clearly represents customary and generally accepted medical practice.[33]

Roles of Regulatory and Licensing Bodies: The Maintenance of Standards

Throughout North America and the United Kingdom, a hue and cry for professional accountability has translated into utilization review by public agencies and by lay member involvement on key committees and governing authorities of regulatory bodies. The shift, according to Southgate and Dauphinee,[34] is from one of establishing standards for entry into practice to one of monitoring practice performance, with further assessment by peers when practitioners are identified as being at risk, followed by feedback, remediation, and support.

Again in the United States, the Federation of State Medical Boards, representing the state and territorial licensing bodies, continues to express concern about the content of certified CME. Thirty-nine of fifty US states now require evidence of CME for reregistration of the medical license.

Funding

Funding issues, key to the survival of CME providers, pose serious and real challenges given the cost-recovery nature of the global practice education enterprise, the sizable pharmaceutical industry co-payment, and the influence of entrepreneurial educational providers. We will consider several forces currently at play here, recognizing that there are many others and that we are defining, not quantifying, these forces.

First, the extensive financial support for CME from pharmaceutical and device companies will continue, most likely without significant change. In analyzing pharmaceutical company expenditures, the share devoted to marketing (including support of education) and advertising is very large—one company reports that more than 30% of its budget is committed to marketing.[35] Overall, the distinction between promotion and education may prove to be a major issue as more "for-profit" providers enter the field and as positive financial return becomes a requirement for most CME providers.[36] Here we raise a question in order to capture the essence of the forces at play: Will the interests of making a profit from CME activities align more readily with the sales goals of pharmaceutical and device companies than has been the case up until now? Further, to what extent can ethical decision-making processes be applied when weighing the financial aspects of CME activity and program support against the promotion of products that may be potentially unnecessary, overly expensive, useless, or even harmful?

Second, for those and a variety of other reasons (electronic education initiatives, rapid turnaround time, accreditation), the for-profit providers of CME will probably grow in numbers, further increasing financial pressures on already-existing providers of CME. Financial incentives offered by the for-profit providers to attract scientific expertise might also reduce the semi-volunteer professional time given by these experts to medical societies and associations. One solution is the possibility of increasing alliances between the for-profit and not-for-profit CME providers. If such alliances are made, differences between them will blur as will the issues of pharmaceutical or medical device industry support.

Third, funding sources for ongoing educational support may derive from a variety of other sources. For example, physicians will (more than ever) need to seek help in locating credible CME as they face a rapid expansion of immediately available content. The roles of medical schools in CME/CPD will need to be clarified. It is likely that physicians will increasingly turn to their medical professional organizations to find such support, financed by their professional dues and other association revenue. In their search to meet these needs, these organizations may turn to new types of partnerships with delivery providers and industry due to the costs and risks associated with certain new directions, eg, online ventures.

Forces for change are persistent, expanding, and rapid. Those engaged in CME/CPD must be flexible, adaptable, and vigilant to assure renewal and their very survival.

Accreditation

The process of accreditation for CME in North America has a profound influence on the provision and direction of CME in both the United States and Canada. The shift in emphasis from process documentation to outcomes orientation, the current direction of the

US Accreditation Council for Continuing Medical Education's (ACCME) "New System," is expected to have an impact.[37]

In contrast, the Canadian accreditation system asks accredited CME providers to document research activities in the field—a phenomenon that has produced a substantial proportion of CME research from this country.[38]

Not alone in their quest to raise standards for CME, the United States and Canada have been joined by institutions in Europe. The European Union of Medical Specialists (UEMS) (www.uems.be) has agreed on a charter on CME.[39] The European charter calls for, among other items, a professional coordinating body, a wide range of CME activities to be made available to learners, awarding of credits, and quality assurance of CME provision. Thus, a European Accreditation Council for Continuing Medical Education became operational in 2000 and is now approving selected courses for CME credit. In 2003, the World Federation for Medical Education (WFME) (www.wfme.org) headquartered in Copenhagen, Denmark, is planning to issue a set of "International Standards for Continuing Professional Development of Doctors," the third in a trilogy of Global Standards for Quality Improvement.

Delivery Methods

The Internet will facilitate a profound change in the delivery of CPD as computer access and familiarity become universal, broadcast bandwidth increases, the presentation of information improves, the quality and validity of information is assured, and more learning resources and educational materials become available. Faced with pressures to remain in their own clinical setting, so as to maintain income or meet job standards and with increased demands to justify quality of care, physicians will likely turn to immediately accessible CME resources for CPD. At the same time, geographic boundaries become less important, perhaps meaningless.

The term *just-in-time CME* has joined its semantic cousins *point of need–point of learning* and *practice-based informatics* in the lexicon of CME providers and learners. Systems to instantly retrieve, store, critically appraise, and apply information needed to manage patients are being developed. As mentioned earlier, the AMA in 2000 embarked on a pilot project to relate these searches and inquiries to the process of CME, including CME credit.[40] Scientific publishing houses are rapidly moving to electronic dissemination methods, which make it even more likely that physicians will seek personalized approaches to their own continued learning. Some type of computer literacy will be a requirement for the physician of the future.

Although the traditional didactic lecture is unlikely to be an immediate causal force in changing physician practice behavior, traditional CME programs (conferences, annual scientific meetings, rounds, and other venues) will continue to play a role in CPD for many reasons: clearly new findings and information may be readily transmitted to large groups of physicians in this way, marked by exchange of opinion and dialogue. This single fact, coupled with the human need to socialize and interact with colleagues, makes it likely that face-to-face meetings will continue to be important in CPD.

Driven by professional and informatics forces, the content of some didactic sessions, eg, specialty society annual meetings, will be distributed through electronic means, either immediately or through an archived file, thus making the meeting available to physicians who could not attend. Increasing in scope and concept, the notion of "wraparound" CME is meant to imply the combined use of Internet technology in some aspects (eg, needs-assessment questionnaires, presentation of syllabus and other materials, follow-up reminders, post-course evaluation questionnaires, among other features). This concept is explored in greater detail in section II of this book.

The environmental forces described in the preceding section will affect the CPD of physicians in at least some of the following ways: (1) the content of CME within the process of personal CPD will be expanded, (2) the educational needs determining physician selection of CME will increasingly be learner-based and learner-driven rather than provider-driven, and (3) delivery methods for CME will be expanded and perhaps radically changed. To meet these changes, CME providers will turn to new partnerships and new funding sources and they will look more intensely at the entire continuum of CPD of the physician.

Embracing this change in the environment, a Standing Committee on Postgraduate Medical and Dental Education (SCOPME) was commissioned by the British government. In 1993, this committee formally recommended that the two professions adopt the terms and concepts of "continuing professional development (CPD)."[41] Recognizing the validity of the concept, the AMA in 1999 formally changed the name of its Division of CME to the Division of Continuing Physician Professional Development (CPPD) to emphasize the notion that the larger process for CME is the lifelong continuing development of the knowledge, skills, and attitudes of the physician.[42]

Accountability: Establishing the Effectiveness of CME

Emphasis on educational return-on-investment for support of CME will grow in importance. This emphasis will manifest itself by more extensive collection of evaluation data and in the choice of vehicles used for the delivery of CME, focusing less on didactic formats with more emphasis on learner interaction that has a more definitive effect on changing practice behavior.[43] Physician learning contracts to demonstrate a commitment-to-change practice pattern as a result of knowledge gained from an educational program will grow in importance and become integral to the total educational intervention. Measurement of change in physician practice behaviors and potential improvement in patient outcomes will assume a critical role in decisions made by industry to invest in CME.[44]

FORCES FOR THE HEALTH PROFESSIONAL/LEARNER

Content Needs

To a large extent, but not completely, physicians are aware of their own learning needs, conveyed to them in a variety of ways. Translated into objectives for CME and CPD, they become powerful forces for change in their own right. Physicians may be able to do more for their patients than ever before, but these new attributes will not come without a delicate combination of new skills, knowledge, and attitudes.

New Skill Sets

Responding to societal and other forces listed above, physicians will need to acquire more comprehensive skills to overcome clinical gaps in care especially in challenges associated with managing the elderly and in chronic disease states. These two areas alone will require physicians to spend more time coordinating patient care. An understanding of disease prevention and health promotion and the ability to communicate to and motivate patients to reduce risk-taking behaviors will also be an increasing part of the physician's practice. Physicians will also have to provide patient education to ethnically diverse groups that may not be proficient in English and have differing cultural belief systems. Effective communication skills, in addition to effective clinical skills, will become a requirement for physician success, especially in areas with growing ethnic and cultural diversity. Physicians will be assisted by and will learn from other health professionals in the areas of patient counseling and communication.

In order to survive the new economic challenges imposed by changing medical practice and financing, physicians will have to become more business savvy and more adept at serving as team leaders in association with other health care professionals. It is likely that "physician as manager and leader" education and training offerings will increase so as to develop and increase skills in team management, leadership, cost containment, and related areas.

Physicians face increasing pressures to gain assistance in monitoring and reviewing their practice relative to accepted standards, including an ability to understand and practice evidence-based medicine. Content for professional development will be directed toward the improvement of one's own practice. Learner-directed, practice-based professional development of the physician will become the foundation for a personally derived and directed curriculum of learning and CME. Medical societies and medical schools should move toward providing mentoring and help to plan an individual program of CME/CPD for a single physician, eg, to create the equivalent of a customized CME "home."

In summary, the entire field of health care has not paid enough attention to change per se and the results of such change. What is certain is that change will occur even more rapidly in the future and the skills of organizational developmental professionals will be in high demand.

Knowledge in the New Workplace

In addition to these skills (eg, communication skills, cultural awareness, understanding of medical ethics, team building and leading), changes in clinical practice will require continual updating of knowledge by physicians. For example, the completion of the Human Genome Project brings with it the necessity for physicians to both understand and apply the clinical applications of genetics and also to manage the ethical issues with a humane and professional approach. Academic health centers are expanding their translational research activities, but the need to assist practicing physicians in the translation of new knowledge into practice has never been greater.

As current established skills become obsolete, physicians who survive and thrive will need to adapt and maintain the most flexibility possible with respect to their type of practice, including location. This may have significant generational overtones. A director of CME at a leading US medical school has commented that he increasingly relies on younger faculty members to relate and "connect" with this "new" breed of community-based physician.[45]

Attitudes: New Values in an Era of Patent Empowerment and Patient-centered Care

Medical education activities must be relevant not only to physician needs but to patient needs as well. Although clearly not a new concept, the shift to patient empowerment entails a redistribution of responsibility between patients and physicians, an understanding and valuing of patient beliefs, and, for many clinicians, a sizable change in their attitude toward patient-centered care. Empowered patients take charge of their own health and their interactions with health professionals. A growing body of evidence suggests that active patient participation in health care is associated with better patient outcomes.[46]

The concept of patient empowerment has emerged over decades. Compare this to an era when patients were seen as passive recipients of care judged acceptable by their physicians; this is clearly no longer the norm. Broader societal interests and the need for autonomy, self-direction, and personal responsibility have empowered patients to assume an important role in caring for themselves rather than totally relying on their physicians and the hospital/sickness–care/health care system. The concept of shared decision making entails a broader relationship for the physician with the patient and the need to learn skills to effectively communicate and partner with the patient to achieve more positive treatment outcomes.[47]

Gender, Training, and Practice Style Issues

Gender

US medical school and residency data indicate that, in due course, roughly half of the practicing physician population will be female.[48] This development is already fully in play in most other developed nations. Although studies of practice styles relative to gender indicate that women physicians will likely bring nontraditional practices to the profession, little is written about their learning styles and preferences. All physicians may be less likely to travel to traditional CME offerings, and even those who have previously served as faculty for these activities will be under pressure to remain in their home setting so as not to reduce their income from clinical practice.

Practice Styles

As a result of managing chronic illness and complex biopsychosocial problems such as those seen in the area of geriatrics, physicians will need to collaborate more extensively and effectively with members of multidisciplinary teams. Given the increased emphasis on ambulatory, home, and community-based care, these teams will probably come from different organizations, requiring interteam negotiation and cooperation, which may be completely new skills for many physicians.[49]

New systems to gather data about patient outcomes will exist. Results of patient outcome studies will drive individual physician learning but must also meet the needs of organizations. When self-recognized shortcomings in clinical practice determine an individual's CME and CPD choices, a demonstration of change toward improved quality will become the indicator of successful professional growth. This will forever change the way in which CME providers define, collect and use evaluation data.

Learning Issues

Finally, and most importantly, the practitioner–learner is characterized as the smallest common denominator in this scenario. There are issues at this level that confront the physician directly, bearing significant implications for his or her learning. The preferred learning styles and educational preferences of a physician will rapidly be translated to forces for change in the CME/CPD environment— forces that the future CME provider fails to note at their own peril.

The literature indicates that there are several themes at play in this domain: the nature of undergraduate education, the type of problem to be solved, professional support for learning, and the inherent learning styles and motivations of physicians, coupled with practice realities.

The Nature of Undergraduate Education.   Some early evidence exists that graduates with undergraduate training in those schools with problem-based learning (PBL) curricula are more up-to-date[50] than those trained in traditional, more heavily subject-oriented and didactic curricula. Although studies of the outcomes of PBL versus traditional curricula exist, few examine such long-term issues as learning styles, learning preferences, and literature searching or critical appraisal abilities, nor are these issues coupled to proof of overall clinical competence. Nonetheless, it makes sense for us to argue that those medical school curricula that stress learner-centeredness, medical practice as a focus of learning, self-evaluation and self-reflection, and the use of evidence[51] will graduate as more self-directed and critical learners. These will be potent forces for change in the provision and delivery of CME/CPD.

Problem Type and Learning Style.   The preceding paragraph is not an argument for the existence of a universal, unalterable learning style for physicians, created entirely by the undergraduate medical curriculum or experience, anymore than there is good evidence about generic problem-solving skills independent of knowledge level. Rather, there is evidence that the learning method chosen is contingent on the type of problem encountered in clinical practice. McClaran and her colleagues indicate that physicians are more likely to select formal CME activities when the problem requires technical expertise or communication skills.[52]

Professional Support for Learning.   One advance of CME and CPD providers over the past decade has been the provision of support services for self-directed learning by physicians on the part of some specialty societies, medical schools, and others (a topic explored more fully in section II). Examples of such support include the use of learning portfolios,[53,54] which in turn empower learners, directing and focusing their choices of topic and mode of learning, thus creating forces for change in themselves.

Inherent Learning Styles, Motivations, and Practice Realities.
Finally, there exist individual characterologic tendencies to motivation, self-reflection, and learning that are independent of undergraduate education, residency training, or CME availability and
resources. The level of development of moral reasoning skills and
moral development of the practitioner has been suggested as an
important factor.[55] Potent forces alone, they are coupled to the
practice realities of today's practitioners, wherever they practice. In
many venues, physicians may even become demotivated to learn,
unable to find or make time for formal educational experiences.
Unless practice-based interventions are instituted, these practitioners may drift in clinical competence. Although clearly more appropriate as the subject of Sections I and II in this book, we flag this
last and highly important issue as a major force for (or against)
change in the landscape of CME and CPD.

REFERENCES—CHAPTER 2

1. Center for Health Policy Research. *Physician Socioeconomic Statistics.*
   Chicago, Ill: American Medical Association; 1999.

2. Tuohy CH. Dynamics of a changing health sphere: the United States,
   Britain and Canada. *Health Affairs.* 1999;18:114–134.

3. Davis D, Fox R, eds. *The Physician as Learner: Linking Research to
   Practice.* Chicago, Ill: American Medical Association; 1994.

4. Fox RD, Mazmanian PE, Putnam RW. *Changing and Learning in the
   Lives of Physicians.* New York, NY: Praeger Publishers; 1989.

5. *National Vital Statistics Report.* 47;13, December 24, 1998.

6. Health People 2010 Initiative, CDC and DHHS. *JAMA.*
   2000;283:989–990.

7. Koplan JP, Fleming DW. Current and future public health challenges.
   JAMA. 2000;284:1696–1698 and *JAMA.* 2001;285:411.

8. Institute for the Future. *A Forecast of Health and Health Care in
   America.* Princeton: Robert Wood Johnson Foundation; 1998.

9. Davis, D. Global health, global learning. *BMJ.* 1998;316:385–389.

10. Garrett L. *The Coming Plague: Newly Emergent Diseases in a World
    Out of Balance.* New York, NY: Penguin Books; 1994.

11. Morrison JI. The Second Curve: Managing the Velocity of Change.
    Presented as "Health Care in the New Millennium" at the National
    Leadership Development Conference; March 2000; American Medical
    Association.

12. Collins FS. Avoiding casualties in the genetic revolution: the urgent
    need to educate physicians about genetics. *Acad Med.* 1999;74:48–49.

13. Singer PA, Todkill AM. Bioethics for clinicians: continuing the series.
    Can Med Assoc J. 2000;163:833.

14. *Networking Health: Prescriptions for the Internet.* Report of the Committee on Enhancing the Internet for Health and Biomedical Applications. Washington, DC: National Academy of Sciences; February 2000.

15. The economist survey of government and the Internet—the next revolution. *The Economist.* June 24, 2000.

16. *Physician Characteristics and Distribution in the United States.* Chicago, Ill: American Medical Association; 2000.

17. Greene J. Emerging specialist shortage triggers work force review. *AM News.* January 2001.

18. Cooper R et al. Current and projected workforce of nonphysician clinicians. *JAMA.* 1998;280:788–794.

19. *Hospital Statistics.* Washington, DC; American Hospital Association; 2002.

20. Dudley RA, Johnasen KL, Brand R, Rennie DJ, Milstein A. Selective referral to high-volume hospitals: estimating potentially avoidable deaths. *JAMA.* 2000;283:1159–1167.

21. Sochalski J, Aiken LH, Fagin CM. Hospital restructuring in the United States, Canada and Western Europe. *Med Care.* 1997;35:OS13–OS25.

22. Kaiser L. Technology: redesigning the medical system. *MGM J.* 1992; Nov–Dec; 21–24.

23. Bodenheimer T. California's beleaguered physician groups—will they survive? *N Engl J Med.* 2000;342:1064–1068.

24. Pauly MV. "In boom times, managed care is a bust!" *The Wall Street Journal.* March 15, 2000.

25. US Census Bureau, Current Population Survey, March 1998 and National Health Statistics Group, Health Care Financing Administration. Washington, DC: Office of the Actuary; 1998.

26. Joint Commission on Accreditation of Health Care Organizations. *Striving Toward Improvement: Six Hospitals in Search of Quality.* Chicago, Ill: American Hospital Publishing, Inc; 1992.

27. Berwick DM. Developing and testing changes in delivery of care. *Ann Intern Med.* 1998;128:651–656.

28. Wynia MK, Latham SR, et al. Medical professionalism in society. *N Engl J Med.* 1999;341:1612–1616.

29. Salisbury C. The Australian quality assurance and continuing education program as a model for the reaccreditation of general practitioners in the United Kingdom. *Br J Gen Pract.* 1997;47:319–322.

30. Parboosingh J. Maintenance of certification for Canadian specialists: exploring options. *Ann R Coll Phys Surg Can.* 1998;31:128–133.

31. Tracey JM, Arroll B, Richmond DE. Changes in CME uptake caused by reaccreditation. *NZ Med J.* 1998;111:118–120.

32. *The Physician Recognition Award Information Booklet*, version 3.0, 2001. www.ama-assn.org/cme/. Chicago, Ill: American Medical Association.

33. *New Criteria for Evaluating and Categorizing Clinical Content of Continiuing Medical Education.* Commission on Continuing Medical Education, 2001. www.aafp.org/cme/accreditation/. Kansas City, KS: American Academy of Family Physicians; 2001.

34. Southgate L, Dauphinee D. Maintaining standards in British and Canadian medicine: the developing role of the regulatory body. *Br Med J.* 1998;316:697–700.

35. Angel M. The pharmaceutical industry, to whom is it accountable? *N Engl J Med.* 2000;342:1902–1904.

36. Relman AS. Separating continuing medical education from pharmaceutical marketing. *JAMA.* 2001;285:2009–2012.

37. *ACCME's Essential Areas, Elements, and Decision-Making Criteria.* Chicago, Ill: Accreditation Council for Continuing Medical Education; July, 1999; (www.accme.org).

38. Research and Development Resource Base, Annual Report, Toronto, Canada (www.cme.utoronto.cardrb/).

39. Leibbrandt CC. Charter on CME in the European Union. *Postgrad Med J.* 1996;72:14–21.

40. CME/CPPD Report: Number 5, Spring/Summer, 2001. Chicago, Ill: American Medical Association; 2001.

41. Oxley J, ed. A working paper for consultation on continuing professional development of doctors and dentists. London: The Standing Committee on Postgraduate Medical and Dental Education; 1994.

42. Wentz DK, Paulos G. Is now the time for continuing medical education to become continuing physician professional development? *JCEPH.* 2000;20:181–187.

43. Davis DA, Thompson O'Brien MA, Freemantle N, Wolf FM, Mazmanian P, Taylor-Vaisey A. Impact of formal continuing medical education: do conferences, workshops, rounds, and other traditional continuing education activities change physician behavior or health care outcomes? *JAMA.* 1999;282: 867–874.

44. Casebeer L, Raichle L, Kristofco R, Carillo A. Cost benefit analysis: review of an evaluation methodology for measuring return on investment in continuing education. *J Contin Educ Health Prof.* 1997;17:225–227.

45. Harrison R Van. Personal communication. December 2000.

46. Roberts KJ. Patient empowerment in the US. *Health Expectations.* 1999;2:82–92.

47. Towle A, et al. Framework for teaching and learning informed shared decision making. *Br Med J.* 1999;319:766.

48. AAMC Data Book, Statistical Information Related to Medical Schools and Teaching Hospitals. Washington, DC: Association of American Medical Colleges; January 2001 (p. 22; Table B7).

49. Ryan DP, Cott C, Robertson D. Conceptual tools for thinking about interteam work in clinical gerontology. *Educ Gerontol.* 1997;23:651–667.

50. Shin JH, Haynes RB, Johnston, ME. Effect of problem-based, self-directed undergraduate education on life-long learning. *Can Med Assoc J.* 1993;148:969–976.

51. Fox R. Implications of the model of change and learning for undergraduate medical education. *J Contin Educ Health Prof.* 1996;16:144–151.

52. McClaran J, Snell L, Farnaco E. Type of clinical problem is a determinant of physicians' self-directed learning methods in their practice settings. *J Contin Educ Health Prof.* 1999;18:107–118.

53. Mathers NJ, Challis MC, Howe AC, Filed NJ. Portfolios in continuing medical education—effective and efficient? *Med Educ.* 1999;33:521–530.

54. Parboosingh J. Learning portfolios: potential to assist health professionals with self-directed learning. *J Contin Educ Health Prof.* 1996;16:75–81.

55. Self DJ, Baldwin DC. Should moral reasoning serve as a criterion for student & resident selection? *Clin Orthop.* 2000;378:115–123.

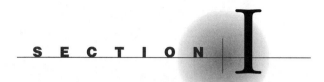

Deciding What to Do

Primary editor: Barbara E. Barnes, MD

A Clinical Thematic: Deciding What to Do

Dave Davis, MD; Robert Fox, EdD;
Barbara E. Barnes, MD; Karen Costie, RN

The Patient Scenario

Marjory Hall has, after some procrastination, made an appointment to see Dr Brucken. He begins the interview by indicating that it has been over a year since she has been in the office. "You're right, Ted," she says, "you know it had to be something pretty bad or I wouldn't be here." She proceeds to tell him about her symptoms, the most frightening being the change in vision that is limiting her ability to work. Dr Brucken listens attentively, knowing that the waiting room is full and that he can spend only 15 minutes with his patient; he wishes it were longer. On examination he detects no eye abnormalities but does note a 20-pound weight loss since her last visit. A blood sugar analysis done in the office is moderately but not dangerously elevated.

"Marjory," says Dr Brucken, "it looks like you have diabetes. We need to run some more tests and I will see you in a week to review the results. In the meantime, try to watch your diet and call me if your symptoms get worse. I don't think you need to be very concerned about your vision—that should get better once your sugar comes down. We'll try to get you an appointment with an ophthalmologist."

While driving home, Marjory has to pull off to the side of the road because she is so distraught. Her mother died from complications of diabetes and she doesn't want to suffer the same fate. She can't understand why Dr Brucken seemed so unconcerned about her condition and why he didn't start some kind of treatment right away. How will she be able to function at work in the next week? Marjory wishes she could speak with a nutritionist and knows she must find some authoritative information about diabetes. She has no idea how she will pay for the lab tests or any prescriptions she might need in the future.

On his way to the hospital for evening rounds, Ted also thinks more about his encounter with Ms Hall. He has seen a lot of new cases of type 2 diabetes recently and he wonders if a community-wide effort to improve nutrition and physical fitness might be in order. Many of his patients are unaware of the symptoms of diabetes and delay seeking medical care until they have significant problems.

In addition, he is not sure about the best way to treat Marjory. He read a recent journal article advocating aggressive dietary management as an initial strategy for patients with mild to moderate hyperglycemia. However, a pharmaceutical company representative just dropped off some literature about the benefits of early use of oral hypoglycemic agents. Ted will definitely need to talk with colleagues and do some reading before Marjory returns to the office.

On reflection, he recalls that the Mountainside Medical Group distributed a practice guideline for the care of type 2 diabetes. He will dig that out of his file and might suggest to his partners that they do an audit of charts to see how well they are complying with the guideline. Dr Brucken has also been meaning to speak with the group practice administrator about establishing a comprehensive diabetes management program. The practice has resisted hiring a nutritionist or nurse educator because most insurance companies do not reimburse these services, but Ted wonders how much his patients' care could be improved if there were better access to these health professionals.

DISCUSSION

The continuing professional development (CPD) professional must be cognizant of the many issues illustrated by this patient encounter. First, it is clear that Ted has to improve his knowledge about this disease. He has not had time to attend formal educational activities addressing the care of diabetes, and the information he has received from journals and the pharmaceutical representative is confusing and may be biased or dated. To determine what he needs to know, Ted can pursue a variety of initiatives, including scanning the literature, consulting with colleagues, and checking out some practice guidelines. In order to see how his performance differs from the standards of the health network and the care being provided by his partners, he and his colleagues may do a chart audit. Will these efforts be sufficient to improve his care of patients with diabetes?

The learning issues that Ted has identified focus largely on the medical aspects of care. However, Marjory has a number of psychosocial and economic issues that must be dealt with as part of the total management of her disease. The scenario indicates that this physician needs to improve his interviewing skills to better identify the emotional issues his patients confront—though he appears unaware of this need. Dr Brucken must learn to more effectively communicate empathy for the stress created by chronic illness and maybe even acquire better skills in this area in the primary care setting.

This case also demonstrates that some of the issues affecting Ms Hall's care transcends the competence and performance of her primary care physician. The medical group has decided that it is not cost effective to offer nutritional counseling and patient education. The group and, in fact, the health care system itself have also placed stringent limits on the amount of time physicians can spend with patients. The problems raised by Ms Hall's clinical encounter provide a basis for discussions between physicians and clinical managers to identify the issues that impact the quality and cost effectiveness of care. For example, the presence of a nutritionist in the practice may lead to increased patient satisfaction, decreased phone calls to office staff, and reduced frequency of hospital admissions. The identification of inefficient office processes and procedures might allow physicians to spend more time with patients. Further, the ability to share experiences among physicians and other personnel can allow best practices to be shared, improving not only the performance of a single individual but that of the practice as a whole.

Although the work of physicians focuses on the care of individual patients, Dr Brucken must also be concerned about the population of diabetic patients in his community, or at least that part of it served by his group. In order to properly diagnose new cases, he needs to be aware of changes in the incidence of disease. If type 2 diabetes is becoming more frequent among, eg, obese adolescents, he might choose to perform screening blood sugars or to be more aggressive in initiating discussions about weight control. Because his community has had an influx of immigrants from Southeast Asia, Ted might want to read more about the incidence of diabetes in this population and particular dietary practices and cultural beliefs that might affect the management of the disease in these patients. Marjory's lack of adequate insurance will also have a bearing on the level of care she receives. A member of the medical profession, Dr Brucken must be knowledgeable about health financing and insurance in order to be an advocate for the needs of his patients.

The chapters in this section are designed to acquaint CPD professionals with the multiple dimensions of needs assessment exemplified by the case study. Beginning with the context within which health care is delivered, Geoff Anderson and Adalsteinn Brown address, in Chapter 3, the population perspective in CPD. They demonstrate why it is important for CPD professionals to take into account factors such as disease incidence, the scope of services employed in the continuum of health care delivery, and the burden of disease on the community while planning educational activities and interventions.

In the modern health care environment, physicians work in a variety of organizational settings including group practices, hospitals, and nursing homes as addressed by Joe Green and Jim Leist in Chapter 6. To operate effectively and provide high-quality care, there must be alignment between the goals of these institutions and the physicians who work within them. In addition, the availability of data on the outcomes and process of care permits physicians to compare their performance with practice guidelines and the practices of colleagues. Gaps between current and ideal performance can form the basis of educational needs assessment. In Chapter 4, Jocelyn Lockyer reviews and assesses the types of data that can be used in the planning of CPD activities.

In Chapter 5, Craig Campbell and Tunde Gondocz discuss how physicians identify knowledge gaps by reflecting on their clinical practice, formulating questions that can be addressed by educational interventions. The authors describe how these inquiries can become the basis for learning portfolios and they review strategies that can be employed by CPD professionals to assist practitioners in the reflective process.

chapter 3

The Population Perspective: Linking CME to Population Needs

Geoffrey M. Anderson, MD, PhD; Adalsteinn D. Brown, DPhil

INTRODUCTION

The core of medical care is the interaction between the individual patient and the provider. This interaction, however, takes place in a larger context defined by the health care system within which the provider works and the population within which the patient resides. Analyses from such a population perspective can produce new and different views of health care and continuing professional development (CPD) needs.

Kerr White, one of the great medical educators of the twentieth century, was the first to point out how physicians' position within a health care system can affect their perspective on population health needs.[1] White integrated data from several sources to show that physicians see only a fraction of the morbidity in a community and that the fraction seen by a physician declines with increasing specialization. Only a portion of the population with a specific health problem seeks care from primary care physicians; a smaller portion visit specialists; and an even smaller portion receive in-patient care.[2] Thus, different types of physicians and surgeons have different experiences with population health needs based on the scope and type of their practice. Analyses of population needs from the provider's perspective, especially from a specialist's perspective, may be misleading. In this chapter, we use the example of chronic back pain to show how different providers may have different perspectives on health care needs. We also show how population-based data and an understanding of care-seeking behavior and referral patterns can inform the development of CPD programs.

In addition to their position along the continuum of care, characteristics of the organization of care may affect physicians' view of population health needs. One such characteristic is the growing reliance on teams of providers. For acute events, such as fractures or many infections, treatment may focus on the correction of one problem with little need for follow-up care. In contrast, treatment for chronic conditions, such as dementia or acute events such as stroke with chronic sequelae, may require a long history of care from a range of providers. Physicians are part of a network of formal and informal providers that includes other physicians, nurses, therapists, community and social service organizations, and patients' families. To the extent that physicians work directly with this network, their understanding of the scope and depth of population health needs will increase. In this chapter, we use the example of stroke care to describe how an overview of all aspects of care can provide a clearer and more useful understanding of patients' needs and can lead to CPD that is focused on teams rather than individuals.

Along with the degree of specialization and the role of physicians within teams, changes in the health care system and the physical or socioeconomic environment can affect physicians' perspectives on population health needs. These changes may alter the underlying health care needs or the referral or care-seeking patterns that make those needs apparent to physicians. Economic incentives common to managed care or other forms of cost control, such as risk contracting, discounting hospital charges, or limiting access to specific treatments, can alter the flow of patients.[3] Incentives to limit access to a particular type of care may lead to reductions in patient exposure to some physicians, although physicians providing a substitute service, in contrast, may see more patients. In this chapter, we use asthma as an example of how the extent of drug benefit coverage can have an effect on the types of patients seen by physicians and how CPD can help providers to understand and adapt to the financial barriers that stand in the way of appropriate care.

Practicing physicians' unique perspective on the need for care has important implications for CPD and their interaction with CPD professionals. To the extent that physicians have a biased perspective on population health care needs, there is a danger that their self-assessed professional development needs and priorities will also be biased. This is understandable; physicians will be most interested in learning about the types of patients they see and in improving what they do for those patients. However, a population perspective can help inform important aspects of professional development and practice including outreach, screening, and attention to the organizational, economic, and environmental determinants of successful clinical care.

CME AND THE POPULATION PERSPECTIVE

The population, or epidemiological, perspective is an understanding of the at-risk population from which patients arise and to which, hopefully, they return.[4] The central element in the analysis of population health needs is the accurate measurement of rates. The numerator is the number of population members at one time suffering from the health problem (prevalence) or who develop the health problem in a specific period of time (incidence). The appropriate denominator for the rate is the population at risk for a particular health problem. Educators and researchers can calculate rates when they have information on the entire population or when they have information on a sample from the population. Understanding population health needs deals not only with experience with the numerator but also an appreciation for the denominator.

Although physicians' biased perspective is as likely to affect the numerator and the denominator, CPD professionals may provide the greatest assistance through the use of epidemiological data on the numerator. Working from the population perspective, we can see that small changes in the numerator will have greater relative effect than changes of the same absolute size on the denominator. Accurate estimation of the denominator is also challenging. Diehr has pointed out that even seemingly simple estimations of the denominator, eg hysterectomy rates, may be complicated.[5] The proportion of women undergoing hysterectomy in a population is properly calculated as the number of women who have the procedure divided by the number of women in the same population with intact uteri at the start of the study. In contrast, in calculations based on routinely collected hospital data, the numerator may reflect repeated hospitalizations for the same woman for complications of surgery, while the denominator will typically include all women in the population, regardless of their eligibility for hysterectomy.[5]

Because of the biased perspective that results from physicians' work environment, the onus for shifting the perspective does not lie with individual physicians. Rather, the onus lies with CPD professionals and others who are responsible for understanding and improving health care performance across the system. If they take a system- or population-based perspective, CPD professionals can help groups of physicians identify untreated, inappropriately treated, and undertreated patient groups that the physicians do not regularly see for inclusion in the numerator. CPD professionals can also help physicians choose areas for professional development that will be of continuing or increasing importance to their own practice.

Example 1: Type of Care

A family physician reads a news brief in the state medical journal describing a recent household survey that found the most common chronic health problem reported by people aged 45 to 64 was back pain. She remembers an earlier article that suggested wide variations in particular surgical treatments for back pain with little impact on patient health status.[6] She phones the head of orthopedic surgery at the closest teaching hospital to see if he believes a course of managing back pain would help improve the appropriateness of surgical treatment. He says the volume of spinal fusion surgery is very low across the local community and does not see much value from such a course.

A few weeks later, she speaks with the chair of the county medical society, another family physician. The chair says that she does not see many patients with back pain, although the ones she does see are often a management challenge and have often already tried self-treatment with bed rest prior to physician consultation. The chair also does not see much value from a course because of the low numbers of patients involved and because her and her colleagues' most common recommendation is for further bed rest.

The next day, the family physician notices three ads for back supports and two ads for chiropractic clinics that specialize in back pain. She decides to do some more research and finds out two additional pieces of information. First, she reads a large study that shows most commonly used treatments to be relatively ineffective for low back pain.[7] She also finds out that low back pain remains one of most common causes of absenteeism on the job.[8] She phones an occupational physician at a local manufacturing plant who confirms this and says that it is his number one problem. He also says that he is frustrated because most of the family physicians in the surrounding community recommend bed rest rather than physiotherapy and other courses that would return patients to work faster. She contacts the chair of the county medical society again and they work with a CPD professional to design a course on better screening and timely treatment of back pain in the primary care setting.

This scenario highlights the point that a common and important problem from a population perspective takes on different characteristics and importance as the treatment sequence moves up from self-care, to primary care, specialist referral, and, ultimately, to inpatient specialist treatment. The frequency and nature of the problem looks very different to providers at different points in the health care system. In most cases, acute back pain resolves without treatment and most patients improve without care over a short period, although the rate of recurrence is also high.[9] Patients may not bother to seek care for their back pain and they improve despite the lack of formal care. Other patients obtain relief with basic self-care or through care provided by other professionals, such as chiropractors or massage therapists. Primary care physicians may focus on the minority of patients who go on to have chronic problems rather than those who get better without intensive therapy.

Specialists will only see a small proportion of patients—the most acute cases with the greatest likelihood of benefiting from surgery or other invasive therapies or those with the greatest self-perceived need for treatment.

Not all causes of health care use will filter through different layers of the health care system. For example, virtually all patients with a hip fracture will present for care by hospital-based physicians. However, even in the case of hip fractures, perceptions of the impact of related diseases such as osteoporosis will be different at different levels within the health care system. Appropriate screening and management of osteoporosis in the primary care population would alter the rate of fractures presenting at the emergency department. The course of particular conditions such as back pain, the constellation of symptoms found in conditions such as depression, and the links between specific clinical events such as hip fractures and risk factors such as osteoporosis can all affect how physicians view the burden of illness and population health needs. It is the role of the CPD professional to better explore the health needs that are out of sight of physicians and to incorporate these needs into education programs. A first step toward such integration is to look to physicians' role within a team providing care to one patient group.

Example 2: Population Served

A neurologist at a teaching hospital is at the meeting of the utilization management committee for the hospital. The committee is reviewing average length of stay information across patient groups and tells the neurologist that stroke patients on her unit have a much longer length of stay than would be expected based on data from similar hospitals across the country. She finishes the meeting and talks to the neurologists who specialize in stroke at her institution. They tell her that they have put a lot of effort into developing and implementing strategies to improve the acute care of stroke patients including a state-of-the-art protocol for thrombolysis. They have also developed a consultation schedule that ensures each stroke patient is seen by a physiatrist before discharge.

She then visits the ward and talks to the head nurse. The nurse says the acute treatment is very good at the hospital but that patients are staying for prolonged periods of time because families do not want to care for the patients at home and because of difficulties in placing the patients in chronic care or long-term care facilities.

She speaks with physicians and managers working at chronic care hospitals in the same community and finds that they have also implemented protocols and can document successful patterns of care for patients but that they do not have sufficient beds to care for the current volume of patients. They also note that they have difficulty in convincing families to accept stroke patients back into the home.

She then speaks with a CPD professional at the hospital about a course to further decrease average length of stay for stroke patients. The CPD professional tells her that he is currently organizing other courses for patient groups where average length of stay is also above the national average but where no protocols have been developed or implemented at the hospital. The CPD professional suggests that she focus her efforts on greater patient advocacy and, if possible, on stroke prevention efforts with community-based physicians.

She then speaks with primary care physicians in the community. They are also following good protocols for secondary stroke prevention but report that they are unable to counsel families about the best care for stroke patients returning from the hospital, in part, because they feel they are unable to access specialists for consultation and advice. After speaking with all three groups of physicians, she works with the CPD professional to develop a program to better integrate the flow of information and consultations between different sectors of the health care system.

This example describes the biased perspective that physicians are prone to because they do not provide all the services that meet patient needs. Each group of physicians is certain it is providing high-quality care to stroke patients[10–12] and is sure that the problems lay elsewhere. In this case, each group is correct, but improved management by other groups is unlikely to reduce length of stay. In fact, high-quality care may actually increase length of stay and the volume of admissions, as more and more patients survive a stroke but require hospital care afterward and are at greater risk for repeat stroke. The care of those with disabilities and the prevention of stroke recurrence place a burden on the institution, the patient, the family, and the community. The idea that care for stroke patients can be easily broken down into components that are and are not the concern of a particular group of physicians is inconsistent with the nature of the condition. The increased length of stay observed in the hospital is not the result of problems with acute care but rather with the coordination of services necessary to support stroke patients outside of the hospital environment.

The importance of looking beyond the bounds of clinical care to better understand population health needs is not unique to stroke. The epidemiological shift in health care needs toward continuing care for chronic conditions as well as changes in the organization of care mean that such issues are increasingly common. Advances in the acute treatment of conditions such as stroke and heart attack reduce mortality rates but may not reduce the overall incidence of chronic sequelae. Providers have turned to vertical integration, or the organization of primary care, specialist care, and long-term care within one organization, as a solution to manage and keep up to date with the shifting needs of their patients. To play an important role in vertically integrated care, physicians must develop a perspective that takes into account the range of health needs of their patients and the resources that can be used to meet those needs.[2]

Nonclinical factors can also affect physicians' perspectives on population health needs, including the organization of care or incentives inherent in care systems. Moreover, patient ethnicity, sex, education, or income may interact with the organization or financing of care to alter the mix of patients seen by physicians and further skew physicians' perspectives on population health needs.[13]

Example 3: Systems and Populations

An emergentologist notes an increase in the number of acute asthma cases he sees in the emergency department (ED) and that the majority of this increase is for low-income children. Unfortunately, a large number of these patients return to the ED with repeat acute asthma attacks, and many children have to be admitted to the hospital for treatment.

The emergentologist talks to some family practitioners and pediatricians in the community. The physicians seem to be aware of the appropriate patient education and drug therapy for asthma—reliance on both bronchodilators and inhaled steroids—although many have heard about a new type of drug called leukotriene-receptor antagonists (LTRA) and are starting to prescribe them as first-line therapy in children.[14]

The emergentologist comes to you and asks if you could provide a course on the management of pediatric asthma in the emergency room. You suggest to him that it might be useful to look at the factors that could be behind the increased ED visits for asthma.

You call up the insurer who covers most of the low-income families in the community. The insurer confirms that it has a drug benefit plan for children but that in recent months it has introduced co-payments on each prescription and a new formulary that reduces drug coverage. You ask the insurer to look at patterns of prescribing bronchodilators, inhaled steroids, and LTRA. The insurer provides only partial payment for LTRA. They have noticed a decrease in the claims submitted for inhaled steroids and bronchodilators.

Your suggestion to the emergentologists is that the best course of action might be to work with primary care physicians to educate them on the key role of inhaled bronchodilators and steroids as first-line treatment for childhood asthma and to work further with the insurer on the relationship between decreased prescription drug claims reductions and increased claims for ED and inpatient care.[15]

This example highlights the importance of identifying the interaction between providers and the population served.[13, 16] The decision to write a prescription is made by the physician; the decision to fill that prescription is made by the patient. When patients face increased costs, especially poor patients, they may not be able to comply with treatment.[17] The parents who routinely fill their child's prescriptions for inhaled steroids and bronchodilators may not be able to afford increased co-payments. If children are switched to high-cost LTRA agents from standard therapy, poor families will be less able than wealthier families to pick up the increased costs.

The primary care physician may not be aware of the change in compliance or the reasons underlying this change. The specialist may interpret an increase in the incidence of a condition as a reason to focus on improving ED treatment rather than on an investigation of the cause of the increase. The insurer may fail to see the link between decreased drug expenditures and the increased costs of ED and hospital care. Few providers may examine broader determinants of compliance and success from asthma therapy.

If health care is going to adequately deal with the health problems of the population, CPD professionals must look beyond the walls of the hospital or the office to define the appropriate numerator and denominator. Many countries have regular health status surveys, which can help define the health needs of the population and clarify areas where further education is needed to describe problems.[18, 19] However, most of these surveys provide information on populations that are similar, but not identical, to the population of interest to specific institutions or physicians. In this case, population needs have to be inferred. With the growing role of managed care plans, there is increasing interest in clearly defining and monitoring eligible populations, and direct information on population health needs is likely to become increasingly common. Organizations such as the National Committee on Quality Assurance already include population-based measures of performance in their accreditation reports.[20] At least part of this growing attention results from concerns that "underservicing" or "underuse" may be a consequence of the economic incentives inherent in managed care.[13] In particular, it is important to realize that specific populations, usually minorities or the poor, are the most likely to be exposed to quality-of-care problems.

CONCLUSIONS

The role of practicing physicians within the health care system gives rise to their unique, but biased, perspective on population health needs. The three examples provided here show how this perspective can affect different physician's understanding of population health needs, regardless of the type of care provided (example 1), the population served (example 2), or the degree to which individual physicians have organized care according to best practices (example 3). The continuing epidemiological shift toward chronic disease, increasing technological capabilities, and changing practice environments and reimbursement systems may further bias individual physician's perspectives on population health needs.

Their responsibility for shifting this perspective lies with the health system as a whole. Even if medical schools increase the amount of time devoted to epidemiological methods and studies within their curricula, CPD professionals can help physicians to understand the population perspective while maintaining their focus on the patients they see every day. Because they aggregate the experience through licensure, survey, or billings data, organizations such as professional associations, insurers, and government can also help promote a population perspective in CPD. Finally, these organizations, along with medical schools and their affiliated universities, can support the development of epidemiological and managerial skill sets for physicians so that physicians can work more closely with CPD professionals and take a more active role in defining epidemiological perspectives on the populations they serve.

If population-based design of health care delivery systems and concerns about underserviced or inappropriately serviced populations are priorities for governments, insurers, managed care organizations, and regional health bodies, these same organizations must support the CPD professionals' access to data and incentives to use this data. CPD professionals must also have access to, or an understanding of, the epidemiological tools and data necessary to support the estimations of rates and other important parameters. Thus, training courses for CPD professionals should include some component on epidemiological methods and data sources.

The format of CPD is also important to surmount the challenge of linking the population perspective to a physician's practice. Education that deals with processes that are under the direct control of the learner can be focused on that learner and specifically directed toward behavioral change.[21] Education that is aimed at improving the coordination and integration of care delivery involves individuals from different professions and organizations working together. In order to have the greatest impact, these sessions should involve providers from across the continuum of care and provide opportunities for them to examine shared populations and overlapping spheres of clinical activity. The preferred model for CPD from a population perspective may include several layers of providers and include more aspects of a quality improvement approach with its focus on teams and processes.[22]

Kerr White's concerns about the biased perspective of practicing physicians and its impact on the health care system remain valid. The challenge facing CPD professionals is to make population health needs a learning priority not only for organizations but also for individuals and to ensure that the education recognizes the role of the physician in the health care team. Failure to successfully incorporate the population health perspective in continuing education will mean that many who could benefit from care will remain underserved.

REFERENCES—CHAPTER 3

1. White KL, Connolly JE, eds. *The Medical School's Mission and the Population's Health: Medical Education in Canada, the United Kingdom, the United States, and Australia.* New York, NY: Springer-Verlag; 1992.

2. White KL. The ecology of medical care: origins and implications for population-based healthcare research. *Health Serv Res.* 1997;32:11–21.

3. Kerr EA, Mittman BS, Hays RD, Siu AL, Leake B, Brook RH. Managed care and capitation in California: how do physicians at financial risk control their own utilization? *Ann Intern Med.* 1995;123:500–504.

4. McWhinney IR. The need for the population perspective at the practice level. In: White KL, ed. *The Health of Populations* (Working Papers–The Rockefeller Foundation). New York, NY: The Rockefeller Foundation; 1980:8–9.

5. Diehr P. Small area analysis: The medical care outcome problem. In: Sechrest L, Perrin E, Bunker J, eds. *AHCPR Conference Proceedings. Research Methodology: Strengthening Causal Interpretations of Nonexperimental Data.* Bethesda, MD: US Department of Health and Human Services; 1990:207–213.

6. Keller RB, Atlas SJ, Soule DN, Singer DE, Deyo RA. Relationship between rates and outcomes of operative treatment for lumbar disc herniation and spinal stenosis. *J Bone Joint Surg Am.* 1999;81:752–762.

7. Cherkin DC, Deyo RA, Battie M, Street J, Barlow W. A comparison of physical therapy, chiropractic manipulation, and provision of an educational booklet for the treatment of patients with low back pain. *N Engl J Med.* 1998;339:1021–1029.

8. Guo HR, Tanaka S, Halperin WE, Cameron LL. Back pain prevalence in US industry and estimates of lost workdays. *Am J Public Health.* 1999;89:1029–1035.

9. Carey TS, Garrett JM, Jackman A, Hadler N. Recurrence and care seeking after acute back pain: Results of a long-term follow-up study. *Med Care.* 1999;37:157–164.

10. Lyden PD. Thrombolysis for acute stroke. *Prog Cardiovasc Dis.* 1999;42:175–183.

11. Holloway RG, Benesch C, Rush SR. Stroke prevention: narrowing the evidence-practice gap. *Neurology.* 2000;54:1899–1906.

12. Rosenberg CH, Popelka GM. Post-stroke rehabilitation. A review of the guidelines for patient management. *Geriatrics.* 2000;55:75–81.

13. Asch SM, Sloss EM, Hogan C, Brook RH, Kravitz RL. Measuring underuse of necessary care among elderly medicare beneficiaries using inpatient and outpatient claims. *JAMA.* 2000;284:2325–2333.

14. Smith SR, Strunk RC. Acute asthma in the pediatric emergency department. *Pediatr Clin North Am*. 1999;46:1145–1165.

15. Stempel DA, Hedblom EC, Durcanin-Robbins JF, Sturm LL. Use of a pharmacy and medical claims database to document cost centers for 1993 annual asthma expenditures. *Arch Fam Med*. 1996;5:36–40.

16. Fiscella K, Franks P, Gold MR, Clancy CM. Inequality in quality: Addressing socioeconomic, racial, and ethnic disparities in health care. *JAMA*. 2000;283:2579–2584.

17. Celano M, Geller RJ, Phillips KM, Ziman R. Treatment adherence among low-income children with asthma. *J Pediatr Psychol*. 1998;23:345–349.

18. Selby JV. Linking automated databases for research in managed care settings. *Ann Intern Med*. 1997;127:719–724.

19. Lillard LA, Farmer MM. Linking Medicare and national survey data. *Ann Intern Med*. 1997;127:691–695.

20. Schneider EC, Riehl V, Courte-Wienecke S, Eddy DM, Sennett C. Enhancing performance measurement: NCQA's road map for a health information framework. National Committee for Quality Assurance. *JAMA*. 1999;282:1184–1190.

21. Davis DA, Thompson O'Brien MA, Freemantle N, Wolf FM, Mazmanian P, Taylor-Vaisey A. Impact of formal continuing medical education: do conferences, workshops, rounds, and other traditional continuing education activities change physician behavior or health care outcomes? *JAMA*. 1999;282: 867–874.

22. Landon BE, Wilson IB, Cleary PD. A conceptual model of the effects of health care organizations on the quality of medical care. *JAMA*. 1998;279:1377–1382.

chapter 4

Performance of Health Professionals to Determine Priorities and Shape Interventions

Jocelyn Lockyer, PhD

INTRODUCTION

High-quality, reliable data that tells physicians how they and their colleagues are doing in practice can be used to identify educational needs. This information can be helpful to practitioners and continuing professional development (CPD) professionals in the design of learning interventions.

Physicians receive feedback about their performance from many sources. The sources are more or less compelling depending on the source of the information, the discomfort the physician perceives with his/her current practices and patient outcomes, and externally and internally generated forces for change.

In some cases, the feedback is informal. Medical colleagues who share care for a patient may ask questions about the patient that call into question the currency of their treatment choices. Case-based discussions at continuing medical education (CME) programs may validate the frequency of follow-up or the need for referral for selected clinical problems. Patients with information from the Internet frequently challenge current thinking and practice.

Feedback can also be formal. It may be part of a regular system of feedback, such as might be provided through a hospital audit process for selected clinical conditions or through recertification processes. It may be received on an ad hoc basis such as the data that would be provided to physicians who use a patient simulator to assess their skills. Similarly, some educational programs have used precourse needs assessments, which give physicians an opportunity to reflect on their knowledge and care practices in advance of a course. Data collected in this way can guide a teacher, be used to redesign an existing course, or be used as the base for initiating other interventions. This information is particularly useful when the target audience is composed of a group of physicians such as a hospital medical staff, insurance company network, or constituents of a peer review organization for which data is available.

A number of questions arise when one considers data. What data is available? How current and precise is the data? Is the data sophisticated enough to help design initial interventions, monitor intervention outcomes so that the interventions can continue to be improved, or enable physicians to have an ongoing system of review? Will the data have to be generated on an ongoing basis? Is it available through other organizations or the efforts of others? How difficult will it be to obtain access to it and to use it? Is the data likely to be compelling enough to convince physicians to change their practices? To what extent are institutional system problems or physician-specific problems identified, given that teams are generally involved in the care of patients?

This chapter will focus on data sources that are available to provide feedback about medical care. Several forms of feedback along with the literature on their use will be described. These include statewide or national clinical performance databases, hospital or clinic chart audit processes or systems, patient feedback programs, multipoint feedback systems, testing in conjunction with educational programs, and competency assessment programs.

USE OF CLINICAL DATABASES

You are the continuing medical education (CME) director for a university CME department. The chair of general surgery has invited you to continue working on a physician-based initiative to increase the use of breast-conserving therapy (BCT) in the treatment of women with early-stage breast cancer. A review of data from the academic medical center reveals the use of breast-conserving surgery is 10% below the national average. Of the five major practice groups, three are below the national average while the other two are significantly above.

The chair envisages a program in which the CME office develops educational strategies for physicians. These strategies would be based of current research on outcome data and national guidelines.

You discuss this opportunity with members of the five practice groups, and they are less than enthusiastic. Some point out that these figures are just "averages" and that if you looked at each patient case by case, there would be a valid reason why the surgeon performed a modified radical mastectomy. Some of the surgeons described the discussions they have had with their patients, which resulted in the patient choosing a more aggressive approach. Others noted that their rates of BCT were low because their patients were regularly referred late to them. You wonder whether it is even possible to develop viable CME initiatives and whether they will have any impact on surgical practice.

The advent of computers has supported the creation of large databases containing information relevant to physician performance. Governments and health care organizations have become increasingly responsive to the need for data. Researchers and program administrators are using data more consistently and in more diverse fields as the data become more readily available, more specific to their needs, and available in formats that are easily accessed and understood. These databases are beginning to address the most common and expensive problems but will expand into new domains such as ambulatory care when mechanisms are found to expedite data collection and dissemination.

The Agency for Healthcare Research and Quality (AHRQ) has funded or sponsored several databases. In particular, the Healthcare Cost and Utilization Project (HCUP), a federal–state–industry partnership to build a standardized, multistate health data system, provides patient-level information in a uniform format. Their Nationwide Inpatient Sample (NIS) has data from more than 1000 hospitals. The State Inpatient Databases (SIDs) has data from community hospitals in 22 states, representing over half of all US hospital discharges. The State Ambulatory Surgery Databases (SASD) has data from ambulatory care encounters in nine states. The intent of the HCUP project is to make the data available to a broad set of public and private users. Other initiatives of the AHRQ include health care quality measurement tools, clinical practice guidelines, and critical analyses of health care practices (see www.ahrq.gov).

Similarly, there are atlases to detect patterns in health care, disease, and mortality. As Gundersen[1] notes, these atlases have been used to detect geographic patterns for the presence of specific types of cancer and, with that data, identify causative agents such as asbestos, which might be responsible for high rates in specific areas. Similarly, the atlases have been used to examine differences in patterns of care such as variations in imaging stress testing, with the data then being used to create and disseminate guidelines to reduce variability. Gundersen[1] provides several Web addresses for obtaining atlases in the United States and the rest of the world for a variety of medical conditions.

Databases maintained by hospitals and health care organizations also provide helpful information. Billing information can be useful in determining the most frequent diagnoses and for comparing costs across individual physician groups. More sophisticated data sources include information included in the electronic medical record. Through data mining techniques, detailed information can be gathered to reflect resource allocation and quality of care. As shown by Anderson et al.,[2] a province-wide prescription database was used to identify and target physicians whose profile for prescriptions for regulated drugs was more than two standard deviations above the mean. Techniques such as small area variation analyses have been used to compare physician practices in one area against practices in other geographic areas. The work done by the Maine Medical Assessment Foundation[3] is particularly notable. They examined the variance in five musculoskeletal injuries and five orthopedic procedures and used feedback to physicians to reduce the variation. More recently, this group has formed the new Outcomes Dissemination Project, which involves physicians in Maine, New Hampshire, and Vermont. They have five specialty study groups that meet three times a year to examine local and national utilization data, guidelines, and research findings. All but one of their groups has made their existence and work known in the broader medical community.[4]

Yet, this data does have its limitations and it must be used judiciously. Codes such as ICD-9, which are used in billing, may be based on symptoms or broad disease categories that may be difficult to interpret in terms of specific disease entities. Occasionally, there are problems related to the quality of the information (accuracy of coding) and timeliness (by the time records are coded and analyzed, the information may be several years old). It is important to understand how and why data are collected and assess whether they are a good match as part of a needs assessment. Lack of consideration for acuity of illness or comorbidities may limit data utility or interpretation. It is also easy to attribute success and failure to the competence of individual physicians or surgeons when it may be more appropriate to look at the institution and its role.

Dupont et al[5] examined breast cancer lymphatic mapping to clarify whether it was surgical skill or the institution that determined mapping failure. Their hypothesis was that mapping failure could be a function of multiple factors, including surgical skills, surgical volume index, and the injection method. All of these factors are under the quality control of an institution. They determined that although there were differences in mapping success across institutions, the disparity lay with the skill of the individual surgeon and not the institution as a whole. In another example of physician profiling, Hofer et al.[6] noted that 4% or less of the variance in the quality of care provided to patients with diabetes was due to differences in physician practice. They found that other issues, including patient factors, were the greatest determinants. More disturbingly, they noted that physicians concerned about their profiles could change their profile results by manipulating their patient populations; they could do this by refusing to care for sick patients, those who have failed therapy, or those who do not adhere to treatment plans. Nonetheless, it appears that skilled CME providers and policy makers can use clinical databases to design CME interventions and improve health outcomes.

CHART AUDIT AND FEEDBACK SYSTEMS

Dr Mary Jones will be attending a course at her university on the management of Alzheimer's disease and other dementias. As part of the precourse activity, she has been asked to complete a chart audit in which she has to record a number of aspects of care provided for five of her patients with dementia. These include the mini mental state examination score, details about activities of daily living, and whether she had discussed guardianship and trusteeship. She asked her nurse to pull five charts. As she goes through the charts, she discovers that she has not done a mini mental state exam for any of the five patients.

Chart audit is the review and assessment of medical records generally using preset criteria and standards against which care is measured. As Jennett and Affleck[7] note, chart reviews can be conducted within all work sites, including hospitals, clinics, offices, and community care sites. Depending on their purpose, chart audits can be done to assess the charts of an individual caregiver or the care provided for a specific condition or procedure over a number of caregivers and institutions. Medical records data, both hospital[8,9] and clinic[10–12] data, have provided the baseline information and impetus for some studies. This data can either be created through self-audit or by third-party audit.

Chart audit offers a number of advantages when assessing performance. It is less expensive and time consuming than methods such as interviewing and video- or audiotaped observation and it is relatively easy to abstract data from charts. Some data are particularly easy to capture in a chart. Rethans[13] found that data related to laboratory, radiology, and medications were most consistently recorded and filed in charts. Data related to the history, counseling, and ongoing monitoring of patient health were least likely to be consistently recorded. Similarly, Peabody et al.[14] hypothesized that treatment plans may be best studied from a medical record because the record is the source that is used to convey treatment orders. Chart audit is not usually considered to be invasive or disruptive to practice. The professional can participate in problem identification and criteria setting, leaving the abstractor to pull the data.

Chart audit does have its limitations. Charts are used primarily by health care professionals to assist them with recall. For this, it is not necessary to record all factors or decisions influencing the management of cases. Thus, records may be incomplete or inaccurate representations of the care encounter. They can be missing relevant information regarding patient symptoms and care options considered but ruled out, as well as issues associated with communication.[7] Other challenges relate to the lack of standardization in chart formats, the varied types of filing systems, difficulties in locating or retrieving all parts of the chart, variations in recording practices, and legibility.[7] Peabody et al.[14] note that institutional structural problems degrade the quality of care as measured by charts, citing orders that are requested by a physician but are lost or delayed. Sample size may also be an issue, with data not being representative of the practitioner's overall patient population or usual standard of care. There are also ethical considerations related to sending outside record abstractors into physician's offices. Patient consent to have records reviewed by an outsider needs to be obtained.

Audit data have been used as a starting point for many analyses and interventions. For example, in a recent study, Laliberte[15] used Department of Defense data to determine whether patient characteristics, rather than surgeon characteristics, were more likely to explain variance in the use of breast-conserving surgery. In another study, Olcott[16] used surgeon data on the risk and cost of carotid endarterectomy to examine the effectiveness of a surgeon-directed institutional peer review process. Similarly, Wigder[17] provided physicians with their own individual and peer data related to their utilization of X rays in accordance with the Ottawa Decision Rule for knee radiography to determine whether this would decrease the percentage of knee injury patients who received an X ray and the percentage of abnormal results.

COMPETENCY ASSESSMENT

> Dr Smith attends a CME program that includes an opportunity to participate in a demonstration of an anesthesia simulator. Dr Smith is an anesthesiologist in a large academic medical center and is anxious to see if the simulator might be helpful in training residents. He participates in a scenario involving a case of malignant hyperthermia. Dr Smith is surprised that he has forgotten the dosage of the pharmaceutical agent used to treat this condition and that he is unable to intubate the simulated patient because of a congenital malformation in the upper airway.

There is increasing pressure to assess physician competency and ensure maintenance of certification. Graduation from medical school and successful passing of specialty examinations is no longer accepted as proof of competency for the life of the practitioner. Recognizing this, most medical specialty boards in the United States have adopted time-limited certification. The complexity of assessing competency is recognized. Physician practices evolve over time. Many physicians will develop areas of special expertise. Others will eliminate aspects of a specialty from their practice profile. Competency may be gradually lost for skills or issues that are not commonly encountered. Examining physicians for the full range of their specialty or at an appropriate depth is very difficult, leading specialty boards to adopt a variety of strategies. Although initial efforts by the American Board of Internal Medicine focused on examination by using a multiple-choice examination format,[18] the new recertification program called Continuous Professional Development is composed of three parts: self-evaluation, secure examination, and verification of credentials. In the self-evaluation, the physician will complete a series of modular examinations taken at home.[19] As Norman[20] noted, a single assessment is unlikely to give all physicians the detailed information needed for appropriate feedback.

Innovative approaches are being tested and adopted to assess competence. For example, the Royal College of General Practitioners in the United Kingdom has developed a direct assessment of interpersonal skills performance using videotaped consultations of actual patient–physician encounters.[21] Physician candidates are advised of the clinical and consulting competencies that are required to be demonstrated. Physicians are required to provide evidence of competence by selecting appropriate patient encounters. Their analysis of their marking systems shows that they can achieve satisfactory levels of reliability. The Royal Australasian College of Physicians has adopted a physician assessment program in which ratings from peers on professional and personal attributes will be sought as part of its recertification process.[22]

In other cases, physicians have undergone knowledge or competency assessment prior to a course, and that data have resulted in the creation of a very targeted course.[23–25] In an Australian study, Ward[23] had physicians answer knowledge-based questions about skin cancer protection, early detection, and management prior to a course; the results were used to modify the presentations. Davis and Suarez-Almazor's[24] used a case study in rheumatology to determine learning needs prior to developing the intervention. A Canadian study by Ward[25] had physicians complete a series of knowledge questions as well as pull information from charts of patients with attention deficit hyperactivity disorder prior to attending an educational program. The data that registrants provided was used to "stream" the learners into high/low skill and to focus the lectures and case-based discussion. That study was helpful in demonstrating that physicians will pull chart data on a limited number of patients. This data can be used to guide an educational program, provided the teachers are flexible. More recently, Peabody et al[14] compared the results of three methods of assessing physician performance—vignettes, standardized patients, and chart abstraction. They found that quality of care could be measured almost as effectively (and certainly less expensively) through the use of questionnaires using clinical vignettes when compared with standardized patients.

Assessment and feedback from standardized patients has also been used. In two studies, Lockyer et al[26] and O'Brien et al[27] showed that physicians would participate in standardized patient or objective structured examination station exercises and that the data from the assessment could be used to design or refine an educational program. Similarly, Armstrong-Brown et al[28] videotaped anesthesiologists during a simulated anesthesia session to determine how completely anesthesiologists check their machinery and equipment, using a checklist of 20 items derived from well-publicized, international standards. That data identified a number of areas for improvement. Unfortunately, the costs associated with such intensive endeavors usually mean that their use is restricted to experimental projects and not used routinely within continuing education.

PERCEIVED PERFORMANCE—MULTISOURCE FEEDBACK

Dr Donaldson, a surgeon, has just participated in a 360-degree (multisource feedback) assessment that his HMO instituted. As part of the review, he was required to get 25 patients to complete surveys about his office, staff, bedside manner, and communication skills. Eight coworkers and medical colleagues also completed forms about his communication skills, technical competence, and collegiality. When he gets his feedback, he is surprised to find that although rated highly for his technical competence, he is well below the mean on all 20 communication items. The feedback on the communication items is consistent, regardless of whether it is reported on the patient, colleague, or coworker surveys. It is equally low for both written and verbal communication.

In reflecting on his scores, his first reaction was to disregard the communication data. After all, his technical performance is what really counts at the end of the day. But he also recalls a recent chat with his department head who had received complaints about his "rudeness" to operating room staff. He also remembers that he had to meet later that day with the HMO manager to discuss what he might say to a patient with a poor surgical outcome who had threatened to sue both the HMO and himself.

The term *multisource* or *360-degree feedback* has been used to describe feedback to a single physician from multiple sources. This type of feedback is common in large organizations in which supervisors, subordinates, peers, and the individual rate him/herself on attributes or skill sets. In some cases, 90- or 180-degree feedback is used (ie, subordinate alone or subordinate and supervisor).

Medical organizations have also adopted multisource feedback. In this case, patients, medical colleagues, nonmedical coworkers (ie, nurses, pharmacists), and the individual physician complete surveys about an individual physician's performance.[19,29-33] The surveyed provide data about such physician attributes as communication skills, collegiality, professionalism, psychosocial skills, self-management, technical competence, office staff, and office systems.[19,29-33] Initial work has shown multipoint feedback to be psychometrically reliable, valid, and feasible. The data generated from such reviews could be used to design educational interventions for groups. Or, as work in Alberta has shown, it can be used by individual physicians to initiate changes in their practices.[31,34]

Multisource feedback can also be done using multiple assessment methods. Norman et al[20] proposed and tested a multiple assessment process as a second stage in a peer review process. In this case, a combination of reference physicians, self-referred physicians, and physicians referred to the licensing authority were assessed using standardized patients, structured oral examinations, chart-stimulated recall, objective structured clinical examination, and a multiple-choice examination. Work by Gerbert and Hargreaves[35] demonstrated that a combination of techniques was superior to any single assessment method. Certainly, as Saturno et al.[36] found, there can be wide variability between self-assessment and peer assessment as well as disparities between self-perceptions and peer perceptions and actual performance. This suggests that caution be used when developing educational programs because physicians may not perceive the same need for educational assistance that the data show.

Multisource feedback is not always comprehensive. It may be useful even when limited to two sources, such as patients and the physician. For example, Clark et al[37] obtained data from both physicians and the parents of children with asthma before randomly assigning physicians to the intervention or control group. That information was used to design an educational program. Limiting data sources can prove to be a problem. Godden and Robertson's[38] follow-up of patients who had temporomandibular joint arthroscopy showed variance in the patients' assessment of outcome and the clinician's assessment of functional capacity, suggesting the need to combine patient information with more objective sources of data when using patient feedback.

Multisource systems may prove to be valuable for both the individual as a quality-improvement technique as well as for providers who have access to large aggregate databases. As the American Board of Internal Medicine[19] and College of Physicians and Surgeons of Alberta[29-31] continue their work using these tools, more information will become available about their potential for both practitioners and providers.

CONCLUSION

New technology, high-speed computer systems, and increased concern about the variability of patient care have enabled the development of new data sources. These data sources can be used to provide individualized feedback to physicians as well as identify patterns of care within and over groups of physicians that may be used to determine priorities and shape educational and systems interventions to improve care.

This chapter has identified several of these. First and foremost is the advent of federal and state databases and atlases. These provide information about variation in care as well as disease patterns. Chart audit systems, in place since the 1920s, allow physicians to compare the care they provide against that of their colleagues. Data from recertification and licensure renewal systems can also identify variance in knowledge and skill. More local systems, such as those provided by patient surveys or educational program data, can give physicians information about specific aspects of their knowledge or skill.

One of the great benefits of these performance indicators in needs assessment is that they can be followed longitudinally as a basis for determining the outcomes of educational interventions. Challenges for the CPD professional involve gaining access to these data sources, justifying the cost in terms of data retrieval and analysis, and understanding how these needs can be incorporated into effective educational interventions. Often, the data are too person-specific or too global to be helpful in designing a course or in marketing the need for the course to physicians.

REFERENCES—CHAPTER 4

1. Gundersen L. Mapping it out: Using atlases to detect patterns in health care, disease and mortality. *Ann Int Med*. 2000;133:161–164.

2. Anderson JF, McEwan KL, Hrudey WP. Effectiveness of notification and group education in modifying prescribing of regulated analgesics. *Can Med Assoc J*. 1996;154:31–39.

3. Keller RB, Soule DN, Wennberg JE. Dealing with geographic variations in the use of hospitals: the experience of the Maine Medical Assessment Foundation orthopaedic study group. *J Bone Joint Surg Am*. 1990;72-A:1286–1293.

4. Schneiter EJ, Keller RB, Wennberg D. Physician partnering in Maine: an update from the Maine Medical Assessment Foundation. *Jt Comm J Qual Improv*. 1998;24:579–584.

5. Dupont E, Cox C, Shivers S, Salud C, Nguyen K, Cantor A, Reintgen D. Learning curves and breast cancer lymphatic mapping: institutional volume index. *J Surg Res*. 2001;97:92–96.

6.   Hofer TP, et al. The unreliability of individual physician report cards for assessing the costs and quality of care of a chronic disease. *JAMA.* 1999;281:2098–2105.

7.   Jennett PA, Affleck L. Chart audit and chart stimulated recall as methods of needs assessment in continuing professional health education. *J Contin Educ Health Prof.* 1998;18:163–171.

8.   Anderson FA, Wheeler HB, Goldberg RJ, Hosmer DW, Forcier A, Patwardhan NA. Changing clinical practice. Prospective study of the impact of continuing medical education and quality assurance programs on use of prophylaxis for venous thromboembolism. *Arch Intern Med.* 1994;154:669–677.

9.   White C, Albanese MA, Brown DB, Caplan RM. The effectiveness of continuing medical education in changing the behavior of physicians caring for patients with acute myocardial infarction: A controlled randomized trial. *Ann Intern Med.* 1985;102:686–692.

10. Perez-Cuevas R, Guiscafre H, Munoz O, Reyes H, Tome P, Liberos V, Gutierrez G. Improving physician prescribing patterns to treat rhinopharygitis: Intervention strategies in two health systems of Mexico. *Soc Sci Med.* 1996;42:1185–1194.

11. Gullion DS, Adamson E, Watts MSM. The effect of an individualized practice-based CME program on physician performance and patient outcomes. *West J Med.* 1983;138:582–588.

12. Jennett PA, Laxdal OE, Hayton RC, Klassen DJ, Swanson RW, Wilson TW, Spooner HJ, Mainprize GW, Wickett REY. The effects of continuing medical education on family physician performance in office practice: a randomized control study. *Med Educ.* 1988;139–145.

13. Rethans JJ, Martin E, Metsemakers J. To what extent do clinical notes by general practitioners reflect actual medical performance? A study using simulated patients. *Br J Gen Pract.* 1994;44:153–156.

14. Peabody JW, Luck J, Glassman P, Dresselhaus TR, Lee M. Comparison of vignettes, standardized patients, and chart abstraction. *JAMA.* 2000;283:1715–1722.

15. Mor V, Laliberte MV, Petrisek AC, Intrator O, Wachtel T, Maddock PG, Bland KI. Impact of breast cancer treatment guidelines on surgeon practice patterns: results of a hospital-based intervention. *Surgery.* 2000;128:847–861.

16. Olcott C IV, Mitchell RS, Steinberg GK, Zarins CK. Institutional peer review can reduce the risk and cost of carotid endarterectomy. *Arch Surg.* 2000;135:939–942.

17. Wigder HN, Cohan Ballis SF, Lazar L, Urgo R, Dunn BH. Successful implementation of a guideline by peer comparisons, education and positive physician feedback. *J Emerg Med.* 1999;17:807–810.

18. Ramsey PG, Carline JD, Inui TS, Larson EB, LoGerfo JP, Norcini JJ, Wenrich MD. Changes over time in the knowledge base of practicing internists. *JAMA.* 1991;266:1103–1107.

19. Lipner RS, Blank LL, Leas BF, Fortna GS. The value of patient and peer ratings in recertification. *Acad Med.* 2002;77:64–66.

20. Norman GR, Davis DA, Lamb S, Hanna E, Caulford P, Kaigas T. Competence assessment of primary care physicians as part of a peer review program. *JAMA.* 1993;270:1046–1051.

21. Foulkes TP, Neighbour R, Campion P, Field S. Assessing physicians' interpersonal skills via videotaped encounters: a new approach for the Royal College of General Practitioners Membership examination. *J Health Commun.* 1999;4:143–152.

22. Paget NS, Newble DI, Saunders NA, Du J. Physician assessment pilot study for the Royal Australasian College of Physicians. *J Contin Educ Health Prof.* 1996;16:103–111.

23. Ward J, MacFarlane S. Needs assessment in continuing medical education: its feasibility and value in a seminar about cancer for general practitioners. *Med J Aust.* 1993;159:20–23.

24. Davis P, Suarez-Almazor M. An assessment of the needs of family physicians for a rheumatology continuing medical education program: Results of a pilot project. *J Rheumatol.* 1995;22:1762–1765.

25. Ward R, Fidler H, Lockyer J, Toews J. Physician outcomes following an intensive educational experience in attention deficit hyperactivity disorder. *Acad Med.* 1999;74:S31–S33.

26. Lockyer J, el-Guebaly N, Simpson E, Gromoff B, Toews J. Standardized patients as a measure of change in the ability of family physicians to detect and manage alcohol abuse. *Acad Med.* 1996;71:S1–S3.

27. O'Brien MK, Feldman D, Alban T, Donoghue G, Sirkin J, Novack D. An innovative CME program in cardiology for primary care practitioners. *Acad Med.* 1996;71:894–897.

28. Armstrong-Brown A, Devitt JH, Kurrek M, Cohen M. Inadequate preanesthesia equipment checks in a simulator. *Can J Anaesth.* 2000;47:974–979.

29. Violato C, Marini A, Toews J, Lockyer J, Fidler H. Feasibility and psychometric properties of using peers, consulting physicians, co-workers, and patients to assess physicians. *Acad Med.* 1997;72:S82–S84.

30. Hall W, Violato C, Lewkonia R, Lockyer J, Fidler H, Toews J, Jennett P, Donoff M. Assessment of physician performance in Alberta: the Physician Achievement Review. *Can Med Assoc J.* 1999;161:52–57.

31. Lockyer JM. Role of Socio Demographic Variables and Continuing Medical Education in Explaining Multi Source Feedback Ratings and Use of Feedback by Physicians [dissertation]. University of Calgary; 2002.

32. Ramsey PG, Wenrich MD, Carline JD, Inui TS, Larson EB, LoGerfo JP. Use of peer ratings to evaluate physician performance. *JAMA.* 1993;269:1655–1660.

33. Wenrich MD, Carline ID, Giles LM, Ramsey PG. Ratings of the performances of practicing internists by hospital-based registered nurses. *Acad Med.* 1993;68:680–687.

34. Fidler H, Lockyer J, Toews J, Violato C. Changing physicians' practices: The effect of individual feedback. *Acad Med.* 1999;74:702–714.

35. Gerbert B, Hargreaves WA. Measuring physician behavior. *Med Care.* 1986;24:838–847.

36. Saturno PJ, Palmer RH, Gascon JJ. Physician attitudes, self-estimated performance and actual compliance with locally peer-defined quality evaluation criteria. *Int J Qual Health Care.* 1999;11:487–496.

37. Clark NM, Gong M, Schork A, Evans D, Roloff D, Hurwitz M, Maiman L, Mellins RB. Impact of education for physicians on patient outcomes. *Pediatrics.* 1998;101:831–836.

38. Godden DR, Robertson JM. The value of patient feedback in the audit of TMJ arthroscopy. *Br Dent J.* 2000;188:37–39.

Identifying the Needs of the Individual Learner

Craig M. Campbell, MD; S. Tunde Gondocz, MSc

INTRODUCTION

Over the past 20 years, research in continuing medical education (CME) has slowly shifted its focus from answering the question, Does continuing medical education work? to understanding how continuing education can assist physicians to identify and adopt new innovations into their practices. *Practice-based learning,* defined as the "process whereby physicians use their practice environment and experiences to identify opportunities for learning,"[1] challenges physicians to acquire the skills to reflect on and select the problems they will address now and to integrate new learning into a highly complex and rapidly changing practice environment. Learning in a technological age characterized by rapid expansion in biomedical knowledge equally challenges physicians to establish and implement their own personal, practice-specific, continuing professional development (CPD) plan and acquire computer literacy and information management skills.[2] The change study authored by Fox, Mazmanian, and Putnam was the first extensive description of the changes physicians identified and implemented in their practice.[3] This study analyzed the personal, professional, and social forces that enhanced or hindered the implementation of these changes. Interviews with physicians who voluntarily enrolled in the Maintenance of Competence (MOCOMP) Program of the Royal College of Physicians and Surgeons of Canada provided evidence of the importance of the process of reflection in the identification of needs and the practice environment in implementing the learning they acquired.[4]

CPD planners seek to design CME activities to address the identified practice-based needs of physicians. Methods for assessing practice-based needs vary considerably, from strategies that determine the expressed needs of individual physicians (perception of need)[5,6] to those that focus on variations in physician performance (eg, adoption of innovations or adherence to established practice standards) or health care outcomes.[7–9] These major areas of the assessment of need are covered in greater detail in other chapters of this book. Although physicians will frequently turn to continuing education professionals to assist them in reviewing and expanding their knowledge and skills, most physician learning is derived from using the practice environment to identify the gaps between current and ideal practice.

The impetus for assisting physicians to use their clinical experiences as a primary source for identifying their needs has been heightened further by environmental changes, such as increasing professional and societal expectations for professional accountability in how physicians maintain clinical competence.[10–12] If they are to respond to these expectations, physicians must acquire new skills and abilities in order to make learning more intentional than incidental.[13] Shifts in the learning environment challenge providers of continuing education to develop new strategies and tools to support the skills and processes that relate to reflective practice and encourage physicians to become reflective practitioners. The assessment of individual learning needs affects not only the nature and effectiveness of learning conducted by physicians but also the formal learning activities they choose to attend.

The chapter will describe:

- theoretical models of reflection, experiential learning, and reflective practice;
- the processes and strategies physicians use to identify their potential needs from their experiences in practice; and
- the ways in which physicians translate these identified needs into manageable problems they can evaluate if they are willing or able to engage in learning activities.

The description of the ideas and constructs developed during this chapter will be illustrated by, and related to, the following case scenario:

Case Scenario—Part 1

Dr Smith is a general internist who has practiced in a rural community setting for more than 10 years. Subsequent to the birth of her second child two years ago, Dr Smith decided to limit her practice to ambulatory medicine. She has had very limited exposure to acute care medical problems, which present to an emergency room, intensive care unit, or acute care hospital ward setting. Dr Smith has been unhappy with having her patients admitted to the hospital under other physicians and the subsequent loss of control and continuity and has decided to apply to a regional hospital for admitting privileges. Although she has read about the acute

care medical problems in journals and has attended local hospital rounds and
occasional medical conferences, Dr Smith remains concerned about her current
competence to assess and manage acute patient care problems and to provide
inpatient consultations for family physicians. Discussion with family physicians
identified a local need for improved access to internal medicine consultants for
patients who are admitted to the hospital. After receiving advice from her local
hospital administration, Dr Smith has decided to systematically review her current
competencies and to contact the university office of continuing education in her
region to help her create a specific learning plan.

The stimulus for engaging in learning often begins when a physician
reflects on her practice and engages in learning in order to find a
solution to a problem, ensure that skills and abilities are up-to-date,
or gain new competencies. Triggers for this stimulus may include an
individual patient whose problem does not fit with the practitioner's
previous experience or knowledge, attendance at formal or informal
continuing education activities, or a general sense of dissonance or
dissatisfaction about perceived competence, performance or health
care outcomes. The motivation to learn may be influenced by previous experiences in learning (positive or negative); perception of the
likelihood of finding an answer to a question;[14] or the relevance of
the problem to current and future professional development. Within
this personal reflection, the standards of care provided by one's
peers may either encourage or place barriers to the pursuit of learning. In the case scenario, Dr Smith, reflecting on her current practice, identified an area of professional development that she wished
to pursue. The uncertainty and anxiety about her abilities to function in a hospital setting are partially fueled by her perception of the
existence of a practice gap: the difference between "what is" and
"what should be." This physician realized that in order to effectively
deal with common acute care problems she would initially need to
create a learning plan that provides her with the opportunity to
manage such problems under supervision.

This case scenario exemplifies one of the major strategies used
by physicians to assess their learning needs: reflection on practice.
How do theoretical models of reflection and reflective practice help
continuing education providers to develop practical strategies for
assessing an individual physician's needs from his or her practice?

THEORETICAL MODELS OF REFLECTION AND REFLECTIVE PRACTICE

The study of reflection and its importance to adult education is certainly not a new idea. Research into the relationship between reflection and learning usually begins with one of several theoretical
models on reflection or reflective practice. It is not our intention to

provide a critique of these models of reflection but to use the models as a basis for understanding the processes by which physicians use their practice environment to identify their needs from a subjective perspective.

The Definition of Reflection

What do we mean by reflection? Jennifer Moon,[15] in her book *Reflection in Learning and Professional Development*, summarizes the common usage of the term reflection to mean, "a form of mental processing with a purpose and/or anticipated outcome that is applied to relatively complicated or unstructured ideas for which there is not an obvious solution."

Brockbank and McGill,[16] in their book *Facilitating Reflective Learning in Higher Education*, define reflection to be "the process or means by which an experience, in the form of a thought, feeling or action is brought into consideration while it is happening or thereafter. In addition, reflection can refer to the creation of meaning and conceptualization from experience and the potentiality to look at things as other than they are." The latter part of this definition embodies the idea of critical reflection that we will discuss later in this chapter. Both definitions imply a strong association with, or involvement between, reflection and learning.

Reflection and Learning

The study of reflection began with the work of John Dewey[17] and Jurgen Habermas.[18] Dewey focused on the process of reflection and its ability to make "sense of the world," particularly when the context for initiating reflection was characterized by doubt, uncertainty, or difficulty. Habermas viewed reflection as a means to acquire and develop knowledge that transformed and liberated the individual in some important way. Both men believed that the notion of reflection was purposeful and central to the generation of knowledge, as long as the individual was willing to learn from experience. However, until Kolb[19] published his experimental learning cycle in 1984 (Figure 5-1), the explicit relationship between reflection and learning remained somewhat contentious.

Kolb's learning cycle identifies "reflective observation" as the critical link between the learner's concrete experiences and the formation of abstract concepts of changes in competence and practice that are subsequently tested in practice. Opportunities for learning stimulated by reflection are not limited exclusively to patient experiences but also arise from participation in formal continuing education, independent personal study, self-assessment of needs, and audits of practice and teaching. Although each stage of Kolb's cycle

FIGURE 5-1

Adaptation of Kolb's Learning Cycle

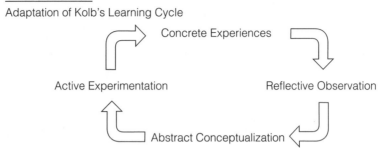

is important, learners may vary in their abilities to function at various stages. We will return to this theory at a later stage in the chapter.

Reflection and Reflective Practice

No individual theoretical construct has had such a profound effect in stimulating interest on the nature of professional practice than that of Donald Schön. Building on Kolb's theory, Schön focused on the issues of reflection and self-direction in learning. His first book, *The Reflective Practitioner*,[20] followed by *Educating the Reflective Practitioner* in 1987,[21] has had a significant influence on research into how physicians use their practice to learn and expand their expertise. Schön was concerned about the limitations of knowledge that professionals acquire during their formal professional education (which he termed *technical rationality*) because the majority of professional work focuses on solving problems characterized by uncertainty, ambiguity, and conflicting values. Schön contended that the education of physicians fails to take into account these situations and inadequately prepares physicians to learn from practice. Schön's theory suggests that professionals (including physicians) use complex and uncertain experiences to generate new knowledge leading to enhanced professional competence and expertise.

Schön's theory makes a distinction between two main processes of reflection in professional practice: reflection-in-action and reflection-on-action (Figure 5-2).

Reflection-in-action results when a physician becomes aware that his knowledge and skills (knowing-in-action) cannot make sense of or understand the unique, unusual, or unexpected features of a case. Reflection-in-action causes the physician to analyze and reconstruct his current knowledge and skills in an effort to understand or resolve the source of the conflict, ambiguity, or uncertainty. Reflection begins when the physician starts to ask key questions of himself. Although there is a debate related to whether these are, in fact, two distinct types of reflection, Schön's theory distinguishes reflection-in-action from other forms of reflection

FIGURE 5-2

Adaptation of Schön's Model Used in MOCOMP Development

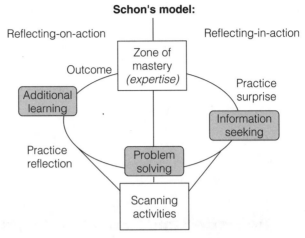

based on its immediacy to the event. Reflection-in-action occurs in the context of actual practice and often stimulates "on-the-spot experimentation" or prompts an immediate search for information to gain greater understanding in an effort to resolve the discrepancy. It is a process of attempting to restructure, understand, and then reframe the situation.

Reflection-on-action is temporally remote from the patient encounter, occurring when the physician reflects on a clinical issue outside the immediacy of work demands in an effort to understand or make sense of what happened. New information sought out as a result of this reflective process is then added to what is already known (or presumed to be understood) and subsequently integrated and validated in professional practice. The resulting change in knowledge and competency is now available when solving similar cases in the future.

According to Fox and Miner,[22] the motivation for physicians to engage in learning is based upon the need to reduce the tension created by the gap that exists between "what is" and "what ought to be." Discrepancy analysis explains the readiness of physicians to learn based upon both intrinsic motivation to enhance mastery of a particular problem and desire to relieve the anxiety generated when things are not as they should be. However, large discrepancies between current and desired practice produce excessive tension and promote an aversion to learning. On the other hand, very small discrepancies are easily tolerated and do not form sufficient basis for motivating a physician to stop and learn. The ability to identify and enhance the motivational level of a learner requires a blending of self-assessment strategies, feedback on actual performance, and removal of barriers to learning in the practice environment.

The critical self-reflections of Dr Smith identified a practice gap between her perceptions of her current knowledge and skills in acute care medicine and the expected standard of performance expected by her peers and colleagues. Despite the relative high levels of anxiety related to the large gap between current and ideal knowledge and competency, she is motivated to undertake learning activities in order to benefit her patients.

Case Scenario—Part 2

Two weeks later, Dr Smith arranged a meeting with the CME provider to discuss the options for a specific learning plan. During the discussion, Dr Smith realized that the area of "acute care medical problems" was too broad and needed to be further refined before a structured learning plan could be created. In listening to Dr Smith, the CME provider recognized that they should focus not only on the acquisition of clinical knowledge and skills but also the enhancement of Dr Smith's ability to function as a reflective practitioner. In addition, in order to make this exercise useful, new learning must be relevant to the clinical environment in which Dr Smith functions. During the discussion, the CME provider began to critically reflect on this physician's practice and began to develop the following questions:

1. What factors or forces in this physician's practice would support or impede learning?
2. What kinds of health care problems are typically referred to general internists in this hospital?
3. What resources are available within the institution for the diagnosis and management of these conditions?
4. What are the accepted professional standards for the management of these conditions?
5. What professional networks exist within the institution to support and enhance reflective practice? Are there regular rounds or meetings with other health professionals that promote the integration of health care and education?[23]
6. Does this physician have the skills to select those problems she needs to solve, frame the problem into a question or problem statement, successfully obtain and appraise information, and integrate new learning into practice?

At the end of the meeting, Dr Smith agreed that she would seek information related to the following questions:

1. In her hospital, what are the top five reasons for family physician consult with a general internist?
2. Are there rounds, journal clubs, or other educational opportunities related to acute care medicine organized within the hospital?
3. What is the extent of radiological and laboratory support provided in the hospital?
4. Does the hospital have a library or access to the Internet for literature searches?
5. What learning strategies have other specialists used to answer questions that arise within an acute care hospital setting?

Because Dr Smith was not currently doing acute care medicine, the CME provider recognized the inherent difficulties of Dr Smith's skills of "reflect-in" and "reflect-on" action related to acute care medical problems. Therefore, they both agreed that Dr Smith would complete an initial two-week clinical preceptorship with a university-based general internist. During this period, she was asked to document all the questions, issues, or ideas that she identified for further learning that arose from her patient interactions. For each question she raised she was asked to describe how she would find an answer. At the end of this experience, they agreed to meet again.

The answers to these types of questions will provide important information to the CME provider in creating a learning plan that accounts for both the nature of the culture within which this physician is planning to expand her professional practice and her skills as a learner. But how can CME providers help this physician to become more conscious of her own approaches to learning and thereby to promote critically reflective learning?

QUESTION-ASKING SKILLS

One strategy to assist physicians to become skilled reflective practitioners is to enhance their question-asking skills. The ability to formulate a question or series of questions is integral to clarifying a learning need and determine if there are sufficient time, resources, and motivation to address it. The process of forming questions enables the learner to clearly determine the difference between current and ideal knowledge and skills, develop a vision of the ideal competencies and behaviors, and reflect on the forces encouraging and impeding change.[3] The clarity and specificity of the question(s) being asked are critical to making this process effective. Once the questions are defined, the ability to reflect can be used to help decide what "I need to know" from "what I don't need to know."

Physicians pursue answers to clinical questions based on perceptions of the urgency of the problem, the relevance of the question to their practice or professional development, and the benefits of information seeking either to themselves or their patients.[21] Through discussion with primary care physicians, Gorman described 12 factors that relate to the motivation to seek further information. His work affirmed the predictions of discrepancy theory, finding that large gaps between current and desired practice resulted in referring the problem to another physician rather than acquiring or enhancing knowledge and skills in order to personally manage the problem. Critical thinking skills required to develop appropriate questions can assist the practitioner in finding the path for the answer.

Question-Asking Skills Development

Asking reflective questions pertinent to professional practice is a skill that can be developed through mentoring and training. King[24,25] designed a tool to help students in large-group learning sessions develop questions by introducing them to a generic stem template (Table 5-1). The stems are effective in generating cognitive prompts to induce analysis, inference, evaluation, comparison, and contrast.[25] The tool functions in a similar manner to how adjectives and action words are used to help in the formulation of cognitive, psychomotor, and attitudinal learning objectives.

Other skills that relate to the development of a question include the ability to:

- find or locate the best resources,
- appraise the information found (did it answer the question),
- evaluate the outcome of new learning for practice, and
- integrate the new knowledge and skills into the physician's "knowledge-in-use."

The work conducted by Gorman[26] and Ely et al.[27] demonstrates some of the characteristics of questions generated by physicians in practice. Gorman studied 154 primary care physicians in Oregon and found that only 88 of the 295 questions (30%) generated in 49 half days of seeing 514 patients were pursued. Ely and coworkers studied a random sample of 103 Iowa family physicians who generated 1101 questions from 2467 patients over two half days. Each physician asked an average of 7.6 questions during the two half days or

TABLE 5-1

A Sample of Question Stems That Help in the Creation of Critical Thinking Questions[25]

Generic Question	Specific Thinking Skills Induced
What are the strengths and weaknesses of . . .?	Analysis/inferencing
What is the difference between . . . and . . .?	Compare–contrast
Explain why . . . (Explain how . . .)?	Analysis
What would happen if . . .?	Prediction/hypothesizing
What is the nature of . . .?	Analysis
Why is . . . happening?	Analysis/inferencing
What is a new example of . . .?	Application
How could . . . be used to . . .?	Application
What are the implications of . . .?	Analysis/inferencing
What is . . . analogous to?	Identification of and creation of analogies and metaphors
What do we already know about . . .?	Activation of prior knowledge
How does . . . affect . . .?	Analysis of relationships (cause–effect)

approximately 3.2 questions per 10 patients seen. The most common question topics were in the areas of drug prescribing (209 questions, 19%), obstetrics and gynecology (96 questions, 9%), and adult infectious diseases (89 questions, 8%). The three most common generic types of questions were, What is the cause of symptom X?, What is the dose of drug X?, and How should I manage disease or finding X?[27] Answers to 702 (64%) of the questions were not pursued, although physicians stated that they might pursue answers to 123 of these questions after the observation period. Physicians spent an average of less than two minutes finding answers to 318 (80%) of the 399 questions they pursued using textbooks or human sources as resources. Literature searches were only performed on two occasions. Although there is incentive for physicians to base their medical decisions on the best available evidence,[27] physicians during practice only pursue "bottom-line" answers by accessing highly digested accessible summaries. Continuing education providers can help physicians find bottom-line answers by enhancing their ability to frame their questions better and find the most appropriate information resources.[27] Ely et al. used these studies to develop and modify a taxonomy of questions[28] to stimulate the organization of clinical questions and develop tools for linking practice questions to answers. Such a system is useful for both practitioners and education coaches to identify, develop, and find resources to answer questions arising in practice.

Case Scenario—Part 3

Dr Smith returns after her two-week preceptorship with a list of diagnoses, problems, and symptoms that family physicians typically refer to an internal medicine consultant. The hospital organizes one round each month for the hospital staff. Each of the general internists is expected to plan and give one of these rounds each year on a topic of their choice. There are no additional journal clubs or interdisciplinary rounds organized through the hospital. However, she discovered that the physicians on the Quality Assurance Committee of the hospital do informally review topics related to the studies being completed. In addition, the local CME coordinator arranges for other consultants to come to their area about six times a year to see patients and give a talk. There is at least one "evening symposium" sponsored by local pharmaceutical representatives. The hospital has two computers available in the hospital's library with Internet access for searching the literature but no full-time librarian to help. The emergency room has a computer with several software programs relating to drug information, poisonings, and some textbooks on CD-ROM. She is now able to describe the radiological and laboratory capability of the hospital that is available to her for the investigation of patients.

During her preceptorship, Dr Smith was able to generate several questions during the investigation and management of patients she evaluated in the hospital with acute renal failure (reflection-in-action). Here is a sample of her questions within this general topic:

1. Acute renal failure management—what's new?
2. What therapeutic strategies are available for managing hyperkalemia?

3. What is the medication of choice to manage poorly controlled hypertension in diabetic patients who are in acute renal failure?
4. What are the latest advances in renal transplantation for patients on chronic hemodialysis?

She discussed the first question with her preceptor and looked up the treatment of hyperkalemia in standard textbooks. She had not pursued the third question to date. Although the fourth question was interesting to her, she decided not to pursue it because she perceived it was not relevant for her clinical practice.

In reviewing these questions, the CME provider concluded that the questions Dr Smith developed were certainly linked to relevant problems in acute care practice, but were these the best questions for her to ask? Why did she ask these questions and not other questions? The questions that she developed certainly varied in focus and complexity. Question 1, although more than a simple topic heading, is a very general question about a broad aspect of acute renal failure. The question is not focused enough to make information gathering timely or succinct. If Dr Smith was looking for specific information regarding the management of acute renal failure, this should have been reflected in the questions she generated. However, the third question was far more specific—it focused on a specific patient population (diabetic patients with acute renal failure) and on one aspect of management (hypertension control). In addition, the question intended to compare and contrast which class of drug was the best (reflected in the medication of choice) for controlling blood pressure in this patient population. The only aspects this question lacked was in defining the level or degree of blood pressure control and specifying the potential clinical benefits of interest (if applicable). If Dr Smith looks for the answer to this question with these appropriate search terms in mind, her quest will likely yield a very workable number of potential articles.

During the discussion with the CME director, Dr Smith noted that the issue of blood pressure control in diabetics with acute renal failure had, in fact, occurred several times over the two weeks. This provided an opportunity for Dr Smith to organize a personal learning project around the control of blood pressure in diabetics with acute renal failure as an example of "reflecting-on-action." Dr Smith agreed to record the resources she used in pursuing this question and the outcomes she identified for her practice. The CME provider suggested that she record the results of this project in a learning portfolio.

Forming Questions That Reflect Educational Needs

The preceptorship provided Dr Smith with an opportunity to be able to take her clinical experiences and identify questions that reflected various levels of needs, from basic factual information to more complex cognitive questions. The search for answers is next guided by the selection of the most appropriate resources and evaluating the relevance of the information found. The importance of asking and answering questions is that this process is personally meaningful[25] and enhances the chance that the information acquired will be turned into new knowledge. Theoretically, when learners develop such extensive cognitive representations of the new material they are more likely to remember it.[25] The personal nature that makes the learning more memorable and meaningful is, after all, one of the goals that adult educators seek. "Adults need to know why they need to learn the information or task."[29] But are all questions equally likely to lead to change simply because they are developed by the individual? According to Campbell et al,[30] the likelihood that a physician will plan to make a change in her practice is influenced by the stimulus for learning. The study examined the relationship between the recorded stimulus for learning and its relationship to the intended outcome of learning for 5708 questions submitted by 317 physicians over one year. Although reading the medical literature was the most frequent stimulus for learning, learning triggered by questions related to the management of more than one patient was 37% (odds ratio 95% confidence interval 1.12, 1.67), more likely than reading to lead to a commitment to change. The authors suggest several characteristics of learning portfolios that encourage a commitment to change, including their ability to stimulate practice reflection and exert an important influence on the effectiveness of workplace learning.

The ability to organize and translate practice needs into manageable questions enhances the effectiveness and efficiency of determining which questions will be dealt with immediately and which questions will be pursued at a later date. Ely et al[28] and Gorman[14] concluded that during practice, family physicians could only focus on what was urgent and when a definitive answer was thought to exist. The pursuit of the urgent is consistent with Schön's concept of reflection-in-action. However, many of the problems that physicians face require a more extensive and critical review of their knowledge and skills. Although the above empirical data would support the value of question-asking skills to enhance the self-directed learning of physicians, there is little agreement about the properties of a good question. In addition, few empirical studies define the context in which questions enhance learning or under which circumstances questions are unnecessary in guiding learning.

Case Scenario—Part 4

The CME provider determined that there is certainly ample opportunity to develop a traditional apprenticeship program under the supervision of an experienced general internist in Dr Smith's local hospital to allow her to gain further experience with the problems she has identified. But what strategies can be considered to support and enhance the ability of this physician to use this experience to learn and to continue to learn after she completes this program and returns to her own practice? Are there any tools that will help her to identify her needs and make her learning more effective and efficient? The questions she developed were certainly linked to relevant problems in her practice, but are they the best questions for her? Why did she ask these questions and not other questions?

While the CME provider began to arrange the logistics for this traineeship, he decided to pursue a review of tools or strategies reported in the literature to support either individualized learning, practice reflection, or question-asking skills. His literature review yielded information related to the role of learning portfolios in aiding physicians to identify and reflect on their needs in practice.

LEARNING PORTFOLIOS AND PERSONAL LEARNING

Learning portfolios facilitate the recording and codifying of practice-based questions that guide personal learning and stimulate practice reflection.[31-34] Portfolios are designed to reflect evidence of personal learning, including the selection of issues for learning, the development of a learning strategy, the conclusions reached, and opportunities for future learning. Although the basic learning process is learner-centered, the facilitation of reflection by a mentor can play an integral role in clarifying learning needs, identifying opportunities for future learning, and both supporting and challenging the learner. Over time, portfolio material represents a collective record and evidence of the content areas and outcomes of learning over time. Portfolio-based learning can be viewed both as an individual learning process and a learning technique. As a learning process, portfolios support the identification of needs from experience and can serve as a tool for the evaluation (formative or summative) of practice performance. The discussion of portfolios as learning tools is the focus of other chapters in this section.

THE IDENTIFICATION OF PERSONAL LEARNING NEEDS: THE ROLE FOR CPD PROFESSIONALS

Continuing education professionals have several potential roles in assisting health professionals to accurately identify their practice-based needs and develop effective and efficient learning plans to address these needs.

Continuing education planners can use several strategies to increase the motivation or readiness of physicians to engage in learning by assisting them to accurately reflect on their current performance and patient outcomes and by reducing inaccurate self-perceptions of their adherence to evidence-based standards. Closing the gap between current and desired performance must be seen as both desirable and important to becoming a better physician. Engaging in pre-tests of knowledge, working through case studies, and reviewing quality assurance data can motivate physicians to learn based on their enhanced perception of need. Continuing education planners have the opportunity to describe the nature and level of motivation by blending traditional testing strategies with technology. For example, self-assessment tests that are Web-based can be linked to online discussion groups with similar physicians and information databases that define practice norms. In addition, providing access to other physicians' questions may raise additional learning needs and provide insight into the most appropriate learning resources as well as expected educational outcomes.[2]

Continuing education planners can assist physicians to improve their questioning skills and provide strategies for the documentation and review of questions that arise in the context of practice. Physicians can be supported in translating the vague uncertainties and ambiguities of practice into questions that are clear and focused. Improved question-asking skills not only assist in defining the problem but also in determining the question's relevance for practice, the probability that it can be adequately answered, and the best resources for efficiently and effectively addressing it. Physicians vary in their ability to "frame problems" and need a mechanism to record or capture the questions that occur to them in practice. Learning portfolios or personal digital assistants are easily adaptable into any practice context. These tools offer the flexibility to quickly record initial thoughts that can be further clarified and modified to determine if a question is worth pursuing now, can wait until a later date, or is not worth pursuing.

Continuing education planners can assist physicians to link learning to common patient problems seen in practice and to their current and potential future areas of expertise. The ability of physicians to describe their practice and the number and type of patient problems that they see will assist in selecting the most relevant problems for learning. In addition, physicians require a clear perception of their current and (potentially) future areas of expertise and the standard of performance they are trying to achieve. The image that physicians have of themselves, their professional roles and responsibilities, and the standards of practice will assist them in defining the best opportunities for learning.

REFERENCES—CHAPTER 5

1. Campbell CM, Parboosingh J, Slotnick H. Outcomes related to physicians' practice based learning activities. *J Contin Educ Health Prof.* 1999;19:234–241.

2. Parboosingh J. Tools to assist physicians to manage their information needs. In: Bruce C, Candy P, eds. *Information Literacy Around the World: Advances in Programs and Research.* New South Wales: Centre for Information Studies: Charles Sturt University; 2000.

3. Fox RD, Mazmanian PE, Putnam RW. *Changing and Learning in the Lives of Physicians.* New York, NY: Praeger Publishers; 1989.

4. Slotnick HB. How doctors learn: physicians' self-directed learning episodes. *Acad Med.* 1999;74:1106–1117.

5. Mann K. Not another survey! Using questionnaires effectively in needs assessment. *J Contin Educ Health Prof.* 1998;18:142–149.

6. Tipping J. Focus groups: a method of needs assessment. *J Contin Educ Health Prof.* 1998;18:150–154.

7. Moore D. Needs assessment in the new health care environment: combining discrepancy analysis and outcomes to create more effective CME. *J Contin Educ Health Prof.* 1998;18:133–141.

8. Jennett PA, Affleck L. Chart audit and chart stimulated recall as methods of needs assessment in continuing professional health education. *J Contin Educ Health Prof.* 1998;18:163–171.

9. Rethans J. Needs assessment in continuing medical education through standardized patients. *J Contin Educ Health Prof.* 1998;18:172–178.

10. Campbell C, Parboosingh J, Gondocz T, Babitskaya G, Pham B. Study factors influencing the stimulus to learning recorded by physicians keeping a learning portfolio. *J Contin Educ Health Prof.* 1999;19:16–24.

11. McLaren B. Task force report in collaboration with the MOPS Evaluation Team. Review of the maintenance of professional standards program. The Royal Australasian College of Physicians, Sydney, Australia; 1999.

12. Pietroni R, Heath I, Burrows P, Savage R, Sowden D, Millard L. Portfolio-based learning in general practice. Report of working group on higher professional education. The Royal College of General Practitioners. Occasional Paper 63. December 1993.

13. Cantillon P, Jone R. Does continuing medical education in general practice make a difference? *BMJ.* 1999;318:1276–1279.

14. Gorman PN, Helfand M. Information seeking in primary care: how physicians choose which clinical questions to pursue and which to leave unanswered. *Med Decis Making.* 1995;15:113–119.

15. Moon J. Reflection in learning and professional development. London, UK: Kogan Page Limited; 1999.

16. Brockbank A, McGill I. *Facilitating Reflective Learning in Higher Education.* Buckingham, UK: Open University Press; 1998.

17. Dewey J. *How We Think?* Boston, Mass: DC Health and Co; 1933.

18. Habermas J. *Knowledge and Human Interests.* London: Heinemann; 1971.

19. Kolb D. *Experiential Learning as the Science of Learning and Development.* Englewood Cliffs, NJ: Prentice Hall; 1984.

20. Schön DA. *Reflective Practitioner.* San Francisco, Calif: Jossey-Bass Publishers; 1983.

21. Schön DA. *Educating the Reflective Practitioner: Toward a New Design for Teaching and Learning in the Profession.* San Francisco, Calif: Jossey-Bass Publishers; 1987.

22. Fox RD, Miner C. Motivation and the facilitation of change, learning, and participation in educational programs for health professionals. *J Contin Educ Health Prof.* 1999;19:132–141.

23. Frankford, DM, Patterson MS, Konrad TR. Transforming practice organizations to foster lifelong learning and commitment to medical professionalism. *Acad Med.* 2000;75:708–717.

24. King A. Inquiry as a tool in critical thinking. In: Halpern D, ed. *Changing College Classrooms: New Technology and Learning Strategies for an Increasingly Complex World.* San Francisco, Calif: Jossey-Bass Publishers; 1994.

25. King A. Designing the instructional process to enhance critical thinking across the curriculum. *Teaching of Psychology.* 1995;22:13–17.

26. Gorman PN. Can primary care physicians' questions be answered using the medical journal literature? *Bull Med Libr Assoc.* 1994;82:140–146.

27. Ely JW, Osheroff JA, Ebell MH, Bergus GR, Levy BT, Chambliss ML, Evans ER. Analysis of questions asked by family doctors regarding patient care. *BMJ.* 1999;319:358–361.

28. Ely JW, Osheroff JA, Gorman PN, Ebell MH, Chambliss ML, Pifer EA, Stavri PZ. A taxonomy of generic clinical questions: classification study. *BMJ.* 2000;321:429–432.

29. Boss BJ. Just use it. *J Interactive Instruction Development.* 1999;11:24–30.

30. Campbell C, Parboosingh J, Gondocz T, Babitskaya G, Pham B. A study of the factors that influence physicians' commitments to change their practice using learning diaries. *Acad Med.* 1999;74:S34–S36.

31. Parboosingh J. Learning portfolios: potential to assist health professionals with self-directed learning. *J Contin Educ Health Prof.* 1996;16:75–81.

32. Westberg J, Jason H. Fostering learner's reflection and self-assessment. *Fam Med.* 1994;26:278–282.

33. Cayne JV. Portfolios: A developmental influence. *J Adv Nurs.* 1995;21:395–405.

34. Sackin P, Barnett M, Eastaugh A, Paxton P. Peer-supported learning [editorial]. *Br J Gen Pract.* 1997;47:67–68.

chapter 6

Determining Needs from the Perspective of Institutions or Organizations Providing Care

Joseph S. Green, PhD; James C. Leist, EdD

SOURCES OF ORGANIZATIONAL NEEDS—AN INTRODUCTION

Physicians have traditionally worked as independent professionals, using their years of training and experience as the primary guide to their individual diagnostic and therapeutic patient-care decision-making. The financial crisis in the health care industry in the United States led to the advent of managed care in the 1990s. "American medicine has led the world in discovery and innovation. Although physicians were trained in and utilized technical advances that made medicine widely available and more effective than ever before, they were unaware of the true cost of these wonderful innovations."[1] Institutions providing health care, such as hospitals, medical schools, physician groups, and managed care organizations, must now account for the cost and quality of that care as never before. Documentation of how care is provided by individual physicians, teams of health professionals, or large groups or departments is now the order of the day. The organization itself is financially, ethically, and legally bound to provide the highest quality, most cost-sensitive care possible to patients. For this reason, health care institutions are studying and attempting to improve identified discrepancies in the systems and processes they use to provide that care. It is within these databases that organizational needs can be found. The new role of the continuing professional development (CPD) office within these health care organizations is to learn to incorporate organizational needs, as determined by analyses of these new data, into their overall vision of facilitating the learning and development of the physicians they serve. This chapter will review some of the tools and strategies that CPD professionals can use to assume this new responsibility.

Case 1

The annual needs-assessment survey of physicians within the institution yielded the same set of data about what individual practitioners "wanted" as it had for years before. The OB/GYNs were interested in some of the new pain medications and innovative laparoscopic and other surgical techniques. That same week, however, the recently named medical director of clinical process improvement shared with the CPD office data that had recently been gathered about inappropriately high C-section rates for the hospital (32%, as compared to national standards of less than 20%). The hospital administration was about to initiate an in-depth analysis of the causes of this problem but thought that an immediate CPD activity should be initiated for the entire department.

Looking at the setting in which physicians practice as a source of educational needs is not a new phenomenon. As early as 1970, Brown and Uhl related continuing medical education (CME) directly to patient care when they developed the bi-cycle model.[2] They proposed that the outer cycle of patient care evaluation be tied to the inner cycle of educational development. This model was an attempt to describe the potential of CPD in an organizational setting such as a hospital. "The work setting can greatly influence the motivation for and attitudes toward continuing education. . . ."[3] A vast majority of the research on needs assessment has focused on the individual learner, because CPD itself has been designed traditionally as clinical education for the individual physician. [4,5] Frankford et al pointed out, however, that fewer and fewer medical school graduates will practice as individuals. More will work in large group practices or in hospitals, academic centers, or in "networks" of some sort. "In such circumstances, it is inaccurate to continue to assume that they learn primarily as individuals . . . instead, it is essential to understand that in a practice world in which financial incentives and management techniques are routinely deployed by organizations to control clinical discretion, physicians now learn and act within organizations."[6] With the advent of the managed care revolution, health care organizations have needed to justify every expenditure in terms of improvements in the quality of care or reductions in the cost of care provided within the institution.

In addition, the work of Senge[7] and others[8–11] on the development and enhancement of organizational learning theory has led to the increasing importance of translating the concepts of needs assessment from individuals to organizations. If health care institutions such as hospitals, medical schools, or medical groups are to become learning organizations, they must start by understanding the learning needs of the organization that directly impact physicians and other health professionals. Garvin[12] described what is unique about learning organizations in that they "have a clear picture of their future knowledge requirements." Most organizations do not take the necessary first step in defining what actually needs to be learned in order to solve identified problems or take advantage of opportunities. Instead, institutions typically move immediately into creating learning solutions. The key task is to study systematically the realities within the organization that have lead to the problems or opportunities in the provision of care. What is required is to analyze both the underlying causes of problems and the results of clinical, pharmaceutical, and medical device research and development to better predict potential opportunities for the improvement of care.

To understand the underlying problems in the provision of care within an organization, two sets of analyses need to be undertaken. The first is finding a discrepancy between the accepted standards of care or levels of institutional performance, as defined by the thought leaders, practitioners, administrators, regulators, payers, and other parties in the health care system, and the current practices of the institution, department, or community of practitioners. This discrepancy between an existing set of circumstances and some desired set[13] could focus on knowledge, attitudes, skills, or system deficits. Once it is clear that such a health care "gap"[14] exists, the second analysis should center on why the gap exists. In order to accomplish either one of these analyses, it is important to look at the sources of organizational needs. Whenever possible, multiple data sources should be used to determine the realities of possible organizational needs. Some of what might be uncovered will be more subjective; other information will be "hard" or objective. The validity and reliability of selected data sources will also vary. Looking at issues that describe multiple perspectives on needs of the organization often requires triangulation[15] in order to reach the most valid conclusions.

Specific methods for gathering organizational needs-assessment data will not be discussed in any depth within this chapter. However, it should be emphasized that organizational needs assessment requires analyzing a variety of data sources rather than relying on the more traditional survey of individual practitioners. The latter tends to yield information about the individual needs and wants of physicians, whereas the former is more useful in identifying and understanding true organizational needs in areas where the institution's performance is not at the highest possible level. There are circumstances, however, when a combination of interviews, questionnaires, observations, cognitive testing, and clinical performance assessment will all play an important part in understanding the realities needed to truly comprehend the institutional problem or opportunity at hand.

How do ideas develop within institutions that suggest that learning activities may be a part of an improvement process? Typically, these ideas come from data sources embedded within the organization. Two types of data are most useful as sources of both problem- or opportunity-based educational needs within organizations. Work setting and health status data describe the specifics of the environment in which the physician works that could affect performance. These data may be epidemiological data that describe the pattern of specific disease states, along with information on morbidity, mortality, and cultural influences on the physicians within the institution. They also describe current practices, standards of care, and demographic descriptors of the physician population serving the organization.[16] Advancements in pharmaceutical and medical devices have opened new opportunities for improving the performance of physicians and the organization. These data come from many sources, most of which are outside the health care institution. The data that are most useful in the context of understanding organizational needs are those that represent new advances, techniques, pharmaceuticals, or devices that are purchased and controlled by the institution.

Work Setting and Health Status Data

Work setting and health status data describe the environment in which the physician practices. Different organizations vary greatly in how they are organized and what realities physicians face as they attempt to apply their craft. Understanding these realities allows CPD offices to gather data that are more relevant to better assess organizational needs. External regulatory bodies establish national standards of care and require institutions to gather quality health care data that is relevant to these standards.

- The Joint Commission on the Accreditation of Healthcare Organizations (JCAHO) accredits hospitals, as well as long-term care settings, home health care organizations, behavioral health care institutions, pathology and clinical lab services, assisted-living groups, and ambulatory care settings. The JCAHO sets standards dealing with issues within these health care organizations, including patient rights; history and physical assessment; informed consent; restraint and seclusion; medications; medical staff credentialing, privileging, and education; infection control; medical records review; and medical staff meeting requirements.
- The Agency for Healthcare Research and Quality (AHRQ) provides a comprehensive clearinghouse of clinical practice guidelines with information on evidence-based practice, outcomes, and effectiveness; technology assessment; and preventive services.
- The National Committee for Quality Assurance (NCQA) collects data from managed care organizations and compares health

plans with report cards. NCQA also collects, summarizes, and analyzes HEDIS (Health Plan Employer Data and Information Set) data to determine national performance statistics and benchmarks related to public health issues such as cancer, heart disease, smoking, asthma, and diabetes.

- The Food and Drug Administration (FDA) regulates foodborne illnesses, nutrition and dietary supplements, drugs, medical devices, and biologics, including vaccines and blood products.

- The Centers for Medicare & Medicaid Services (CMS—formerly HCFA) provide health insurance through government-sponsored programs and perform quality-focused activities such as the regulation of lab testing and quality-of-care improvements.

Most of these data that are collected within the institution or from any of these agencies compare current practices with nationally mandated standards of care. Various committees within the local institution are responsible for monitoring these data. Higher-level organizational committees often discuss trends. Although not easy to obtain, the data are available to CPD offices and/or specific physicians who are called upon to develop local improvements and solutions. Depending on what the organization has done with the surveys mandated by these external regulatory bodies, there may be more or less access to the data involved. Each one of these efforts provides a plethora of information that can be used to determine organizational problem-based needs.

Probably the most relevant health care assessment activities that occur within institutions that provide care are those referred to as *clinical process improvement.* Within the past several years, these activities have also been referred to as *total quality management* (TQM) or *quality improvement* (QI). Within an institution, these activities may be the responsibility of one or more offices, committees, or individuals who access comprehensive patient data, analyze clinical process and outcomes, and apply clinical knowledge in order to improve health care delivery and reduce medical errors. The analyses completed by these groups focus on patient characteristics, such as severity and risk, the process of care, the utilization of resources, and health care outcomes. There are many clinical process-improvement models[17]; however, most of them include some variation of the following steps:

1. **Define the process of care.** This part of the process involves deciding on what needs to be examined, the tools that will be used, the information needed, and the location of the data. Tools that are most often used include:
   - cost profiling data,
   - brainstorming,

- process observation,
- chart review/audit,
- study group,
- cause-and-effect or "fishbone" diagrams, and
- process flow charts.

2. **Display the information.** The next step involves analyzing the data and looking for variations in patterns of care, including average length of stay, average costs, timing of surgery, use of diagnostic tests, use of drugs, etc. Several analysis tools are commonly used:

- *Pareto charts* that account for most of any discovered variation,
- *histograms* that display frequency distributions,
- *scatter diagrams* that portray the relationship between two variables,
- *run charts* that record occurrence of a single variable over time, and
- *control charts* that determine whether a process is within acceptable limits.

3. **Specify outcomes.** These are the clinical outcomes or consequences of patient care. These data can be found in:

- clinical findings of morbidity and mortality,
- functional quality-of-life measures,
- resource utilization data, and
- patient satisfaction information.

4. **Document the process of care.** These processes involve mapping a patient's care and include the development of:

- *clinical pathways:* care maps that organize major activities of a health care team,
- *guidelines:* evidence-based statements developed to assist in physician and patient decision-making, and
- *algorithms:* step-by-step processes used by physicians.

The final two steps in the overall process usually include implementing the revised process and holding the gains. According to Rosenstein, "performance profiling has become an inevitability for healthcare providers . . . to identify potential opportunities for outcome improvement."[18]

"The fundamental learning unit in any organization is a team, not an individual. The basic premise has always been that when we are talking about organizational knowledge, skills and capabilities, they are embedded in working teams. Otherwise, they don't exist."[7] Some organizations are merely an amalgam of individuals providing care; however, in order to survive in today's economic environment, most organizations providing care look at the group of individuals involved. Katzenbach and Smith[19] identified several factors that influence high-performing teams, including the degree of commitment of the members of the team to learning and improving. Much of the data that are gathered compare groups or teams with one another or with other institutions. The groups might be floors in a hospital, all interventional cardiologists, or a clinical business unit such as cardiac services that would include multiple teams providing care. Whenever data indicate that a gap exists between current and ideal performance of a team, there is the possibility it is a function of learning needs. Some times these teams are organized to provide more effective care and other times they also form natural "communities of learners."[10] Activities such as morbidity and mortality conferences focus entirely on learning by studying mistakes or complex patient problems. Whether the team includes two physicians and a nurse providing emergency services or the entire medical staff of a hospital, the focus is on the performance of the team, not on the individual care provider.

Some organizational cultures support change and improvement; others do not. Schein suggests that growth stages of an organization determine the degree to which organizations are motivated to support change.[20] Organizations that are committed to learning understand that learning is the essence of enhanced intellectual capability obtained through institution-wide opportunities for continuous improvement and occurs only through the shared insights, knowledge, and mental models of members of the organization.[10] Prather suggested that physician motivation and organizational readiness were the keys to positive change within an institution.[1] In these organizations, most of the committees appointed and policies and procedures developed involve opportunities for a better understanding of how the institution and its members can learn from reflecting on practice. These groups and documents become invaluable as data sources for institutional needs.

Epidemiological data that focus on patterns of disease within the institution also provide valuable clues as to potential problems in the provision of that care. Whether the information deals with higher-than-normal mortality rates in the operating room or increased infection rates on a particular patient floor, organizational learning needs may often be uncovered. Data sources include infection control data, mortality statistics, patient safety reports, morbidity information, medical error rates by clinical service unit, seminal event analysis, and pharmacy and therapeutics committee minutes. Also, HEDIS data (as previously mentioned) are available related to compliance rates for childhood immunizations, breast cancer screening, control of high blood pressure, beta blocker treatment after heart attack, cholesterol management, antidepressant medication management, smoking cessation, flu shot history, and well-child visits.

Additional information that may shed light on patient care patterns relates to personal data about the population of patients served by the physicians within the institution. Cultural information and attitudes about health care of certain population groups are often collected and analyzed. These data might include information about patient age, sex, economic background, or education and are typically compared across physician groups to uncover patterns of insufficient or inappropriate care.

There is other information available that focuses on the characteristics of physicians involved with the organization. These data include such things as age, years since residency, specialty training, research interests, educational patterns and accomplishments, responsibilities on committees, publications, learning-style preferences, and presentations. This information may be available on individuals in an institutionwide faculty or physician database or as part of summary data in departments, groups, or clinical service units. This type of information can be very valuable in attempts to uncover causes to identified problems or possible target audiences for educational activities. Davis and Fox discuss the importance of these characteristics as they relate directly to motivation to learn, self-efficacy, goal-setting capability, curiosity, professionalism, resistance to change, adoption of innovation, and self-directedness in the pursuit of knowledge.[21]

Finally, traditional quality assurance (QA) data have yielded discrepancies between actual and ideal organizational performance; however, the more recent quality-improvement approaches have been far more effective in this effort.[22,23] The reason these latter efforts have proven more fruitful is that the process focuses more on determining the root causes of identified problems. Solutions are not proposed until this analysis is complete. Often, the needs that are identified do not lend themselves to educational interventions, but rather suggest the need for system solutions.[24,25]

Case 2

An urgent meeting has been called and the individuals are willing to come to your office. The three include a surgeon, an infectious disease specialist, and the nurse who staffs the Infection Control Committee at the hospital. They tell the CPD Office that they have several journal articles that clearly articulate the national standards for rates of infection, morbidity and mortality related to the placement of central venous line catheters. They indicate that they also have just completed a quality-improvement study of physicians within the institution and that the infection rates are significantly above those acceptable standards. After some interesting dialogue, it is clear that part of the reason for the higher infection rates has to do with the fact that both the residents and attendings do not understand the appropriate methodology for insertion of these catheters. It also becomes clear that every incident of unnecessary infection is costing the institution thousands of dollars and could lead to the loss of life. They have come to the CPD Office to get help in the form of an educational intervention aimed at the residents, followed by the practicing physicians who either do or oversee this procedure.

Advancements in Pharmaceutical and Medical Devices

Advancements in an organization's capabilities in terms of purchase and control of pharmaceutical products and medical devices are critically important for assuring improvements in the quality of care as well as cost-effectiveness within the institution. There are several ways that new-development information reaches a CPD office. Commonly a pharmaceutical representative offers to fund a CPD activity, usually based on their desire to disseminate information about a new drug or new FDA-approved or off-label use of that drug. This may represent an opportunity for the institution to improve either the quality of care or cost of care provided by physicians within the organization. There is also the possibility that the offer is not in the best interest of the organization. In order to sort out organizational needs related to managing the adoption of new developments, several resources are very useful as potential partners for the CPD office:

- The Pharmacy and Therapeutics Committee (P&T Committee) of the institution may provide monthly data on new drugs approved for the formulary of the organization. The approval is based on the scientific evidence available to the committee on effectiveness, safety, equivalence, and cost. The P&T Committee often mandates informational newsletters or formal CPD activities to prescribing health professionals in order to deal with the quality or cost-related institutional needs uncovered by these new developments.

- Web sites, such as HealthEconomics.com, deal directly with the cost-effectiveness of pharmaceuticals.

- The US Department of Health and Human Services publishes *HHS NEWS*, which has focused on the dissemination of off-label uses of drugs and the changing regulations about the process.

- The Web site FDCreports.com provides news on the pharmaceutical, medical device, and diagnostic industries. Its "Pink Sheet" describes all the drugs that have received FDA approval on a monthly basis.

- New devices and diagnostics are covered in other publications, such as the "Green Sheet" (weekly pharmacy reports), the "Blue

Sheet" (health policy and biomedical research), and the "Gray Sheet" (medical devices, diagnostics, and instrumentation).

■ Drugs that are being developed by pharmaceutical companies are followed and described in *R&D Insight*, an online publication by Adis Business Intelligence. It provides in-depth clinical profiling of each new compound, along with a rating for therapeutic value.

■ The Pharmaceutical and Research Manufacturers of America (P*h*RMA) represents the country's research-based pharmaceutical and biotechnology companies. This professional organization provides useful information on the new developments in the industry that might directly affect the quality or cost of care provided within the institution.

■ CenterWatch is a weekly clinical trials listing service that provides invaluable data on the results of recently completed and ongoing clinical trials.

Case 3

As a member of the Pharmacy and Therapeutics (P&T) Committee, you are attending the monthly meeting when a unanimous vote occurs about a new drug being put on the formulary. Before it is approved, however, it is given a level 3 rating, meaning that no physician will be authorized to prescribe it without first going through a mandatory CPD activity and then passing an exam about the drug. The drug, thalidomide, is extremely toxic, but recent research has shown it to be very effective if used for the appropriate patients and prescribed within the labeling restrictions approved by the FDA. This has developed into an organizational need because the implementation and management of risk is thrust on the institution rather than only on the individual. Both the pharmacy and the credentialing office will need to be involved. The question on the table is how the committee, with the help of the CPD Office, can better understand the nature and scope of this critically important need.

Comments on Case Studies

Case 1. Although the department of OB/GYN's eagerness to solve this problem with a CPD activity is understandable, it is probably incorrect. The positive side is that CPD professionals are engaged in dialogue with the clinicians and have established a relationship that can be a basis for good work. The task of the CPD office is to encourage the department to initiate their root cause analysis before deciding on any possible solutions. Even though CPD seems like it will be part of the solution, it is too early to decide whom the target audiences are and what their educational needs might be. The office might also suggest that others be asked to be a part of the analysis, such as the nurses in the labor and delivery departments and perhaps the researchers at the institution. The CPD office may also ask to be a part of the committee that will be doing the analysis. Offering to set up these meetings is a good way to get or stay involved.

Case 2. In this case, clinicians are willing to come to the CPD office with real data about organizational problems; this is an important opportunity to assist in this valuable quality-of-care analysis. Suggesting that the committee gather pre-CPD data on the target audiences in order to validate the organizational problem will help make the eventual learning activity even more responsive to the individuals and the institution. After studying the data, it may become clear that someone else needs to be involved as learners or that some other aspect of the central venous line placement needs to be highlighted. Alerting senior executives within the organization about the possible cost savings might also help to secure the necessary resources to complete the project by studying the impact after the educational intervention.

Case 3. This case offers a hint at the value of being at the table for the process of making plans and decisions on the part of the P&T Committee. This is particularly valuable when it is time to decide how physicians within the organization are going to be held accountable for appropriate prescribing behavior. A useful strategy may be to involve some members of the proposed target audience to assist in validating the pre-test, as well as providing useful suggestions about the proposed content and methodology. Linking the entire process to the institution's credentialing function guarantees more credibility for the CPD Office and its educational contribution.

CONCLUSIONS

This chapter has presented cases, concepts, and examples. Some discussion of the implications of each is in order, by way of drawing conclusions. The following sections provide a brief discussion of this material in an effort to draw out the meaning for practitioners and others interested in the emerging body of literature on integrating organizational needs with CPD programs and services.

One of the major reasons that CPD offices are not as involved as they should be in the myriad of quality-improvement activities is because the individuals responsible do not normally think of CPD professionals as being able to "bring something of value to the table." Their view is that they study about the nature of identified organizational problems and that knowing this is enough. The other part of that reality is that often times the CPD office is in a position only to suggest educational solutions without any knowledge of the nature of the problems. What is needed is to create partnerships between the two functions. When this happens, it can be very effective for the organization. The practice of getting out of the CPD office and in on the various health care decision-making processes is another key concept in effective organizational needs assessment. Again, however, most senior executives in health care organizations do not naturally think of the CPD office as needing to be involved in these various committees. A major task is to convince these leaders that the CPD office can be part of the solution for organizational problems. It is also helpful to invite some of those involved in analyzing health care to join the CPD's advisory committee or board. When the CPD office does get involved in a successful quality improvement effort, it is essential to document the role that CPD played so that it can be used later to convince others of the value. Another tactic is to let those who come to the CPD office seeking credit know of how your office might have been better able to help had the office been involved earlier in the process. Helping physicians understand what they don't know is a unique part of the organizational needs-assessment process. Because the institution has certain risks and responsibilities, it does not translate automatically into a "felt need" on the part of physicians. Involving members of the physician target audience early in the assessment process helps with this reality. Understanding health care quality data and data analysis techniques is becoming more and more important for the CPD office, even though it does not mean that the office needs to undertake this effort alone. Establishing key partnerships within and outside the institution is what is most helpful. Keeping track of who within the organization is responsible for all of these quality functions and meeting with them whenever possible is the only way to get that important invitation to the table.

In the future, the CPD office needs to try to become a formal part of every relevant quality function within the institution. More connection between the CPD office and the credentialing function is also on the horizon. Changing the nature and membership of the CPD Advisory Committee to include as many of these other individuals as practical should also be considered. Establishing an informational database on the physicians within your institution, as well as one on the new developments within the pharmaceutical and device industry pipelines, is going to prove very helpful for the CPD office. Other parts of the organization will hopefully realize the value the CPD office brings in understanding the nature of organizational needs and opportunities. Finally, routinely taking the CPD message to others throughout the organization is going to be critically important for obtaining the support needed to sustain this effort. Formal presentations at departmental grand rounds or informal periodic meetings with specific leaders will assist in this process.

Practical Tips and Suggestions for the CPD Office

The following are additional tips and suggestions that will assist the CPD office in carrying out this important organizational needs assessment function.

- *Gain the confidence of executive leadership.* Be engaged and share valuable educational accomplishments of the CPD Office when a dialogue occurs about problems, opportunities, or solutions that contribute to health care quality or cost reductions for the institution.

- *Develop in-house clinical expertise.* To understand the implications of organizational quality data for education, CPD offices must add individuals to their staff, train existing staff, and/or seek an internal physician/clinical consultant.

- *Seek risk-takers.* In every organizational setting, there are physicians and others who quickly grasp the potential of CPD to assist in the task of improving institutional performance. They will help their colleagues evaluate and understand the potential that exists within the CPD office to contribute to the larger organizational mission.

- *Work with physician champions and educational influentials.* In any initiative, the CPD office undertakes identification of physician champions who take up the cause and provide expert insight. These educational influentials[26] are also best positioned to seek out other colleagues to join in this rewarding journey.

- *Obtain external funding.* Identify funding sources (foundation, local voluntary health care organization, community public health office, or pharmaceutical or device manufacturing company) to study and respond to a specific problem or opportunity. These strategic partnerships assist in energizing the individuals within the institution who need to be involved and provide additional credibility for the CPD office.

These tips, along with a strategy for incorporating organizational needs into the overall mission of CPD, allow for greater improvements in organizational performance. This, in turn, promises to improve patient care and health outcomes, as well as organizational efficiency. Without attention to the organization as a source of action and information related to needs, the opportunity to integrate players engaged in the process of planned and purposeful change is lost.

REFERENCES—CHAPTER 6

1. Prather SE. *The New Health Partners*. San Francisco, Calif: Jossey-Bass Publishers; 1999.

2. Brown CR, Jr, Uhl HSM. Mandatory continuing medical education: sense or nonsense? *JAMA*. 1970;213:1660–1668.

3. Green JS, Gunzburger LK, Suter E. Interaction of continuing education clients and providers: increasing the impact of education. In: Green JS, Grosswald SJ, Suter E, Walthall DB, eds. *Continuing Education for the Health Professions: Developing, Managing, and Evaluating Programs for Maximum Impact on Patient Care*. San Francisco, Calif: Jossey-Bass Publishers; 1984.

4. Moore DE, Green JS, Jay SJ, et al. Creating a new paradigm for CME: seizing opportunities within the health care revolution. *J Contin Educ Health Prof*. 1994;14:261–272.

5. Barnes BE. Evaluation of learning in health care organizations. *J Contin Educ Health Prof*. 1999;19:227–233.

6. Frankford, DM, Patterson MS, Konrad TR. Transforming practice organizations to foster lifelong learning and commitment to medical professionalism. *Acad Med*. 2000;75:708–717.

7. Senge P. *The Fifth Discipline: The Art and Practice of the Learning Organization*. New York, NY: Doubleday Currency; 1990.

8. Watkins K, Marsick V. *Sculpting the Learning Organization: Lessons in the Art and Science of Systemic Change*. San Francisco, Calif: Jossey-Bass Publishers; 1993.

9. Schein EH. Three cultures of management: the key to organizational learning. *Sloan Management Review*. 1996;38:9–20.

10. Marquardt MJ. *Building the Learning Organization*. New York, NY: McGraw-Hill; 1996.

11. Confessore SJ. Building a learning organization: communities of practice, self-directed learning and continuing medical education. *J Contin Educ Health Prof*. 1997;19:5–11.

12. Garvin DA. *Learning in Action*. Boston, Mass: Harvard Business School Press; 2000.

13. Knox AB. Clientele analysis. *Review of Educational Research*. 1965;35:231–239.

14. Fox RD. Discrepancy analysis in continuing medical education. *Mobius*. 1983;3:37–44.

15. Webb E. Unconventionality, triangulation and inference. In: Denzin NK, ed. *Sociological Methods*. Chicago, Ill: Aldine; 1970.

16. Levine HG, Cordes DL, Moore DE, Pennington FC. Identifying and assessing needs to relate continuing education to patient care. In: Green JS, Grosswald SJ, Suter E, Walthall DB, eds. *Continuing Education for the Health Professions: Developing, Managing, and*

Evaluating Programs for Maximum Impact on Patient Care. San Francisco, Calif: Jossey-Bass Publishers; 1984.

17. Gaucher EJ, Coffey RJ. *Total Quality in Healthcare: From Theory to Practice.* San Francisco, Calif: Jossey-Bass Publishers; 1993.

18. Rosenstein A. Provider profiling: Improving outcomes of care. *J Outcomes Manage.* 1996;3:10–17.

19. Katzenbach JR, Smith DK. *The Wisdom of Teams.* New York, NY: HarperCollins Publishers; 1993.

20. Schein EH. *Organizational Culture and Leadership.* San Francisco, Calif: Jossey-Bass Publishers; 1988.

21. Davis D, Fox R, eds. *The Physician as Learner: Linking Research to Practice.* Chicago, Ill: American Medical Association; 1994.

22. Berwick DM, Godfrey AB, Roessner J. *Curing Health Care: New Strategies for Quality Improvement.* San Francisco, Calif: Jossey-Bass Publishers; 1990.

23. James BC. Implementing practice guidelines through clinical quality improvement. *Frontiers Health Serv Manage.* 1993;10;3–37.

24. Mager R, Pipe P. *Analyzing Performance Problems or 'You Really Oughta Wanna'.* Belmont, Calif: Fearon Publishers; 1970.

25. Eisenberg J. Continuing education meets the learning organization: the challenge of a systems approach to patient safety. *J Contin Educ Health Prof.* 2000;20:197–207.

26. Stross JK, Bole GG. Evaluation of a continuing education program on rheumatoid arthritis. *Arthritis Rheum.* 1980;23:846–849.

SECTION II

Deciding How to Facilitate Continuing Professional Development

Primary editor: Dave Davis, MD

A Clinical Thematic: Deciding How to Facilitate Continuing Professional Development

Dave Davis, MD; Robert Fox, EdD;
Barbara E. Barnes; MD; Karen Costie, RN

The Clinical Scenario

After thinking about his patient Marjory and the broader subject of diabetes, and after considering his educational needs in this area, Ted decides to bring this topic to the monthly meeting of his local "quality circle." This is a group of 8 to 10 physicians, some of whom are in the Mountainside Clinic, some in the local hospital's department of family practice, who have met regularly for several years.

Growing out of the department's quality assurance committee, this is an interesting group, one whose members (not all of the department, by a long shot) represent a cross-section of interested, educationally aware, and self-directed learners. They share common qualities. First, they often attend, but just as often express general dissatisfaction with, large-group didactic continuing professional development (CPD) events such as those produced by the medical schools and large hospitals. In this context, they complain about the costs involved in losing practice time, the dependence on the "expert" speaker, and other problems. Despite these complaints, many still attend these events and often report back to the quality circle what they've learned, using them for at least two functions: to socialize and for information-scanning. Second, they use other resources frequently and well: journal articles, Web searches, and self-assessment programs, to name a few. Third, they are, by and large, "well connected," ie, they frequently speak to other primary care team members, physicians, specialists, each other, even community members. And fourth, they are aware of their practice patterns and styles and are open to evaluation.

With all of these elements in play, the group operates as one part journal club, one part quality-assurance mechanism (eg, by asking physicians to bring their charts or quality problems), and one part CPD experience, with members often bringing useful printed material, articles, and other resources to help satisfy questions of practice. Sometimes, when complex or fact-intensive problems arise, the group invites a specialist resource person. And, the group has become important to Ted and the other members. He'd tell us that he gives up the first Monday evening of every month only because these are friends and trusted colleagues who often provide support and help in making decisions.

The group first deals with several issues from last month: one of Ted's colleagues reports on his review of new guidelines for low back pain; another gives a brief overview of current antidepressants and where the "new" SSRIs (selective serotonin uptake inhibitors) fit in the picture; finally, the group leader reports on a utilization review report regarding mammograms that she found of interest.

Turning to the group for current questions and issues arising from patient care, Ted presents Marjory's case and learns from his colleagues about:

- *the new American Diabetes Association clinical practice guidelines for screening (although he has received them, he hasn't had a chance to read them yet);*
- *similar problems other doctors in his group have experienced with diabetics management (eg, "I don't think I can influence a patient's lifestyle or diet.");*
- *some clinics that have developed their own flow charts and reminders for diabetic management to help the physician or his/her nurse follow the elements in care, like a routine prenatal form. This has helped their group improve the quality of care delivered and has even interested the managed care organization that funds 80% of their practice;*
- *community resources (nutrition counseling, motivational groups, diabetes self-help groups); and*
- *how some of his colleagues have used educational materials for their patients (eg, Agency for Health Care Research and Quality [formerly the Agency for Health Care Policy and Research] low back pain guideline for patients).*

DISCUSSION

This scenario allows us to raise many questions about learners and continuing professional development (CPD) activities. What are the qualities that make these learners effective? What might a CPD provider do to increase the effectiveness of this group? What other means exist to deliver information in a timely and relevant fashion about diabetes? What about the organization that this group represents? What about physicians *not* represented by this group?

This scenario also allows us to examine the learning issues at a number of levels—those relating to the individuals who comprise the quality circle, those that operate in groups like this and others, those that affect (and are situated in) the practice of the Mountainside Group, those physicians and other health care workers not in this learning circle, and finally those issues that affect the community in which these individuals practice and live. This section of the book related to CPD methods begins with the smallest common element—the individual learner—and moves progressively through larger clusters and dimensions of practice. And, although specific to this group, they also can be generalized to any learning situation.

Individual Learners

While we do not know much about the backgrounds of the other individuals in Ted Brucken's group, we do know a bit about the group and its issues, from an earlier section. These issues are common in the practice of most physicians: practice and resource allocation restraints, time pressures, governmental regulations in and guidelines for the delivery of health care, and, perhaps above all, a knowledge (or at least information) explosion, unprecedented in practice. We know that whatever we do in CPD, learning activities must fit the time and other restraints under which physicians operate.

Moreover, we know a bit about Ted Brucken: in mid-career, with training in family practice, and a reasonable "traditional" undergraduate education, Ted's (and his colleagues') pursuit of answers to questions in diabetes permits us to understand this process from two perspectives.

First, there are many issues that pertain to Ted as an individual and as a learner. For example, we have already seen that Ted has the ability to reflect on his practice (in this case, later in the day following his diagnosis of Marjory's diabetes) and to extrapolate his concerns to his practice population. Explored in greater detail by Karen Mann and Mark Gelula in Chapter 7 on self-directed learning, other individual learning issues include his (and his group members') motivation to learn, his past experiences (both clinical and educational), and his ability and willingness to evaluate his gaps in knowledge or skills. In addition, the pressures and restraints of practice affect learning and its effect on outcomes. Understanding the factors and principles that apply in this and other scenarios is key to understanding the learning process.

Individualized Learning Strategies

Second, from the perspective of the CPD professional or the continuing medical education (CME) provider, there are clearly other means by which physicians like Ted can learn, not dependent on the presence of other learners. For individuals who practice in a more solo manner, for those who are isolated by geographic or other reasons, for those not predisposed to group learning, other strategies are commonly used. Calling these methods "individualized learning strategies," in Chapter 8 John Parboosingh and his colleagues outline methods such as self-assessment programs, mailed materials, and learning portfolios that are applicable to the individual-as-learner. Further, in Chapter 11 Barbara Barnes and Chuck Friedman examine the question of educational technology, which is readily applied to the question of individualized learning methods.

Group Learning Strategies

Third, we are fortunate to see what appears to be a well-functioning learning group operating at the Mountainside Clinic. Most of us would acknowledge that such highly operational, practice-based groups are desirable but less common than the mainstay of traditional CME—the large conference, course, or refresher program, generally held in locations away from the practice setting. Long the hallmark of the CPD professional, such courses are examined in detail in Chapter 9 by Linda Casebeer and her associates on group learning, along with an exploration of tools to augment this process—small-group learning, problem-based strategies, distance education methods, and workshops.

Organizational Learning

Fourth, although we know a fair amount about the quality circle (we could call it a community of learners or a small group) described above, there are many issues about which we don't know very much, those about the health care (and therefore educational) system in which Ted and his colleagues operate. What about the organization of the Mountainside Group? Does it have educational rounds or other activities? What about the local Ranier County Hospital or the Central-North health care system? And what about the local community in which all of these elements are situated? In Chapter 10, Nancy Bennett and Bob Fox examine the broader question of organizational learning, exploring principles, concepts, and practices in what appears to be a new and sizable challenge for CPD professionals. These concepts and practices are as important to the understanding of CPD as the principles of the individual learner.

Technology and Learning

Fifth, while our scenario only alludes to educational technology (mentioning Web-based searches), clearly this book would be deficient if it did not include reference to the effect of computer-based learning, the Internet, Web-based CME resources, simulations, and a host of other resources provided to us by new technologies and connectivity. Barbara Barnes and Chuck Friedman explore these issues in Chapter 11 on technology-based education.

Practice-Based Strategies: Audit and Feedback

Finally, there are other elements to the learning and change experience represented in our scenario by practice-based strategies, not generally thought of as educational, but clearly important methods in the CPD providers' "toolbox." Often described as audit and feedback, reminders, utilization reports, and other measures, they serve to help in facilitating change in the practice site and in providing feedback to physicians about their performance. Not generally construed to be educational in the traditional sense, we make the case that they nonetheless promote and support change. These tools are described in greater detail in Nancy Bennett and Dave Davis' Chapter 12 on reminders, audit, and feedback.

Other Issues

There are many other ways to look at this next section, critical to examining and developing a toolbox of educational strategies to be used in CPD of physicians. These are explored in greater detail within the chapters themselves and in the conclusion of the clinical thematic in the final section.

How to Facilitate Self-Directed Learning

Karen V. Mann, PhD; Mark H. Gelula, PhD

Linda Sanchez, a family physician who has been practicing for about 10 years, has developed an interest in health promotion behaviors that will decrease the risk of heart disease and stroke in middle-aged and elderly patients. She contacts you to find out whether your office has any courses coming up that will fill the bill. She talks a little about her needs, but she is unable to find a particular course that will give her what she wants. She says to you, "I've tried to gather some information, but my current strategies don't seem to be working. I don't know where to start."

A pediatrician, William Gilchrest, finds that the incidence of teenage pregnancy is reported to be on the rise in the geographic area of his practice. Although he has some adolescent patients, he generally doesn't address issues of sexuality because it makes him uncomfortable to do so. You know this isn't directly addressed in a course and it never brings a large enough registration to be fiscally viable. How can you help?

In a stairwell conversation, Dr Hugh Elwood, a physician you know fairly well, tells you he has been uncomfortable with his treatment of patients with type 2 diabetes. A general internist, this physician has felt extremely comfortable in the general treatment of diabetes, but lately this self-assurance has begun to dwindle. Although he has spoken to no one about his concerns, he has become increasingly aware of the recent research and published findings with respect to appropriate levels of HbA1c. What is more, he is being besieged by pharmaceutical representatives who "make me feel as if I have fallen behind. They certainly appear to know more now than I do." He is questioning not only his knowledge about the treatment and management of this disease but his competence as a practitioner. What role is there for you?

After overhearing a conversation in the doctor's lounge, a physician remarks to a colleague that he is completely inundated at his practice and cannot keep up with current literature, let alone participate in conversations like the one just overheard. You happen to have overheard both conversations. Is there a role for you as a continuing professional development professional?

A colleague calls you. She has a physician in her local rural hospital who has had some credentialing difficulties. The credentialing committee at her hospital has determined that both an in-depth review and retraining are necessary for the physician to meet their requirements. Unfortunately, your colleague does not have the resources to help the physician meet these requirements. Is this a self-directed learning issue? Is there a place in it for you?

Each case represents a facet of the variety of activities that may be encountered by the continuing professional development (CPD) professional. Each case represents an opportunity to assist a physician explore the many paths of self-directed learning (SDL). In this chapter, we will explore SDL and its implications for continuing professional education providers. We will provide background information on SDL, as well as approaches that will encourage the reader in ways to provide assistance in SDL. Interspersed throughout the chapter are references to one of the six case vignettes previously described. We hope that reference to these cases will provide a link between the abstract and the concrete, providing the reader with grounded ideas that may be used immediately.

INTRODUCTION

Although much of the literature in continuing professional education addresses formal continuing medical education (CME), it is increasingly acknowledged that attendance at formal CME events is probably analogous to the tip of the iceberg, representing only a small portion of the ongoing learning undertaken by physicians. Further, for some time, CME providers and practicing physicians have recognized that active engagement in self-planned learning activities represents more effective learning than the passive learning that has often characterized formal CME. Finally, the value of learning stimulated by and using practice as a resource places SDL firmly at the center of ongoing professional development. As CME providers and educators, we want to support our learners in their ongoing learning and development. To do so, we need to understand the concepts and principles underlying SDL.

Malcolm Knowles[1] established a definition of SDL that guided work in this area for two decades. That definition is:

> a process in which individuals take the initiative, with or without the help of others, in diagnosing their learning needs, formulating goals, identifying human and material resources for learning, choosing and implementing appropriate learning strategies, and evaluating learning outcomes.

As our understanding of SDL has grown, more recent definitions, such as the following by Hammond and Collins,[2] reflect the complexity of the phenomenon:

> A process in which learners take the initiative, with the support and collaboration of others, for increasing self- and social-awareness; critically analysing and

reflecting on their situations; diagnosing their learning needs with specific reference to competencies they have helped identify; formulating socially and personally relevant learning goals; identifying human and material resources for learning; choosing and implementing appropriate learning strategies; and reflecting on and evaluating their learning.

Recall Dr Gilchrest, the pediatrician in case 2 who is disturbed by the increase of teenage pregnancy in his practice area. Dr Gilchrest's concerns are typical of many physicians who select a self-directed learning path. As suggested by Hammond and Collins,[2] he is motivated by his social awareness and through a critical analysis of his practice demographics.

DEFINING AND DESCRIBING SELF-DIRECTED LEARNING IN ADULTS

Our knowledge of SDL has characterized this ability both as a set of personal attributes and as the acquisition of specific skills. In the former, self-direction is seen as a goal toward which individuals strive. The achievement of self-direction, in this sense, reflects a humanistic orientation, such as that seen in models of personal development described by Maslow[3] and Brockett and Hiemstra.[4] These models imply personal growth and achievement of a desired level of personal development, along with the acceptance of personal responsibility for one's learning, personal autonomy, and individual choice.

The second perspective of SDL considers it the ability to organize learning and instruction, wherein the tasks of learning are predominantly in the learners' control. Early understandings described learners moving linearly through a series of steps to reach their learning goals (eg, Knowles[1]); later models view the SDL process as more iterative, involving opportunities and interactions in the environment, the personality characteristics of learners, cognitive processes, the context of learning, and opportunities to validate and confirm SDL collaboratively. Examples of this are seen in several models clearly described by Merriam and Caffarella.[5] Also included are models of instruction such as those of Grow[6] and Hammond and Collins,[2] which present frameworks to assist educators in the integration of SDL into formal educational settings. The emerging model of practice-based small-group learning also recognizes the more complex nature of ongoing SDL learning in practice.[7] Brockett and Heimstra[4] have combined both personal self-directedness and skills in self-direction as factors in what they term "self-direction in learning."

Candy[8] has clarified and expanded the field of SDL significantly. He describes four dimensions in self-directedness: personal

TABLE 7-1

Skills and Competencies of the Lifelong Learner

The lifelong learner would:

- be methodical and disciplined
- be logical and analytical
- be reflective and self-aware
- demonstrate curiosity, openness, and motivation
- be flexible
- be interdependent and interpersonally competent
- be persistent and responsible
- be venturesome and creative
- show confidence and have a positive self-concept
- be independent and self-sufficient
- have developed information-seeking and retrieval skills
- have knowledge about, and skill at, learning generally
- develop and use defensible criteria for evaluating learning.

autonomy, self-management in learning, learner control of instruction, and the independent pursuit of learning. Reviewing the plethora of studies exploring SDL, Candy identified and condensed approximately 100 traits associated with self-direction (Table 7-1).

Generally, self-direction in learning is not limited to specific settings; it is a natural process of human life and can occur inside or outside of formal settings. Further, SDL does not exclude formal activities such as lectures or courses. It is the learner's choice of activities to meet a particular learning goal that denotes self-direction; many combinations of learning activities may occur. Two early studies that examine why adults participate in continuing education can assist us in understanding SDL. The first study by Tough[9] found the following four salient factors:

- There are usually multiple reasons that adults undertake a learning project.
- Adult learners seem to frequently be motivated by the pragmatic desire to apply the knowledge or skill gained through their learning.
- There are three patterns common in starting learning projects: a specific identified learning need, curiosity about a topic, and a general desire to learn.
- Most participants enjoy learning, and this enjoyment typically has a key place in the motivation to maintain a learning project.

Houle[10] also studied adult students in continuing education to explore why adult learners are so active and discovered three main groups of learners:

- *goal-oriented learners* who use learning to achieve specific objectives (eg, learning to do colposcopies or learning to use a new generation of antibiotics), often involving discrete learning episodes;
- *activity-oriented learners* who participate primarily for the sake of the activity itself, rather than to develop a skill or learn a specific subject matter (eg, joining a group); and
- *learning-oriented learners* who enjoy learning for its own sake and who have a desire to know as much as possible about something and to grow through learning. Learning is constant among this group.

LEARNING MODELS

SDL is consistent with a number of perspectives on understanding learning, including the social learning, humanist, cognitive, and constructivist approaches. Each approach, discussed below, is supportive of SDL and helps us understand the process.

1. *The social learning approach* (social cognitive theory) views individuals as inherently self-regulating; therefore, self-direction is considered a natural evolution and activity. In this approach, people learn and change in a dynamic environment that influences the goals they set and the outcomes they achieve. Social learning theory relies on individuals being able to set goals and evaluate their own progress toward them. The CPD professional working in this orientation would focus on helping the individual set goals, determine ways to meet these goals, and monitor progress and achievement. This approach also emphasizes the need for individual learners to develop self-efficacy or confidence in their ability as self-directed learners as well as autonomy.

2. *The humanist approach* views learning as leading to higher levels of personal development and focuses on encouraging personal growth. In this view, helping learners become self-directed means helping them to assume responsibility for their learning. Both the humanist and the social learning approaches incorporate the notions of competence and autonomy as keys to effective self-direction.

3. *The cognitive perspective* emphasizes the importance of perception and meaning. It recognizes the need to build a rich, interconnected base of existing knowledge, which allows for the continuing incorporation of new learning. Cognitive models are

the most common approaches to understanding learning and they focus on how knowledge is acquired and used. This perspective supports helping learners to identify knowledge deficits, select the best resources to address any knowledge deficits, and use approaches that enhance the meaning and relevance of learning.

4. *The constructivist perspective* recognizes the unique personal and social construction of knowledge built by individual learners based on their personal experience, prior knowledge, and cultural, social, and other characteristics. For the CPD professional, this approach helps explain why learners will choose varied resources and paths to reach apparently similar learning goals.

Taken together, these different perspectives highlight the complex nature of SDL. They also offer ways to inform our approaches to those undertaking these activities as they understand and become managers of their own learning.

HOW DOES SDL OCCUR AMONG PHYSICIANS?

Two major understandings of SDL in physicians have been drawn from studies grounded in their actual experience. The first is a model of change and learning described by Fox, Mazmanian, and Putnam,[11] which was developed from interviews with more than 300 physicians who described more than 700 incidents of personal learning and change. The second understanding also derives from empirical studies of practice in several professions, conducted by Schön[12,13] who describes a model of learning from experience that he called "reflective practice." A third explanation of how learning occurs from experience, developed by Kolb[14] and drawn from the general educational literature, is also helpful in understanding physician learning. For those who wish to understand these models in depth, the full works are recommended.

THE MODEL OF CHANGE AND LEARNING

The "change" model[11] uses an inductive approach to understanding change based on the actual experience of physicians. In this model of learning, physicians are motivated to learn and change by forces that may be professional, personal, and social. In the study from which the model was developed, the most common forces for change were professional, including the general desire for competence or the perception that the clinical environment was pressing for change. All or any of these forces may be in constant interplay in the physician's life and practice; at some point, their effect is sufficient to raise ideas of change. Once the physician is aware of the need to change, he or she begins to develop an image of how the changed practice would look. Development of this image requires gathering information and may often involve attending CME events. This process enables physicians to develop a standard to assess their existing skills against those required and to analyze the gap that needs filling. It is the process of analyzing and describing the gap that provides the point of departure for planning, developing, implementing, and assessing learning activities. Changes made may range from minor accommodations of routine practice to major transformations and usually involve a wide variety of resources, including, but not limited to, formal CME. The process of change involves three stages: preparing to change, making the change, and sustaining the change.[15]

Geertsma[16] and colleagues also identified three stages in physician learning:

1. Deciding whether to take on a learning task to address a problem.
2. Learning the skill and knowledge anticipated to resolve the problem.
3. Gaining experience in using what has been learned.

More recently, these stages were re-examined by Slotnick,[17] who, while interviewing 32 physicians, added a fourth category that takes into account prior awareness acquired by "scanning the practice environment."

Several studies have provided validation for the change and learning model. A study of Canadian radiologists[18] confirmed that physicians use a variety of resources in adopting an innovation and that the characteristics of a change influence its adoption. For the CPD professional, this model helps us to understand that the resources needed to make a change are often outside the realm of formal CME and may include colleagues, other educational programs, and other professionals. Another study, conducted with general practitioners in the United Kingdom (1997),[19] confirmed that multiple factors are necessary in initiating and maintaining change. Work by Parboosingh and colleagues[20,21] have further validated the variety of stimuli for SDL among specialists.

REFLECTIVE PRACTICE AND LEARNING FROM EXPERIENCE

The notion of learning from experience has been with us since Dewey.[22] Many authors have written about the value of experience as a basis for learning, for reviewing and integrating learning, and for determining ongoing learning needs. Two approaches that have been used in medical education are described here.

Schön's Approach

Schön[12,13] studied several professional groups, from which he described a cycle of learning from experience that incorporates five stages. These are:

1. "Knowing-in-action," which represents the composite of the physician's existing knowledge and skills, much of which may be tacit, or beyond the physician's mindful awareness. Most of physician practice occurs in this area.

2. An encounter with a "surprise," where the physician's usual "knowing-in-action" is not matched with the situation, starts the reflective cycle. For example, a usual treatment approach is ineffective or a presenting problem is unusual, leading the physician to the third stage.

3. "Reflection-in-action," where the physician literally thinks on her or his feet about what is different about the situation and what alternate approaches to understanding and solving the problem are available.

4. Some of these approaches will be considered and rejected. Schön called this the "experiment" stage, although not in our usual sense of the term. In most cases, the approaches are tried in the physician's mind before one is selected.

5. The fifth and last stage of the cycle is arguably the most important, in that when the physician can look back and "reflect-on-action," new directions for learning can be identified. It is through this process that new learning can be effectively incorporated into the physician's "knowing-in-action," returning to the beginning of the reflective learning cycle.

Schön's model assumes that there are various levels of reflection and that the process of encountering the need to change is serially reviewed as the event, or analogous events, unfolds. For a physician who encounters a patient who does not respond to a drug regimen as expected, that lack of response triggers a reflective response. Even after acting with this patient, the physician will probably continue to reflect on why the regimen failed, even as he or she prescribes the same drug for other patients, reads the literature, and consults colleagues. Jennett and colleagues describe this process as informal self-directed learning.[23]

Kolb's Learning Cycle

Kolb[14] describes a four-stage learning process (Figure 7-1), recognizing, like Schön, that learners advance their learning through experience:

1. *Concrete experience.* In this first stage, the physician may encounter a situation in patient care that differs from expected

FIGURE 7-1

Kolb's Learning Cycle

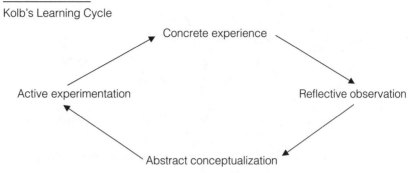

practice; eg, a child presents with severe otitis media and no history of illness or current fever. Interested and surprised by this, the physician has a moment of interest and concern.

2. *Reflective observation.* Following the patient encounter, the physician may reflect further on the experience, go to the computer to consult an online text, or consult with a partner. Or the physician may do nothing different at the moment but may investigate this experience later.

3. *Abstract conceptualization.* Kolb defines this process as one in which learners reconsider their experiences and previous learning based on reflection. Thus, the self-directed physician may identify a blood test or a new antibiotic or see a general principle emerging that can help with this problem. This process parallels the "experiment" in Schön's conceptualization of learning.

4. *Active experimentation.* In this stage, new approaches, or "experiments," are employed that may be small trials, a new question asked, or a departure in some way from traditional practice. These approaches immediately become new concrete experiences and an opportunity for further reflection.

In summary, the CPD professional works with physicians to help them move from their concrete experience (stage 1); reflectively discuss their issues of concern (stage 2); find sources for reconceptualization and generalization (stage 3); and help prepare them for future action or a new approach to the next relevant learning experience (stage 4).

ENGAGING THE PHYSICIAN IN CHANGE AND LEARNING

There is considerable literature describing general processes of change. One specific model that may be relevant is the transtheoretical or "stages of change" model.[24] Although this model evolved from the stages of change observed in persons trying to change addictive behaviors, educators have also found the model to be helpful in thinking about change.[25] The model describes five stages of "readiness" to change that represent an iterative approach to initiating and maintaining change. These are:

1. *Precontemplation.* The individual sees no need for change.
2. *Contemplation.* The benefits and barriers to change are considered.
3. *Preparation.* Individuals decide to change and begin to plan for change.
4. *Action.* The change is established and maintained.
5. *Maintenance* of the new behavior.

The stages-of-change model may help to understand where physicians are in the process of change and learning and therefore to direct interventions toward helping them move through the cycle of change.

Summary

The models of change and of experiential learning introduced here share commonalities that are helpful to us as CME providers. They all describe a series of stages in the process of change. They are also iterative and emphasize that making a change may involve moving back and forth through the stages and cycles before actual change occurs. Lastly, they all involve a central role for reflection, integration of the new learning into practice, and reintegration of older knowledge reconsidered through reflection-in-practice and reflection-on-practice.

CAN WE IDENTIFY AND MEASURE SELF-DIRECTEDNESS?

Physician competence is an ongoing process. Physicians are continually confronted with the challenge of new information, such as breakthroughs in understanding genetics, new manifestations of disease, new techniques, new drugs, new problems, and new skills in areas such as communications and ethics. By attempting to incorporate these changes into practice behavior, physicians may become aware that they are no longer as competent in some areas as they wish.

As a result, several challenging questions arise for the CPD professional: Is the physician ready to change? What are the forces driving the physician's desire to change and learn? How can I recognize self-direction and readiness for change?

One of our early vignettes provides useful insight into these issues. Uncomfortable with his treatment of type 2 diabetes,

Dr Elwood (in case 3) is also reluctant to formally do anything about his problem. Yet, he does "catch you" in the stairwell, revealing a readiness to consider ways to address his concern. The question is then, To what extent will Dr Elwood be ready to take on change? Considering his readiness to change may provide you with information, as well as help to trigger this change effort and guide your interventions.

If a physician like Dr Elwood is considering whether a change would be beneficial for patients, we might provide the opportunity to talk about the relative benefits and disadvantages of changing this aspect of the physician's practice. Alternatively, if the physician has decided that change is required, the role for the CPD professional is to help in the assessment of the resources needed and the actual preparation for change. The task for the CPD professional is not to measure a physician's degree of self-directedness but to identify the factors to support physicians moving toward the changes they wish to make.

Comprehensive measures of self-directedness are not plentiful; however, two scales have been used sufficiently to achieve validation.[26,27] The self-directed learning readiness scale (SDLRS) was developed by Gugliemino[26] to assess the degree to which people perceive they possess the skills and attitudes conventionally associated with SDL. Analyses of the scale have revealed these underlying factors: openness to learning opportunities; self-concept as an effective learner; initiative and independence in learning; informed acceptance of responsibility for learning; love of learning; creativity; future orientation; and ability to use basic study and problem-solving skills. This 55-item scale has been widely used but is criticized mainly because it relies on self-report rather than objective measures and may not measure SDL with acceptable validity.[28]

The Oddi continuing learning inventory (OCLI)[27] is a 26-item scale developed to identify clusters of personality characteristics that relate to initiative and persistence in learning over time. Four main clusters have been found within the inventory to explain continuing learning, including self-confidence, the ability to work both independently and through involvement with others, avid reading, and the ability to be self-regulating.

Although it may be possible to measure readiness for SDL, measuring change readiness appears more problematic. Bligh[29] found three dominant factors that contribute to a readiness to learn: enjoyment of and enthusiasm for learning, a positive self-concept as a learner, and a factor suggesting the possibility of reproducing an orientation to learning. These are very similar to the factors noted by Tough[9] and Houle[10] described earlier.

In addition, Fox[30] has developed a change readiness inventory for physicians in CME. This inventory allows respondents to characterize their current state of knowledge and goals through a series of objectives strictly related to a specific disease process. An individual working with Dr Elwood (case 3), for instance, could benefit by using an instrument like the change readiness inventory. The area of identifying and measuring SDL and change readiness still holds many unanswered questions. As work in the field continues, however, these instruments will undoubtedly provide us with valuable tools.

INFLUENCES ON THE CAPACITY FOR SELF-DIRECTION

Learners will have different abilities and experience in SDL. Several factors, both within the learner and in the surrounding environment, will affect the capacity of the learner to be self-directed. These factors include

- *The learner's view of the learning task.* We know that an internalized, or intrinsic, motivation to achieve personal goals is more enduring than motivation evoked by externally determined goals or rewards. Certainly, the self-direction evident in the plethora of learning activities undertaken by adults demonstrates clearly the power of the learning goal and the learner's view of learning.[10,31]

- *The learner's view of themselves as learners.* Learners who view themselves as competent learners, able to learn in a variety of learning situations, are more likely to be self-directed, independent learners. For CPD professionals, future generations of learners who are graduates of medical curricula that emphasize SDL may perceive themselves as very competent independent learners. New approaches to CME may also lead to new expectations by those physicians currently in practice. The work by several current researchers who are examining the effectiveness of small-group and problem-based learning strategies[7,32,33] with practicing physicians in a CME context has led to previously inexperienced physicians now having experience with PBL, small-group collaborative learning, group problem-solving, and the SDL that occurs within and resulting from these activities.

- *The learner's mastery of the subject matter.* In this view, as learners build a knowledge base and skills in a particular area, the capacity to be self-directed is enhanced. Some believe that this basic knowledge is essential for effective physician SDL. Others suggest that, unless the task is completely unfamiliar to the physician, there are few situations where the knowledge relevant to engage in a learning task or to address a problem is completely lacking. Learners who feel lacking in certain background knowledge may feel less confident about undertaking

SDL activities. Our task as CPD professionals is to help them develop a strategy that they feel is manageable.

■ *The learner's ability to reflect on learning and experience.* Much professional knowledge and acumen in medicine are thought to be tacit and embedded in practice.[12] Others describe this as "situated" learning, which cannot be easily separated from the context in which the knowledge is used. The clues that help the physician to frame the problems of practice and develop solutions are only available in the actual context of practice. Schön has described this as "knowledge-in-action," which grows and changes dynamically as a result of practice experience. Learners must practice and develop skills in reflecting on their learning so they can identify additional learning needs and set goals accordingly.

■ *Access to colleagues and communities of learners.* Situated learning generally occurs in experiences rooted in practice, but, increasingly, the importance of learning from participation in small groups or communities of learning is understood.[34,35] Learners benefit from involvement with people who express opinions and ideas beyond their current experience or expertise. By working with peers, learners are motivated to try new procedures or to achieve ways of thinking that were previously beyond their abilities. This is described in Vygotsky's[36] terms as their "zone of proximal development." In small-group settings, physicians can learn by both listening and participating. This may be one reason that the traditional doctors' lounge is such a valuable place for learning. Its rich environment of give-and-take allows even the peripheral listener to acquire new information and can promote subsequent reflection-in-action and reflection-on-action.

THE PROCESS OF CONSULTATION

Planning a self-directed curriculum involves a series of activities that often occur informally between the physician and the CPD professional. In moving to a more systematic approach, we may be informed by a model of process consultation[37] that is continuous and based on emergent needs. Schein[37] defines process consultation as "a set of activities on the part of the consultant that help the client to perceive, understand, and act upon the process events that occur in the client's environment in order to improve the situation as defined by the client." The process is concerned with the human issues (the essential needs and interests of the physician), the process (the interaction with the consulting CPD professional), and the long-range effectiveness (outcomes). These issues are offset by tasks (educational activities to be undertaken), content (based on needs identified during the process consultation activities), and expediency (how drastic is the need?). A key to Schein's perspective of process consultation, making it a useful model for CPD professionals, is that the process consultant is seen as a skills and values resource rather than a content resource. The consultant's assistance, then, focuses on supporting physicians in solving their own problems, rather than solving the problems for them. Schein would assume that the physician is an able and active partner in the process.

SUPPORTING NATURAL PROCESSES OF LEARNING

Using Effective and Appropriate Motivational Strategies

Understanding the processes of physician learning and change[11] suggests two important aspects of motivating learners. The first is to help learners identify gaps between needed skills and current capabilities; the second is to help learners visualize an image of change to see how it might look to do something differently. This visualization of change can lead to defining goals or it may follow from the statement of broad goals that can help clarify what planning and resources will be required. Moreover, based on the belief that supporting autonomy will enhance motivation, and may also further enhance motivation through building self-efficacy, providers should be mindful of the importance of their support of the learner's attempts at self-direction and feedback on progress.

SUPPORTING EFFECTIVE SDL

We often view SDL as synonymous with independent learning; however, the defining characteristic of SDL is its direction by the learner. Indeed, a key role of the provider may be to link the learner with appropriate learning methods. Problem-based (practice-based) small-group learning[7] involves having practicing family physicians in ongoing learning groups follow a process that tries to incorporate the key aspects of PBL as reported in undergraduate learning (ie, learning from relevant problems that stimulate learning and general discussion). It also involves having access to appropriate information to direct to learners in their discussion of questions that may arise in case discussions. Where Internet links are available, the CPD professional can provide Web site addresses for learners. Interactive learning is now accessible through several forms of distance learning, including Web-based and videoconferencing modes. The provider also has an important role in linking the learner to appropriate, relevant resources at all stages of the SDL process.

THE SDL CURRICULUM

The steps below are essential in planning the self-directed curriculum and work best if a process-consultative approach is taken.

1. **Determining needs.** Whether identified through the process consultation stage or as a result of extant quality-improvement data, needs-assessment activities are key to determining what is to be learned. Goals are set from needs assessment, outcomes are established, and the processes by which these are achieved are designated. We noted earlier that, as more graduates of programs that emphasize SDL enter practice, some of the skills of SDL might become more widely present and normative among the profession. Traditionally, physicians and other professionals have had limited experience in the self-assessment of learning needs. Methods and opportunities are becoming increasingly available for physicians to engage in ongoing and periodic self-assessment. We know that physicians respond to areas of deficient knowledge by referring difficult problems, attending CME events, and reading journals, as well as through discussions with colleagues and by the acquisition of new skills.[17] CPD professionals can, however, help in the systematic assessment of needs. For example, the increased use of computerized patient records allows physicians to review, for example, patients with diabetes under their care and to look at both the process of care (eg, referrals for patient education) and outcome events, such as re-admissions to the hospital.

   When the CPD professional enters into discussion with physicians about their learning needs, the experiential model provides a useful framework against which needs, goals, and actions can be assessed. Physicians have frequently not consciously reflected on their experience; however, the questions that they raise, the concerns they have for their patients, and their interest in solving a problem all reflect the ongoing learning that occurs. By conducting a conversation with physicians guided by Kolb's model, we are able to help them identify what has been experienced, what reflection has occurred, and what conceptualization or generalizations may be drawn.

   Physicians respond most commonly to perceived needs, stimulated by caring for a particular patient, through a "surprise" that challenges usual practice, anticipation of needed skills generated by reading, in conversation with a colleague, by overhearing conversation among other physicians, or through formal CME events. For many, however, those self-directed needs may be subjective and may not reflect objectively determined actual needs. They may also exclude unperceived needs. The CPD professional can assist with SDL both by raising the learner's awareness that unperceived needs may exist and by making available tools for more reliable and valid self-assessments. Examples of these methods might include a reflective diary or portfolio, practice audit, or computerized tests. The key is to assist the physician to develop a self-management strategy, rather than to respond to ad hoc events.

2. **Setting learning goals.** The very nature of practice, especially for generalists, involves addressing various patient problems, suggesting that the development of long-term goals may require the collection and analysis of several sources of information. In the task-centered, hypothetico-deductive world of the physician, the need to solve individual patient problems may give rise to goals that are more short term in nature. Learners need assistance in developing longer-term goals, within which shorter-term goals can be more systematically developed. One method of developing these goals is through the use of learning "partners," as described by Charles Campion-Smith,[38] where physicians work in pairs to assist one another with the development of goals and with other steps in the SDL process, eg, evaluation of achievement. This kind of partnership works well beyond the setting of goals and into actual learning. The work of activity theorists and of Vygotsky,[36] described earlier, suggests that one physician of the pair inevitably leads, pulls, or pushes the other to a new perspective or greater understanding. This can lead to acceleration of learning and change.

3. **Developing a curriculum.** Once the learning goals have been set, physician-learners must develop a curriculum to attain them. The word *curriculum*, in this sense, includes the "package of knowledge," skills, and attitudes required to meet the goal. There may be no formal curriculum; often the curriculum may be an informal working plan that evolves through the process consultation phase, changing as physicians encounter new ideas and methods or find answers to problems that have plagued them. The CPD professional can serve as a listener, respond to learners' plans of self-devised curricula, or assist more actively in determining the content and sequence of the plan if learners wish. In this way, the CPD professional may serve as a process consultant, both advising and serving as a sounding board for physicians in exploring their own ideas.

4. **Selecting learning resources.** The identification and matching of learning resources to a learner's needs is an important task for the CPD professional. Understanding the physician's preferred learning methods and their effectiveness in meeting the learning goals is the primary consideration for the CPD

professional and will probably require a significant amount of discussion and consultation. Applying learner preferences to identify resources, the availability and accessibility of the resources, and their effectiveness and efficiency with respect to learners' goals are important aspects of the CPD professional's contribution. Learners should be encouraged to select from both formal and informal CME resources and may need assistance to consider and weigh possible alternatives, such as clinical traineeships, formal CME courses, home-study modules, study groups, and online study.

5. **Choosing outcomes.** Perhaps most difficult is the learner's task of selecting appropriate signposts of progress and valid indicators that goals have been met. If a review of some aspect of practice has triggered the new learning, a similar review, repeated at an appropriate time after the learning, may indicate successful learning and change. It is important for the provider to assist in the selection of outcomes that are relevant and valid indicators of change. Further, where the desired goal may be long term, learners may wish to identify indicators along the way. For example, if a physician wishes to decrease the incidence of influenza complications among senior patients, an appropriate signpost might be the establishment of a means to identify those who should receive a flu vaccine. Other outcomes may include the use of portfolios,[39] in which the physician can assemble evidence of progress toward and achievement of goals, to be reviewed either alone or with the CPD professional.

    Linking learning to outcomes and indicators of change provides the learner with important feedback, as well as the opportunity to plan a strategy and recruit reinforcers to inform and facilitate progress. As noted above, it is critical that the physician has selected valid outcomes and criteria by which to judge their attainment. An additional strategy for the provider may be that described by Mazmanian and Mazmanian[40] regarding the commitment to a specifically stated change. This commitment of the learner to a personal learning contract can have the effect of enhancing motivation and strategies to accomplish the stated change.

6. **Providing coaching.** The analogy of the "coaching" role for the CPD professional is intended to convey the role of "showing how" and "supporting." Process consultants do not coach content but they do offer support and suggestions for the process of SDL. Coaching learners through the various steps of the process may be a critical role for the provider. By providing feedback on progress and specific assistance, the provider can

assist learners to gain confidence not limited to specific knowledge, skills, and attitudes but also in the process of SDL. By both supporting learners' autonomy and providing opportunities for the development of learners' self-efficacy, the CPD professional can facilitate SDL processes and enhance learners' persistence. As goals are met, the CPD professional can assist in the identification of new goals.

An important role for the provider can be to ensure that the learner has access to feedback and to reinforcement for efforts. Feedback can come from a variety of sources, including the provider, patients, and colleagues and through a review of data.

Case 5, in which a physician is identified as needing in-depth review and subsequent retraining, represents an opportunity for the CPD professional to assist in the identification of a program to meet the physician's needs and to help him with a commitment contract. For CPD professionals, such contractual functions may become increasingly important activities.

OVERCOMING BARRIERS TO SDL

Despite thoughtful efforts by the CPD professional, barriers to SDL may continue to exist within the physician-learner. Furthermore, barriers may be created by the system of health care delivery and by perceptions of patient demands. They may even exist with the CPD professional whose system and goals are often apparently in conflict with the encouragement of SDL.

Learners' challenges may generally be related to a lack of skill and confidence at any level of the SDL process, as well as to barriers such as lack of time, lack of remuneration, and competing responsibilities. Similar barriers exist for the CME provider, who requires the knowledge and skills to assist learners, as described above. The provider may also face the challenge of lack of time and competing responsibilities already incorporated in the work of directing a CME office. An even greater influence may be the competing goal of attracting learners to formal events and the value placed on this particular goal in the institutional milieu. It can be argued that, as the literature indicates, at least 70% of ongoing physician learning is done independently of formal courses.[41] In this view, the role of the CME provider in improving the effectiveness of ongoing activities, and increasing the amount and quality of the SDL is even more essential.

Some physician-learners may be unfamiliar with the use of systematic SDL and may therefore lack confidence in undertaking it. CME providers have opportunities to influence the educational methods used in formal CME, such as problem-based learning;

by using these methods, they can foster competence among physician-learners.

SOME REMAINING QUESTIONS ABOUT SDL

Although there is widespread agreement that SDL can and should be enhanced, there is less agreement concerning reliable ways to assess its impact. Several measures have been identified that should relate to and arise from the outcome indicators the physician-learner has selected. For example, the learning portfolio offers a method of assessment that, as yet, requires further development. Although Snadden and Thomas[39] have reported on the usefulness of the portfolio, Pitts et al[42] found the reliability of peer assessors of portfolios to be insufficient for any summative judgments.

Other measures of SDL progress have been reported. A particular example is the PC Diary, a software based program to record self-directed learning.[21] To date, the analyses provide an excellent description of the questions raised by those who use the diaries and indicators of those patterns of reflective learning that tend to be associated with change. There are as yet no published reports linking reported change with changes in physician behavior measured objectively and in health care outcomes.

Further questions about SDL require our continued attention. For instance, how prepared are learners to undertake SDL? How can we develop and use the most effective strategies? What is the importance of the role of a group of colleagues in learning and change?

Finally, ethical considerations imply that we are always conscious of the need to match the ends and means of our practice. For example, as we encourage and expect physicians to assume responsibility for their learning, our means must include the support and preparation required for them to assume control over their educational activity. We must recognize the implications of this and our ethical obligations both to the learner and society to ensure that the outcomes of physician-directed learning contribute positively to health care outcomes.

REPRISE: A REVIEW OF THE INITIAL CASES

This chapter began with five cases describing situations where SDL might be effective. We will briefly revisit each one to synthesize the ideas presented in this chapter.

First, what about Dr Sanchez? Traditionally, the CPD professional might have suggested some courses that Dr Sanchez might not have been aware of. A more physician-centered approach might be to work with Dr Sanchez through an online search procedure. Often physicians are not aware of the variety of resources that are available beyond the standard Medline literature search. A critical issue for the CPD professional is to identify the limits of involvement with the physician. How can the provider's involvement foster SDL and facilitate learning opportunities for the physician? Dr Sanchez and the CPD professional may conduct a reasonably good needs assessment by working together in the online search environment. Once she has identified some sources for further work, the CPD professional would be effective in establishing a contract for other support as necessary. This contract should include expectations for Dr Sanchez's personal progress. Such contracts appear to be most effective when written.

Second, understanding Dr Gilchrest's learning needs regarding sexuality is central to our work. The explicit activities of the CPD professional here are based on those understandings. A process consultation effort would be helpful here. It is likely that Dr Gilchrest will find ideas and support from the literature. In addition, he may be bolstered by the support of a group of physicians and other health care providers who share his concerns and who may meet regularly to discuss their concerns, solve patient problems, do research, or produce patient and family education materials.

Third, employing a survey like the change readiness inventory may help in approaching Dr Elwood; however, survey approaches are only the start in this consultation effort. The provider might also work with him to design a self-paced computerized learning program on appropriate levels of HbA1c. Dr Elwood can get feedback on his efforts through follow-up with the participants to determine the extent to which they are using the information the program offered. This academic detailing activity may spur Dr Elwood toward other kinds of study and research.

Fourth, the challenge in this case lies in engaging and motivating the physician. CPD professionals are very often able to identify opportunities where their expertise may be helpful to a physician colleague. Neither their efforts, nor those of the physician, are likely to succeed, however, unless the physician becomes actively engaged. Such engagement demands an open discussion with the CPD professional and requires that the CME provider have excellent listening and interaction skills.

Fifth, an interesting and challenging element in the last case about credentialling difficulties is that it is systemic in character and appears to involve a wide range of learning needs. Finding solutions requires balancing the needs of the hospital, the credentialing process, and the individual physician. Although SDL is at the heart of the case, so too are the demands of the system. In this case, the CME provider may be instrumental in bringing relevant resources together to develop collaborative approaches to assist the physician in remedying identified deficiencies.

SUMMARY

SDL is a complex phenomenon. It is both a process undertaken by the physician and a system of practice supported by the CPD professional. Supporting SDL must include cognizance of the complexities of individual physician practices within the context of hospital systems or modern health care organizations. Understanding SDL provides insight into the means by which we, as providers, may facilitate opportunities for learning by making resources available to physicians. There are many facets to the process of physician learning, and the CPD professional must be attuned to their potential in order to make the best of the opportunities in their work with physicians in SDL.

REFERENCES—CHAPTER 7

1. Knowles MS. *SDL: A Guide for Learners and Teachers*. New York, NY: Associated Press; 1975.

2. Hammond M, Collins R. *SDL: Critical Practice*. New York, NY: Nichols/GP Publishing; 1991.

3. Maslow AH. *Toward a Psychology of Being*. 2nd ed. New York, NY: Van Nostrand Reinhold; 1968.

4. Brockett RG, Hiemstra R. *Self-direction in Adult Learning: Perspectives on Theory, Research and Practice*. New York, NY: Routledge; 1991.

5. Merriam SB, Caffarella RS. *Learning in Adulthood. A Comprehensive Guide*. 2nd ed. San Francisco, Calif: Jossey-Bass Publishers; 1999.

6. Grow G. Teaching learners to be self-directed: a stage approach. *Adult Educ Q*. 1991;41:125–149.

7. Premi J, Shannon S, Hartwick K, Lamb S, Wakefield J, Williams J. Practice-based small-group CME. *Acad Med*. 1994;69:800–802.

8. Candy PC. *Self-direction in Lifelong Learning*. San Francisco, Calif: Jossey-Bass Publishers; 1991.

9. Tough A. Why adults learn: a study of the major reasons for beginning and continuing a learning project. *Monographs in Adult Education*. Vol 3. Toronto, Ont: Ontario Institute for Studies in Education; 1968.

10. Houle CO. *The Inquiring Mind*. Madison, Wis: University of Wisconsin Press; 1961.

11. Fox RD, Mazmanian PE, Putnam RW. *Changing and Learning in the Lives of Physicians*. New York, NY: Praeger Publishers; 1989.

12. Schön D. *The Reflective Practitioner*. New York, NY: Basic Books; 1983.

13. Schön D. *Educating the Reflective Practitioner*. San Francisco, Calif: Jossey-Bass Publishers; 1987.

14. Kolb DA. *Experiential Learning: Experience as a Source of Learning and Development.* Englewood Cliffs, NJ: Prentice-Hall; 1984.

15. Putnam RW, Campbell MD. Competence. In: Fox RD, Mazmanian PE, Putnam RW, eds. *Change and Learning in the Lives of Physicians.* New York, NY: Praeger Publishers; 1989.

16. Geertsma RH, Parker RC, Whitbourne SK. How physicians view the process of change in their practice behavior. *J Med Educ.* 1982;57:752–761.

17. Slotnick HB. How doctors learn: physicians' self-directed learning episodes. *Acad Med.* 1999;74:1106–1117.

18. Fox RD, Rankin R, Costie KA, Parboosingh J, Smith E. Learning and the adoption of innovations among Canadian radiologists. *J Contin Educ Health Prof.* 1997;17:173–186.

19. Allery LA, Owen PA, Robling MR. Why general practitioners and consultants change their clinical practice. *BMJ.* 1997;314:870–874.

20. Parboosingh IJ, Gondocz ST. The maintenance of competence (MOCOMP) program: motivating specialists to appraise the quality of their continuing medical education activities. *Can J Surg.* 1993;36:29–32.

21. Campbell C, Parboosingh J, Gondocz T, Babitskaya G, Lindsay E, DeGuzman RC. Study of physicians' use of a software program to create a portfolio of their self-directed learning. *Acad Med.* 1996;71:S49–S51.

22. Dewey J. *How We Think.* Boston, Mass: DC Heath and Company; 1933.

23. Jennett P, Jones D, Mast T, Egan K, Hotvedt M. The characteristics of self-directed learning. In: Davis D, Fox R, eds. *The Physician as Learner: Linking Research to Practice.* Chicago, Ill: American Medical Association; 1994.

24. Prochaska JO, DiClemente CC. Stages and processes of self-change of smoking: toward an integrative model of change. *J Consult Clin Psychol.* 1983;51:390–395.

25. Parker K, Parisk SV. Application of Prochaska's transtheoretical model to continuing medical education: from needs assessment to evaluation. *Ann Royal Coll Physicians Surg.* 1999;32:590–596.

26. Gugliemino LM. Development of the SDL readiness scale. (Unpublished doctoral dissertation) Athens, Ga: University of Georgia; 1977.

27. Oddi LF. Development and validation of an instrument to identify self-directed continuing learners. *Adult Educ Q.* 1986;36:97–107.

28. Crook J. A validation study of a self-directed learning readiness scale. *J Nursing Educ.* 1985;24:274–279.

29. Bligh JG. Independent learning among general practice trainees: an initial survey. *Med Educ.* 1992;26:497–502.

30. Fox R. Using theory and practice to shape the practice of continuing professional development. *J Contin Educ Health Prof.* 2000;20:238–246.

31. Tough A. *The Adult's Learning Projects: A Fresh Approach to Theory and Practice in Adult Learning.* 2nd ed. Toronto, Ont: Ontario Institute for Studies in Education; 1971.

32. Zeitz HJ. Problem-based learning: development of a new strategy for effective continuing medical education. *Allergy Asthma Proc.* 1999;20:317–321.

33. Doucet MD, Purdy RA, Kaufman DM, Langille DB. A comparison of problem-based learning and lecture format in continuing medical education on headache diagnosis and management. *Med Educ.* 1998;32:590–596.

34. Lave J, Wenger E. *Situated Cognition: Legitimate Peripheral Participation.* New York, NY: Oxford University Press; 1991.

35. Chaiklin S, Lave J, eds. *Understanding Practice: Perspectives on Activity and Context.* London: Cambridge University Press; 1998.

36. Vygotsky LS. Mind in society: The development of higher psychological processes. In: Cole M, John-Steiner V, Scribner S, Souberman E, eds. Cambridge, Mass.: Harvard University Press; 1978. Cited in JV Wetsch. *Vygotsky and the Social Formation of Mind.* Cambridge, Mass: Harvard University Press, 1985.

37. Schein EH. *Process Consultation Volume 1: Its Role in Organization Development.* Reading, Mass: Addison Wesley Publishing Company; 1988.

38. Campion-Smith C. Interprofessional Learning in Primary Care: the Dorset Seedcorn Project. World Conference of Family Doctors. Dublin; June 1998.

39. Snadden D, Thomas ML. Portfolio learning in general practice vocational training—does it work? *Med Educ.* 1999;32:401–406.

40. Mazmanian PE, Mazmanian P. Commitment to change: theoretical foundations, methods, and outcomes. *J Contin Educ Health Prof.* 1999;19:200–207.

41. Nowlen PM. *A New Approach to Continuing Education for Business and the Professions: The Performance Model.* New York, NY: MacMillan; 1988.

42. Pitts J, Coles C, Thomas P. Educational portfolios in the assessment of general practice trainers: reliability of assessors. *Med Educ.* 1999;33:515–520.

chapter 8

Individualized Learning Strategies

John T. Parboosingh, MB; Mary Carol Badat, MAd Ed;
Douglas L. Wooster, MD

> Janet Nguyen has been chair of her National Specialty Society's Continuing Professional Development (CPD) Committee for one year, with little progress in helping her committee members understand the shift from continuing medical education (CME) to CPD or in getting her committee off its favorite subject—the society's annual conference. Today, however, she has been successful in getting her colleagues together for a full-day retreat, and she is hopeful that she'll achieve her objective. As she explains to her group, this includes establishing a specialty society CPD agenda that allows for the development of individualized learning strategies that could be made available to society members, throughout the year and in their practice settings. She has invited a CPD consultant to speak to the group about individualized learning strategies.

What are individualized learning strategies? How can a continuing professional development (CPD) committee create or obtain these learning resources and encourage society members to use them?

INTRODUCTION

Physician organizations, such as medical academies, associations, and specialty societies, traditionally offer members an array of educational services. In addition to scientific meetings and workshops, they offer the members a variety of other educational formats, including peer-reviewed journals and newsletters to support their self-directed learning. Physicians in the twenty-first century, faced with the rapid turnover of medical information and technologies, are seeking new ways to manage their information needs. They have high expectations that national and regional organizations will increase their educational services to meet the needs of their members. This chapter is about how physician organizations may enhance their educational offerings by providing individualized learning strategies and by encouraging their members to include them in their learning plans.

Organizations play a significant role in motivating physicians to engage in lifelong learning. Although some physicians express the desire to self-manage their learning, others are reluctant to move away from traditional educational methods (outlined in Chapter 9). To physicians in practice for more than a decade, continuing medical education (CME) means attending lectures. It will take time, and a shift in the locus of control, for many physicians who were trained in teacher-dominated educational environments to plan their own learning.

Recent studies suggest that participating in an organization or peer group influences the value that the individual physician places on lifelong learning. The studies support the argument that effective physician organizations, by fostering communities of practice,[1] encourage networking among peers and, with the help of mentors and role models, support physicians as they try new learning experiences. Studies undertaken in the United Kingdom[2] and North America[3] show that the quality of resources that physicians use to update their practices is determined to a great extent by the practice communities in which they function. Their findings are consistent with Nowlen's[4] concept that the value practitioners place on professional development is a function of the culture within which they practice and their personal development as individuals. Nowlen described the model as a double helix; one strand of the helix carries the values and culture of a given professional while the other strand carries the individual's skills, values, and past experiences. Professional practice is described as an intertwining of these two strands.

The potential of physician organizations and the continuing professional development (CPD) professionals who work within them to enhance the value physicians place on lifelong learning compels us to learn more about how these organizations influence their members. As learning organizations, they do so by creating and sustaining an environment that encourages continual learning and renewal of standards and the democratization of knowledge, which leads to improved performance and health outcomes for their patients. By rewarding role modeling and mentoring, learning organizations, in a non-threatening manner, create the peer pressure that motivates members to aspire to high standards of learning. These activities are perceived to be more effective and less threatening than regulations and mandatory policies.[3]

In addition to motivating members to value lifelong learning, learning organizations reward those who contribute to the creation of new knowledge that leads to enhancement of performance.[5]

Physicians instinctively form small groups or communities of practice where they network with peers and mentors and learn practical ways of putting innovations to practice.[6] Eraut[7] refers to this as the creation of tacit knowledge; Coles[8] perceives it as the generation of practical wisdom. Whatever term is used, this information is essential for physicians to apply evidence-based advances in medicine to their practices. The concept of organizations promoting best practices by fostering communities of practice is old, but academicians have only recently studied it.[9]

This chapter will review the ways that a physician organization may assist its members to plan and implement individualized learning strategies. The term *individual learning strategy* is used here to define the process whereby physicians identify a need or an opportunity to update their practice; select, with or without the help of others, the learning resources they need; assign time to learn with a busy daily schedule; integrate the newly acquired competence into their practice; and, finally, reflecting on the new learning, evaluate its worth to their practice.

We will explore how the individual physician can influence the standard of CPD activities of a group of peers and, also, how group activity can influence the learning habits of individual physicians in the group. We will show how an organization can offer self-learning tools, such as self-assessment programs and simulators, as a service to its members. We will describe how learning contracts and learning portfolios may be used to assist members and enhance the effectiveness of mentors as they guide small groups of practitioners intent on integrating an innovation into their practices. We will touch on strategies such as academic detailing and clinical traineeships, not generally the focus of professional societies, to round out our exploration of individualized learning methods. The chapter will conclude with a discussion of how computerized learning tools provided by specialty societies and other physician organizations can assist individuals and groups to focus and manage their individualized learning strategies.

SELF-ASSESSMENT PROGRAMS

The CPD consultant provides a brief description of individualized learning strategies. Dr Nguyen reminds the committee that the research literature suggests that educational strategies that empower individuals to identify their practice needs and select their own learning methods are more likely to enhance practice than traditional CME. The CPD consultant informs the committee that self-assessment is a key component of individualized learning strategies.

Specialty societies have a long tradition of offering self-assessment tests that members use to assess their knowledge and decision-making skills. More recently, CD and Internet technology provide opportunities for the development of self-assessment programs (SAPs) that assess a physician's competence to perform a specific procedure. Advanced multimedia computer technology, such as virtual reality, can be used to train and evaluate physicians on a wide range of invasive surgical and endoscopic procedures and to assess other patient–physician interactions. Simulators and telerobots are available commercially and are being used for tele-mentoring.[10] It is not farfetched to expect that in 10 years specialists will learn, practice, and be evaluated for maintenance of certification on simulators.

The Role of Self-assessment Programs in Physician Learning

Self-assessment programs help physicians to answer the question they constantly ask themselves, "Am I keeping up-to-date in my practice?" Essentially, self-assessment programs enable physicians to compare their knowledge and decision-making to that of their peers; set national standards of practice; assist members to identify their strengths and weaknesses; and provide a means of focused self-directed education.[11] Self-assessment programs are perceived by physicians to provide cost-effective education. The costs to users are significantly less than the costs of attending traditional CME and there is the added advantage that physicians can set the pace for learning to fit with their practice and personal schedules. In addition, a specialty society may use the information obtained from physician users to identify learning needs for group learning activities, such as seminars, and to select areas of practice that warrant the development of self-audit tools.

Developing Self-assessment Programs

Assessing Knowledge

High-quality self-assessment programs should assist physicians to undertake a "knowledge inventory" that will inform them of what they know and what they don't know. Knowing what we don't know, according to Pencheon,[12] helps physicians to legitimize learning by inquiry and undertake focused educational projects.[13] It follows that self-assessment programs should be based on the practitioners' needs, since the extent to which an identified knowledge gap will motivate a physician to acquire new knowledge will depend on the desired outcome for the knowledge and the individual's readiness to apply it to practice.[14]

The program should have an identifiable sponsor, which in the case of the society would be its CPD committee. The authority indicates the program's legitimacy, quality, and relevance to the practice of potential users.

Assessing Other Dimensions of Competence

Self-assessment programs are often designed to address components of competence other than knowledge. In some programs, the demonstration of knowledge, comprehension, application, analysis, synthesis, and evaluation of the outcome leads to a definitive assessment by the program of the participant's ability to handle a specific clinical issue[15] (Table 8-1). Matching the question format and content to this taxonomy can be helpful in the preparation of the program items. Carefully crafted items can test comprehension, application, and synthesis of information as well as knowledge. This leads to a deeper level of assessment, which is more useful to a practitioner than an assessment of knowledge alone.

Increasingly, self-assessment programs are using multimedia, computer simulations, and in-house simulators similar to those used in the aircraft industry to test the user's competence to perform a function or skill. In each case, program design consists of matching question format (or sets of tasks to be performed) with the knowledge, skills, and attitudes of the competence or behavior to be tested. Inferences are made regarding the participant's knowledge and skills from an analysis of their test responses.

Developing Quality Questions

There are three classes of items (questions) in self-assessment programs: trivial, discriminating, and motivating. The program itself may represent three levels of competency: introductory, qualifying, or mastery (Table 8-2). Most items in self-assessment programs are of the discriminating type. This class of item provides a clearly defensible "best answer," which serves to identify if the participants possess a specific knowledge, skill, or attitude. Motivating questions are used to introduce new knowledge or controversy. The "best answer" allows opportunity for interpretation or further qualification. It should prompt the learner to read more around the topic or

TABLE 8-1

Components of Competence That May Be Assessed by Self-Assessment Programs

1. **Knowledge:** Recallable information
2. **Comprehension:** Meaningful manipulation of knowledge
3. **Application:** Complex integration of information
4. **Analysis:** Identify relevance of information
5. **Synthesis:** Develop abstract relationships
6. **Evaluation:** Assess appropriateness

TABLE 8-2

Levels of Competency That May Be Assessed by Self-Assessment Programs

1. **Introductory:** Items are factual knowledge; basic comprehension, rudimentary applications (eg, basic pre-test; introducing issues)
2. **Qualifying:** Discriminating items requiring knowledge and skills, comprehension, application and analysis (eg, end of training or registration examination; assessing for safety)
3. **Mastery:** As for qualifying plus in-depth analysis, synthesis, and evaluation (eg, self-assessment program for consultants; motivating further study)

discuss the issue with a knowledgeable colleague.[16] The layout and character of the items will also be adjusted depending on whether this is an introductory program, a qualifying program, or a mastery program. An introductory-level program would be appropriate for a focused self-assessment program involving an area of new knowledge, for a beginning trainee, or as a follow-up to a basic-level seminar. There are generally fewer questions, the class of question is trivial or discriminating, and only the knowledge domain is assessed. Mastery programs probe expertise at a high-level consultant range. The items are usually discriminating and motivating. All levels of the taxonomy of knowledge, skills, and attitudes are addressed to identify a deeper understanding of the subject area. Self-assessment programs prepared by specialty societies should be aimed at the mastery level.

New Technologies in Self-assessment Programs

There are a variety of interactive computer-assisted models in use today. Early examples consisted of text-based programs with directions to listen to an audiotape or view a video and answer the questions. This type of program is moderately inexpensive to develop and can test skills and attitudes as well as knowledge. It is an effective way of presenting specific intervention maneuvers, such as techniques for inserting catheters for measuring central venous pressure or carrying out a lumbar puncture.[17] Video- and audiotape-based self-assessment programs are used, for instance, to assess clinical decision-making based on physical signs and heart sounds.[18]

Computer-based simulations may be simple extensions of the videotape- or audiotape-based models. They may be combined with a computer-based instructional program directed to a specific skill or knowledge area.[19,20] Images or sound clips can be accessed in a random fashion on a CD-ROM, allowing choices in a multiple-choice question to be linked directly to additional information about a case or clinical problem. Also, participants can retrieve expert comment from the CD-ROM in response to the answer.

In addition, these models enable adaptive testing, a technique that presents participants with questions of increasing difficulty as they gain competence.

Computer-based simulators, similar to flight simulators, present the most sophisticated forms of computer-based testing. Such programs are available in several specialty areas, for instance, anesthesiology, laparoscopic surgery, or ultrasound scanning. In the ultrasound and surgery models, participants are able to use the probe or the surgical equipment in a plastic model or a virtual-reality setting. Feedback is provided from the simulator to represent the results one would encounter in the actual procedure with a patient. This allows participants to modify their approach as they perform the procedure. Simulator programs evaluate and store performance characteristics and provide feedback as participants learn and manage clinical problems. Anesthesiology simulators are computer-based self-assessment programs that have the capability of testing the physician's response to different clinical problems.[21,22] The simulation range covers the spectrum of clinical problems, from basic problems that are suitable for first-year trainees to complex patient situations with multiple complications and problems being presented throughout the simulation.[23–25]

Skills labs and objective structured clinical examinations (OSCEs) represent another type of self-assessment program that, although used most frequently in undergraduate medical education, is also provided by some national specialty societies for practicing physicians. They use a variety of formats, including standardized patients, animal preparations, and plastic models.

Web-based Technologies

Self-assessment programs can be incorporated into Internet CME programs.[26–28] Quality indicators, such as the sponsor or authority, may be difficult to determine. There are many society and university sites that contain links to adjudicated sites or provide reliable programs.[28–30] In addition, there are criteria regarding the appearance and resources linked to Web sites,[31] but these are less important than the scientific content. A scoring system has been developed to help identify high-quality Web-based self-assessment programs (Table 8-3).[32]

Barriers to Developing Self-assessment Programs

Developmental and maintenance costs, both financial and human resource costs, present the major barrier to specialty societies developing high-quality self-assessment programs. The costs are moderate for a text-based program and higher for computer-based models. The development of a skills lab or simulator-based

TABLE 8-3

A Scoring System for Internet Self-Assessment Programs Sites

Educational Principles:

Recognizable source
—University
—Specialty societies
Stated objectives
Graded levels of participation
Feedback allowed to program
Evaluation provided to participant
Free of corporate bias
'Accredited' activity

Delivery:

Overall style and quality ('readability')
Speed of loading/Ease of navigation
Quality of images

Scoring: 1 point per item.

program is a costly exercise, which is best performed in concert with already established programs. The preparation of quality items requires both clinical expertise and skilled item writers.

Feedback

Feedback to Learners

The feedback to the participant may be either direct or extended. Direct feedback provides the participant with the answer key and a total score. In addition, it usually provides the best answer, a discussion, and supporting references for each item. Extended feedback provides the individual with an evaluation of the performance data. A performance analysis is provided, broken down into specific areas. This inventory of strengths and weaknesses allows the participant to develop personal learning projects and focus their reading or identify courses or meetings that are most relevant to their needs. In addition, the individual's performance can be compared to a benchmark that may be set by the writers of the program. This "norm-referenced" score can be set to the best learner, the expectations of experts, or the results of a peer group. Although it is not always germane to know how well or how badly one performed as compared to one's peers, there is a clear quality-control aspect in knowing how one's performance compared to expected benchmarks set by the program.

Physicians most often use self-assessment programs in the same way they used examinations during training to test what they know or can do. The ability of the programs to identify what physicians don't know and need to learn more about is less well known or utilized. The performance analysis is the most powerful stimulus for developing personal learning projects or other educational activities based on the self-evaluation process (Table 8-4). Advanced types of

TABLE 8-4

An Example of a Performance Analysis Provided to a Vascular Surgeon on Completion of a Self-Assessment Program

Performance Analysis	Registration Number: zzz		
Subject	Your Score	Total Score	Percentage Correct Items
Overall	144	250	58
Basic Science	20	31	65
Clinical	124	219	56
Diagnosis	27	39	69
Treatment	16	29	55*
Drugs (incl anticoagulants)	14	23	61
Complications	23	43	53*
Outcomes	13	29	45*
Vascular Lab	18	22	82
Anatomy	6	10	60*
Systems Aorta (AAA)	11	24	46*
Carotid	24	32	75
Renal	1	3	33*
Extremity —upper	8	15	53
—lower	10	19	53*
Veins	20	28	71
Procedures CEA	7	10	70
EV	6	6	100
EAB	3	5	60
FP	4	11	38*
Grafts	3	6	50*
Sympathetomy	1	4	25*
Miscellaneous Popliteal Artery	9	11	88
Miscellaneous Aneurysms	12	16	75
Vasculitis	6	9	67
Trauma	8	13	62
Diabetes	1	6	17*

*The result falls below the norm for that category.

feedback that can be provided to the participants include progressive questions or adaptive testing, online resources, prepackaged literature searches, and access to expert comment. These options allow learners to delve more deeply into a specific area of study within the self-assessment program. Although these options are generally not available in text-based programs, they are certainly feasible in programs provided on a CD-ROM or via the Internet.

Feedback to Program Planners

Program planners obtain important information from participants in the responses to individual items, assuming that participants return their answers for marking. The types of feedback relate to specific questions, the overall strengths and weaknesses of participants as a group, and the appropriateness of the material presented in the program. For example, a scatter of answers to a particular item suggests that the question is ambiguous or the choices are poorly constructed. Equally, questions that are most frequently answered correctly serve little purpose, as they do not assist in discriminating users based on their knowledge or behaviors. In addition, if the responses to one particular area within the program are unexpected, the relevance of that area, the quality of those questions, or the depths of the questioning needs to be reviewed. Self-assessment programs should include a questionnaire for participants to provide information on its usefulness to their professional development and suggestions for future editions.

Summary

High-quality self-assessment programs can provide a cost-effective CPD tool for specialists. Knowledge, skills, and attitudes can be assessed and a knowledge inventory developed. Feedback on a practitioner's performance provides objective needs assessment, which can direct learning activities such as focused reading, personal learning projects, and mini-practice audits that will be directly relevant to improving a specialist's clinical practice. Specialty societies can create the culture and peer pressure for its members to use self-assessment programs to drive lifelong learning in practice. They can also use the information gained from such programs to develop other educational activities. It is important to remember:

- Self-assessment is a key component of individualized learning strategies.
- Virtual reality environments will enable self-assessment to be integrated into practice.
- Self-assessment motivates the learning project and evaluate its worth in practice.

LEARNING CONTRACTS

The CPD committee members express concern that busy physicians will have difficulty assigning time in their busy schedules to undertake self-directed learning projects. The consultant suggests that the committee, as part of its new strategy, assist society members to use learning contracts for this purpose. Dr Smith, a member of the CPD Committee, recalls how he was introduced to learning contracts. Last year, he attended a lecture on the effectiveness of administered folic acid to reduce neural tube defects in newborn infants (NTD). During the question period, he listed a number of concerns and questions about providing folic acid to his patients. Folic acid, for instance, has to be administered before conception while most patients present in early pregnancy. Will a diet of green vegetables reduce the incidence of NTD? Dr Jones, the lecturer, offered to assist Dr Smith and his partners in the coming months to learn more about the use of folic acid to prevent NTD and to explore the barriers to introduction in greater depth. He helped the group to develop a learning contract and an implementation plan to introduce a protocol to administer folic acid to all women of childbearing age in their practice.

"The chief mechanism used as an enhancement of self-direction is the learning contract. In adult education, contracts have been proposed as the most effective technique for assisting students to diagnose their learning needs, plan learning activities, identify and select resources that are relevant and appropriate, and become skilled at self-evaluation."[33] Can learning contracts support learning strategies developed by individuals or groups of physicians?

Definition

A learning contract is a tool for identifying needs, setting goals, selecting resources, and developing and carrying out a planned learning activity. Although learning contracts are usually negotiated between an individual and a facilitator or a group of learners and a facilitator, the contract can be made between a learner and himself or herself. Anderson and colleagues describe learning contracts as "negotiated learning agreements." The term is used interchangeably with *contract learning* and sometimes used synonymously with *learning plan*. Some may differentiate between learning contracts and learning plans, arguably stating that learning plans are "less formal and focused more on short-term goals."[34]

Although contract documents vary in complexity and style, the framework assures that the stages of the learning process are clearly defined. These include the following items (applied to the case study):

■ the learning objectives (eg, to identify women at risk and reduce the incidence of NTD);

- strategies (eg, to introduce community-based pre-pregnancy counseling) and resources (current literature, community health educators);
- evidence that the objectives have been met (an evaluation plan);
- the evaluation of such evidence (eg, results of monitoring rates of NTD);
- the completion date and the estimated time to develop, implement, and evaluate the project; and
- the expected role of the facilitator (eg, Dr Jones).

Learning contracts have become a core component of learner-centered programming in higher education, training, and professional development. They are used in nursing and medical undergraduate and graduate education but are not a common feature of CME.

The Use of Learning Contracts

By Physician Organizations

Learning contracts may assist physicians to learn more efficiently and to assign time for practice-based learning. Mentors within societies frequently assist physicians to adopt new practices, as in this case, through the use of informal learning contracts or plans. Contract learning requires a reappraisal of the traditional roles for both the learner and the instructor. The learner must assume control and responsibility for his/her learning experience; the role of the instructor shifts from imparter of knowledge to facilitator of learning.[35] Programs of this nature often require training of some type for the facilitators. Establishing institutional support for this type of individualized programming is difficult. Mentors or educational influentials willingly give their time to assist colleagues but, by their nature, tend to work informally.

Learning contracts can be used to support traditional CME. For example, the physicians in the above case study could obtain a standardized learning agreement form from the specialty society's Web site. But information and communication technology based CPD management systems recently offered by some specialty societies provide protocols that enable users to develop their own learning contracts and implementation plans and interact more efficiently with mentors. Electronic learning portfolios and online learning systems such as Pedia*Link*™ (described below) may increase physician awareness of the value of planning their learning.[36] In the next phase of development of Pedia*Link*™, communicating with pocket organizers and e-mail will offer physicians the option to be reminded of upcoming deadlines for completing learning projects.

By Physicians

How may learning contracts assist physicians to set learning objectives?

For the practicing physician, the challenges encountered daily on the job present identifiable needs that, when viewed through the lens of a learning contract, can be focused into objectives that are relevant both personally and professionally.[37] Formulating a learning contract requires significant self-reflection. Determining needs and developing clearly focused objectives is one of the more difficult tasks when constructing a learning agreement, but the time invested in self-examination can lead to a much deeper level of learning. It is important to provide guidelines and facilitation to aid learners in setting clear and achievable goals. Sample contracts and guiding questions for setting objectives are helpful materials. Using today's technology, the learning team and their mentor may complete the forms and submit them to a database on the society's Web site. Such a topical database of learning contacts could serve as a needs-assessment tool for the society.

How can learning contracts assist physicians to identify resources and formulate learning strategies?

Learning contracts may encourage the use of a wider range of learning resources than individual learners would otherwise consider. This can promote greater creativity in developing strategies for learning and new perspectives for the learning task at hand. For instance, peers, patients, and mentors in the workplace may become sounding boards, offer ideas and feedback, and assist in the demonstration/evaluation process. Because time is such a premium for physicians, it makes sense to take direct advantage of the workplace as a learning environment.[38] Documentation of the learning process is inherent in contract learning and advantageous to both the learner and mentors or facilitators. It is an effective way to provide recognition, enhancement, and documentation of the problem-solving processes inherent in the physician's daily efforts to better care for his or her patients.

By the CPD Consultant

What is the role of the education consultant?

In the case described here, the group of physicians, nurses, and health educators embark on their project, consulting with their mentor at regular intervals via e-mail and possibly at a monthly conference call. The education consultant may offer the group the society's information services, for instance, to provide a practice guideline on the prophylactic administration of folic acid or suggest access to the local university library resources.

The education consultant could be the recipient of learning contracts completed by society members and be responsible for posting them on a dedicated corner of the society's Web site where they can be a resource (and provide motivation) for other members.

In circumstances such as those described in our case, the extent to which a signed contract with a mentor motivates a physician group to complete a predetermined task is a function of the peer influence generated within the group and a measure of its success as a community of practice. Physician organizations provide the umbrella and create the culture that drives small groups of members working together toward a common goal, which is most often geared toward raising standards of practice. These groups run the risk of failure and the feelings of frustration expressed by busy physicians. Physician organizations have the opportunity to foster the formation of working groups and facilitate interaction between peers and mentors using tools such as learning contracts. In the next section, we describe the use of learning portfolios, which may be viewed as "expanded learning contracts" designed to assist physicians to manage learning in the workplace.

LEARNING PORTFOLIOS

Definition

Learning portfolios were introduced to students in the visual arts in the 1970s with the intent of engendering feelings of self-control and ownership over their learning. A learning portfolio to most educators is a collection of evidence that demonstrates the continuing acquisition of knowledge, skills and attitudes, understanding and achievements reflecting the current stages of development and activity of the learner.[39] This definition focuses on the role of the learning portfolio as a dossier of achievements of a learner collected over time, in which case the term is synonymous with learning diary or journal. The application of information and communication technologies (ICT) has produced *e-learning portfolios*, which have the potential to influence learning behaviors to a greater extent than paper diaries.

What Role Do Learning Portfolios Play in the Learning Process?

Assisting Physicians

Initial reports from physician users suggest that learning portfolios, particularly the electronic versions, help them to focus learning on their practice needs.[40] For instance, they report that reflecting on patients' problems more often stimulates learning projects that lead to changes in practice than does attending traditional CME programs.[41] Learning portfolios guide practitioners to create learning plans based on practice needs and perceived areas of expertise. Graphically expressed learning plans, available in electronic versions of learning portfolios are meant to guide diary users to select learning projects based on their predetermined plans.[42]

The ability for users to communicate with colleagues undertaking similar projects is enhanced in electronic versions of learning portfolios when users have the capability of transferring learning items to a central database that can be accessed by peers.[42] This capability encourages sharing of references and other learning resources and the identification of mentors and resource persons.

The Role of the Professional Society

Studies that show the inefficiencies in traditional teacher-centered CME suggest a need for physicians to take charge of their learning. This can be done by using practice experiences to identify what to learn, selecting learning resources, and setting learning plans based on individual learning preferences and unique schedules. The specialty society can influence the quality of CPD activities undertaken by its members by fostering their use of learning portfolios. Specialists in Canada are able to submit portfolio items, termed personal learning projects, for credit in the Maintenance of Certification program of the Royal College of Physicians and Surgeons of Canada. A Web diary is available for them to record learning projects on an Internet portal.[43] Specialty societies in Canada sponsor workshops to assist their members to use personal learning projects to upgrade their learning skills. Speakers in the plenary sessions at the society annual meetings are encouraged to conclude their presentations with a discussion of possible learning projects that members could undertake. In the future, we predict physicians will leave these sessions and access e-learning portfolios through personal digital devices. Portfolios have the potential to encourage physicians to participate in learning activities and promote the society's educational activities.

Learning portfolios and learning diaries have the potential to encourage physicians to move from counting hours of participating in CPD activities to counting items of learning or personal learning projects that they generate from their education and practice experiences. In this context, portfolio items or personal learning projects are analogous to problem based learning in the undergraduate curriculum, in that it is learning that results from the process of working towards the understanding or resolution of a problem, be it a real problem in practice or one presented in a CME session or an article.[44]

The CPD committee, in its endeavor to promote individualized learning strategies, may wish to provide its members with access to a searchable database of learning projects submitted by learning portfolio users. Such databases of learning projects support communities of learners and motivate those working on projects, such as those described above, to share their experiences with peers. Information on learning projects can be posted on the society's Web site or newsletter and used at workshops to help physicians to set standards for their CPD activities. Analysis of data from the central database can provide users with information on their learning habits. For instance, analysis of the data generated from users in one study suggests that certain stimuli to learning are more likely to lead to commitment to change practice compared with others.[45] Such feedback to groups can generate active discussions on learning practices, a subject that physicians rarely discuss among themselves. Also, by describing the interface between the competencies of practitioners and the needs of their patients, a database of learning projects may be used to create learning objectives for society-sponsored continuing education programs. Small-group education sessions can be designed for specific physician members to meet with peers who are undertaking similar learning projects.

The specialty society that fosters the use of learning portfolios is providing a sophisticated educational service for its members who, we predict, will use them increasingly as evidence of lifelong learning in practice, which is required for purposes of licensure and maintenance of certification.

COMPUTER-SUPPORTED LEARNING ENVIRONMENTS

The CPD Committee, exploring the pros and cons of individualized learning strategies, sees a significant role for the society to use information and communication technologies (ICT) to promote individualized learning strategies to its members. The CPD consultant describes some recent developments in the application of ICT in this field.

Pedia*Link*™ is an online system offered by the American Academy of Pediatrics to assist pediatricians to direct, focus, and manage their CPD.[36] The system tracks and provides feedback on the quality of the pediatrician's learning cycle, from the identification of practice needs, through the development and implementation of learning plans, to the introduction of changes in practice, based on newly acquired knowledge and skills. Pedia*Link*™ provides physicians with online multimedia self-assessment tools to identify gaps in their knowledge and a searchable database to deposit questions they raise in practice and topics they wish to pursue. The system uses Unified Modeling Language System (UMLS) to scan the academy's extensive online learning resources, including a course calendar and recommends appropriate learning resources. Pedia*Link*™

assists the user to develop a learner plan and set deadlines for completion of learning projects. It keeps track of CME hours and provides users with a transcript of credits. Pedia*Link*™ prompts users to create a vision of the outcomes of learning projects and keeps a database of changes they intend to make to their practice as a consequence of their learning activities. The system provides access to online sources of medical literature and may be expanded in coming years to provide access to academy-appointed mentors and librarians. Pedia*Link*™ is an individualized learning strategy designed for pediatricians and offered by their national society. In addition, it provides documented evidence of lifelong learning from needs identification to integration of new knowledge into practice. The planners of the system, looking to the future, are creating "performance dashboards" that enable individual users to select their peer group and compare their learning activities with those of their peers.

As learning and professional practice become closely intertwined in the twenty-first century, it is predicted that physicians will learn with peers, and other care providers with whom they work, in communities of practice. Communities of practice are defined as, "Cohorts, representing a variety of formal and informal, internal and external professional groups, teams, associations and societies; through participation in which the identity of the individual professional as a learner and knowledge seeker develops."[2] Specifically, they do so by creating and sustaining an environment that encourages continual learning and renewal of standards and the democratization of knowledge within teams of caregivers, which leads to improved performance and health outcomes for patients. It is predicted that ICT will play a significant role in supporting multidisciplinary teams in the care delivery units of the future.[46]

Knowledge Forum® is an example of ICT designed to support team learning.[47] Knowledge Forum® participants read and build on each other's notes. Tracking cognitive processes, such as literature review and reflection, Knowledge Forum® encourages participants to create high-level syntheses of their work while background operations record those processes automatically. The computer system provides the organization and support for the complex array of individual and group discussions and development of ideas that constitute a working knowledge-building community. The knowledge-building functions have the potential to bring together groups of physicians and other caregivers in the service of knowledge advancement. It provides the medium for knowledge sharing and telementoring. We predict that software of this type will, in the future, assist specialty societies and other organizations that bring experts together to set standards and create practice guidelines as well as motivate health professionals to focus learning on their practice needs.

ALTERNATIVE INDIVIDUALIZED STRATEGIES

Although this chapter has focused on individualized strategies of most use to specialty and other professional organizations, there are a number of other methods that are tailored to the physician's needs. These will be described briefly here in order to provide closure to this aspect of the tools available to the CPD professional. They include academic detailing and clinical traineeships. Additional mention will be made of opinion leaders, a strategy targeted toward individual communities but often focused on the work of specialty societies, the natural home of such clinician educator–leaders.

Academic Detailing

Academic detailing is a method derived from other disciplines, such as agriculture, in which the physician is visited by a health professional in order to educate him or her about an aspect of practice. Modeled after the successful "drug rep" visit employed by the pharmaceutical industry, the health professional is often a pharmacist but can also be of other disciplines, eg, nursing.

Clinical Traineeships

Most often falling under the rubric of the medical school, the clinical traineeship represents a focused and individualized effort on the part of a clinician to return to the teaching/learning environment in a structured manner, often called a mini-residency or preceptorship. Here, for a period of days or months, the learner is immersed in educational and clinical endeavors, such as attending ward rounds, admitting and working up patients, presenting and reviewing cases with respected staff colleagues, and learning new procedures. Physicians undertake clinical traineeships for a variety of reasons, most commonly to learn a new competence for which they see a need in their practice or to see what's new since they left residency training.

A clinical traineeship provides the optimum environment for a physician to acquire a new competence. Clinical traineeships are usually arranged on an informal basis, which probably explains why there are few studies in the education literature. Especially where the acquisition of a new skill is the centerpiece of the traineeship, a well-balanced clinical traineeship will ensure that the physician not only acquires the skills to do the procedure but also the background knowledge about the skill, including the evidence for its effectiveness. In addition, the academic environment provides opportunities for the physician to discuss its use with other learners and mentors and gain practical tips (tacit knowledge) that will assist in the introduction of the new procedure in practice. A relationship with a mentor, initiated during a clinical traineeship, can provide the foundation on which the physician, on return to practice, communicates with the mentor as he or she gains experience with the new procedure. Traditional methods of communication can be complemented by information and communication technologies in the form of telementoring.[48] Telementoring provides the opportunity for the mentor to facilitate the process whereby the physician, gaining experience with a new procedure during a traineeship, moves through the stages of competence, from "novice" to "advanced beginner" to "competent" and finally "master"[49] in his or her home environment. Although clinical traineeships are popular with physicians,[50] they are less frequently used than other methods of CME.[51] Physicians must take time away from practice and pay for travel and accommodation in a different location. Most teaching units, already feeling the effects of a reduced patient load, are obliged to give opportunities for hands-on experience to residents. Although there may be more opportunities for hands-on experience in community hospitals and for physicians on staff who are willing to be preceptors, there often are administrative barriers to obtaining privileges to practice in these institutions.

SUMMARY: TRANSLATING EVIDENCE TO PRACTICE

Physicians depend on self-directed learning strategies to keep current and maintain standards in practice. The learning is typically stimulated by questions raised while reflecting on their management of patients and their perception of practice needs. Reading the literature, networking with peers, and seeking help from mentors are their most useful learning resources. Studies show that they are often used in combinations,[52] but assistance from a mentor, often during a traineeship, is the most frequently used learning resource when a new procedure is being learned.[53] The informal nature of such projects makes it hard to study objectively without interfering with the learning habits of the individual. Yet, the increasing demand for rapid learning by physicians who are pressured to adopt proven practice innovations is providing the incentive for research into innovative ways of making learning more efficient.

The learning strategies reviewed in this chapter cannot operate by themselves. They simply enhance and embellish the physician's basic self-directed learning strategies. For instance, self-assessment programs and simulators can only assist physicians who are motivated to plan their learning based on objective assessments of their learning needs. Physicians who choose to learn how to use a new endoscopic instrument by taking a traineeship with a mentor rather than attending a course provided by the makers of the instrument are demonstrating their skills in selecting appropriate learning resources.

The research agenda must focus on seeking a better understanding of the natural processes of learning from practice as well as developing new technical aids to learning. Only physicians who have insight and spontaneously reflect on their performance will use simulators and computerized learning environments.

At the beginning of the chapter, we point to studies that suggest that factors in the environment in which physicians work and the colleagues they respect influence the value placed on learning and the likelihood that individualized learning aids will be used. Specialty societies provide a unique venue for this research.

REFERENCES—CHATPER 8

1. Wenger ET, Snyder WM. Communities of practice: the organizational frontier. *Harvard Business News.* Jan–Feb, 2000.

2. Report of the Standing Committee on Postgraduate Medical and Dental Education, UK. Strategy for continuing education and professional development for hospital doctors and dentists. *Med Educ.* 2000;34:421–423.

3. Fox RD, Mazmanian PE, Putnam RW, eds. *Changing and Learning in the Lives of Physicians.* New York, NY: Praeger Publishers; 1989.

4. Nowlen P. *A New Approach for Continuing Education for Business and the Professions.* New York, NY: Macmillan; 1988.

5. Senge PM. *The Fifth Discipline: The Art & Practice of the Learning Organization.* New York, NY: Doubleday; 1990.

6. Confessore SJ. Building a learning organization: communities of practice, self-directed learning and continuing medical education. *J Contin Educ Health Prof.* 1997;17:5–11.

7. Eraut M. *Developing Professional Knowledge and Competence.* London, UK: The Falmer Press; 1994.

8. Coles C. Credentialing through the natural process of CPD: what more do we need? Paper presented at Credentialing Physician Specialists: A World Perspective, June 8–10, 2000. Chicago, Ill.

9. Wenger E. *Communities of Practice: Learning, Meaning, and Identity.* Cambridge, Mass: Cambridge University Press; 1998.

10. Schulam P, Docimo S, Salch W, Breitenbach C, Moore R, Kavoussi L. Telesurgical Mentoring: Initial clinical experience. *Surg. Endosc.* 1997;11:1001–1005.

11. Davidoff F. The American College of Physicians and the medical knowledge self-assessment program paradigm. *J Contin Educ Health Prof.* 1989;9:233–238.

12. Pencheon D. "I don't know": the three most important words in education. *BMJ.* 1999;318.

13. Hammond M, Collins R. Self-directed learning to educate medical educators. Part 1: How do we use self-directed learning? *Med Teacher.* 1987;9:253–260.

14. Parker K, Parikh SV. Application of Prochaska's transtheoretical model to continuing medical education: from needs assessment to evaluation. *Ann Roy Coll Phys Surg Can.* 1999;32:97–99.

15. Drumheller SJ. *Handbook of Curriculum Design of Individual Instruction.* Englewood Cliffs, NJ: Educational Technology Publications; 1971.

16. King A. Designing the instructional process to enhance critical thinking across the curriculum. *Teaching Psychol.* 1995;22:13–17.

17. Braslow A, Brennan RT, Newman MM, Bircher NG, Batcheller AM, Kaye W. CPR training without an instructor: development and evaluation of a video self-instruction system. *Resuscitation.* 1997;34:207–220.

18. Harrell JS, Champagne MT, Jarr S, Miyaya M. Heart sound simulation: how useful for critical care nurses? *Heart Lung.* 1990;19:197–202.

19. Anderson JG, Jay SJ. Dynamic Computer Simulation Models. *J Contin Educ Health Prof.* 1997;17:32–42.

20. Prolla JC, da Silva VD, Muller RL, Muller RL. Imagequest: a model self-assessment and self-teaching program for cytopathology. *Acta Cytologica.* 1997;41:1497–1499.

21. Chopra V, Engbers FH, Geerts MJ, Filet WR, Bovill JG, Spierdijk J. The Leiden anaesthesia simulator. *Br J Anaesth.* 1994;73:287–292.

22. Chopra V, Engbers FH, Geerts MJ, Filet WR, Bovill JG, Spierdijk J. The Leiden anaesthesia simulator. *Br J Anaesth.* 1994;73:293–297.

23. Norman J, Wilkins D. Simulators for anesthesia. *J Clin Monit.* 1996;12:91–99.

24. Byrne AJ, Jones JG. Responses to simulated anesthetic emergencies by anesthetists with different durations of clinical experience. *Brit J Anaesth.* 1997;78:553–556.

25. Devitt J, Kurrek M, Cohen M. Can a Simulator Based Evaluation Be Used to Assess Anesthesiologists? *Anesthesiology.* 1998;89:A1172.

26. www.science.widener.edu/~withers/inform.html

27. www.love2learn.com

28. www.cme.utoronto.ca/evaluating_sites.html

29. www.clearinghouse.net/ratings.html#eval

30. www.acc.org

31. www.omni.org

32. Wooster DL, Samson L. Personal communication. 2001.

33. Brookfield S. *Understanding and Facilitating Adult Learning.* San Francisco, Calif: Jossey-Bass Publishers; 1986.

34. Anderson G, Boud D, Sampson J. *Learning Contracts.* London: Kogan Page Limited; 1996.

35. Solomon P. Learning contracts in clinical education: evaluation by clinical supervisors. *Med Teacher.* 1992;14:205–210.

36. Sectish TC, Floriani V, Badat MC, Perelman R, Bernstein HH. Continuous professional development: raising the bar for pediatricians. *Pediatrics.* 2002;110:152–156.

37. Malkin KF. A standard for professional development: the use of self and peer review; learning contracts and reflection in clinical practice. *J Nursing Manage.* 1994;2:143–148.

38. Parsell G, Bligh J. Contract learning, clinical learning and clinicians. *Postgrad Med J.* 1996;72:284–289.

39. Parboosingh J. Learning portfolios: potential to assist health professionals with self-directed learning. *J Contin Educ Health Prof.* 1996;16:75–81.

40. Campbell C, Parboosingh J, Gondocz T, Babitskaya G, Lindsay E, DeGuzman RC. Study of physicians' use of a software program to create a portfolio of their self-directed learning. *Acad Med.* 1996;71:S49–S51.

41. Campbell C, Parboosingh J, Gondocz T, Babitskaya G, Pham B. Study of factors influencing the stimulus to learning recorded by physicians keeping a learning portfolio. *J Contin Educ Health Prof.* 1999;19:16–24.

42. Parboosingh J. Chapter 10. Tools to assist physicians to manage their information needs. In: Bruce C, Candy P, eds. *Information Literacy Around the World: Advances in Programs and Research.* New South Wales: Charles Sturt University Centre for Information Studies; 2000:121–136.

43. www.mainport.org

44. Seifer SD. Recent and emerging trends in undergraduate medical education-curricular responses to a rapidly changing health care system. *West J Med.* 1988;168:400–411.

45. Campbell C, Parboosingh J, Gondocz T, Babitskaya G, Pham B. A study factors that influence physicians' commitments to change their practice using learning diaries. *Acad Med.* 1999;74:S34–S36.

46. Parboosingh J, Jennett P, Longpre A, Russell A. Evaluating technologies for team learning in health sector workers: a review and synthesis of the literature and recommendations for future research. A Report to the Office of Learning Technologies, Project 21001R,

2001, Human Resources Development Canada, Government of Canada, Ottawa.

47. Scardamalia M, Bereiter C. Technologies for knowledge-building discourse. *Commun ACM.* 1993;36:37–41.

48. www.uthscsa.edu/hetcat/Tele023.html

49. Dreyfus SE, Dreyfus HL. A five-stages model of the mental activities involved in directed skill acquisition. Operations Research Center, 80-2, University of California, Berkeley, 1980.

50. Kantrowitz PM, Rezler AG. A personalized miniresidency program at the University of New Mexico School of Medicine: a seven-year perspective. *J Contin Educ Health Prof.* 1991;11:197–204.

51. Curry L, Putnam WR. Continuing medical education in maritime Canada. The methods physicians use, would prefer and find most effective. *Can Med Assoc J.* 1981;124:563–566.

52. Campbell C, Gondocz T, Parboosingh J. Documenting and managing self-directed learning among specialists. *Annals Royal College Phys Surg Canada.* 1995;28:80–87.

53. Fox RD, Rankin R, Costie KA, Parboosingh J, Smith E. Learning and the adoption of innovations among Canadian radiologists. *J Contin Educ Health Prof.* 1997;17:173–186.

chapter 9

Learning in Large and Small Groups

Linda Casebeer, PhD; Robert M. Centor, MD; Robert E. Kristofco, MSW

Dr Jones, chief of neurology and a long-time contributor to continuing medical education (CME) events, comes to you with a proposal to hold an all-day learning event titled "Advances in Neurology for Primary Care Physicians" to highlight new research from the university and bring in well-known speakers for the event. A pharmaceutical company marketing a new drug for Parkinson's disease has promised a grant for the event. Dr Jones has signed a hotel contract for the 500 participants he expects to come from the entire region. He would like to plan an evening at the art museum following the day of CME for participants and spouses. He anticipates large revenues will accrue to his department from this course. He has come to you for assistance with CME credit and event planning, including promotion of the activity.

INTRODUCTION

Requests, just like this one, to develop new continuing medical education (CME) courses are frequent in the CME offices of hospitals, medical schools, and specialty societies. Motivations to develop a new CME course include the desire to:

- disseminate new research in their field,
- teach physicians, often in the most cost-effective mode (large group),
- attract more referrals from physicians in the area,
- generate revenue from registration fees and pharmaceutical grants, and
- contribute to promotion and tenure.

Sometimes, course development coincides with both the perceived and actual needs of targeted physicians. However, the course subject is often more important to the potential course director than to participants. Potential physician participants have competing educational needs and opportunities. Practicing physicians are accustomed to receiving and discarding a large number of mailed brochures promoting courses. The CME office may be left with a course director's good idea, the costs of promoting and planning the course, but few paying participants. Or the CME office may be left with a large physician attendance at a conference with little evidence of improved performance or health care outcomes.

By understanding more about large- and small-group learning strategies, continuing professional development (CPD) professionals can serve as educational design consultants to course directors to ensure a more successful learning experience. This chapter will provide the CPD professional with an explanation of why physicians attend courses, schemes for categorizing formal group instructional strategies, effective group instructional strategies, and a summary of the role of the CPD professional in facilitating effective group learning. For the purposes of this chapter, CME group learning will refer to live, planned, group educational events such as courses, conferences, rounds, small-group discussions, and workshops.

PHYSICIAN INFORMATION-SEEKING AND FORMAL CME

Throughout their careers, physicians seek information from a variety of sources. Rounds, conferences, and symposia are important to physician lifelong learning. Hundreds of millions of dollars are committed to the development and implementation of formal CME activities annually.[1] Costs include the CME providers' and grant supporters' direct costs as well as physician participant (opportunity) costs for course registration, travel, and time away from office and family.

When asked about their motivations to attend formal educational activities, most physicians indicate keeping up-to-date with advances in medicine and maintaining professional competence as their prime reasons. Physicians also attend such activities to obtain CME credit for relicensure. The decision to attend may also be influenced by social or recreational benefits.[2,3] In addition to these reasons, physicians seek information to deal with uncertainty in the clinical encounter: surprise, stress, and cognitive dissonance in this context may lead to information seeking.[3]

In contrast to these more extrinsic motivations, three intrinsic forces behind health professionals' attendance at continuing education events have also been identified: a need to do their jobs differently, opportunity to network, and validation of current practice.[4] It has been suggested that physicians experience three stages in seeking information and making changes: preparing to make the change, making the change, and solidifying the change. Putnam and Campbell have reported that physicians use different information-seeking strategies in various phases of change. By providing expert opinion, formal CME activities help physicians prepare to make changes while they may be used less frequently in solidifying them.[5]

Trends in physician information-seeking are changing. Results of an annual national survey of a sample of 1000 US physicians demonstrated that 100% reported traveling to attend at least one CME meeting in 1993. In 2000, 34% of respondents did not attend any meetings requiring travel. Compared to 1993, respondents reported that they relied more on local CME events and CD-ROM and Internet programs.[2]

CATEGORIZING FORMAL GROUP INSTRUCTIONAL STRATEGIES

A speaker with slides in a lecture hall may personify "CME," but clearly this represents only one type of large-group instruction. It may be helpful to consider categories of group instruction and the planning criteria used to make choices among them. For the purposes of this discussion, group instruction is defined as any live instruction that occurs between a faculty member and at least two learners. Group learning includes lectures, panel discussions, small-group workshops, hands-on laboratory sessions, games and simulations, outreach visits to group practices, and distance learning activities.

Whenever there are groups of learners gathered, group instruction can be categorized by:

■ group size (how many learners are present) and
■ group interactions (how the learners work together).

Group Size

In CPD, groups are usually categorized as large group (lecture) or small group (discussion). Workshops of intermediate size and a variety of formats fall between the large and small groups.

Group Interactions

Types of interactions that occur as a function of the learning process are another way to categorize group instruction. In group settings, communication may be one-way (eg, a speaker lecturing to an audience) or two-way (ie, the instructor and the learners interact in some type of dialogue). As group size increases, two-way communication becomes more difficult and more unlikely. One-way communication strategies are known as expository strategies, or those designed for exposition of information. Small-group strategies incorporating high levels of interaction are known as exploratory strategies, or those in which faculty members facilitate learners' explorations of a topic.

The lecture has a long tradition in medical education, but it is not the only one-way communication method; others include panels, symposia, and colloquy. In a panel, three to six speakers discuss a topic in front of an audience. A symposium includes three to six speakers each addressing a large audience on the same topic. A colloquy is made up of six to eight people, both experts and representative members of the audience, who discuss a topic in front of a large group. Although each method may be modified to include audience question-and-answer sessions at the end of the formal presentations, these forums would be classified as methods using primarily one-way communication.[6,7]

In small-group instruction, communication is more frequently two-way or multiway, meaning learners learn from each other and from the instructor. Small-group instructional methods include: group discussions; research seminars used to present and discuss research findings and conclusions; workshops used for the development of skills; and workshops incorporating brainstorming, games, and role-play devoted to the solution of real-life problems.

TYPES OF LEARNING

Expository Versus Discovery Learning

Expository learning is exposition or communication by an expert of information that is received in a passive way (usually listening to a lecture) by the learners. Lecturers first present information concerning a general principle or rule; this general information is followed by illustrations of the rule. Learners are left to infer a particular application from the general principle and are expected to make their own leaps to applying the information to real-world situations.

Discovery learning is based on learning by experience and follows a different sequence of events than expository learning. Learners begin by acting in a particular instance. In medical education, a physician may manage an individual patient case, either in real life or in a simulated fashion. The learner processes and reflects on the experience of managing the patient. In understanding a particular case, the learner is then led to generalize and anticipate the effects of his/her actions in similar circumstances and then moves from the particular instance to understanding general principles. The learner may examine data from a group of patients or a large population to see if the general principle is applicable to a broader group. Finally, the learner is expected to act in a new circumstance and apply the principles learned from this process.[7]

Independent, Competitive, or Cooperative Learning

Group learning strategies may also be classified as competitive learning, independent learning, or cooperative learning. Competitive learning strategies set a standard that learners must meet, and data are supplied on other learners' performances. In medical education, the practice of audit and feedback is an example of a competitive learning strategy.

Independent learning occurs when learners are not concerned with others. This is the case in a lecture, since participants each learn independently and are neither cooperative nor competitive. In fact, learners in a large-group lecture learn largely as if they were in an individual learning situation, receiving little from other learners and contributing little to their learning. When a learner learns independently, the learner is left to reflect on his/her own. When CPD professionals plan large-group learning activities, they assume that individual physician learners who have little training in identifying and meeting their learning needs can, in fact, accomplish this independently.[8]

Cooperative learning is usually facilitated in small groups. Cooperative learning strategies involve exploratory and analytical discussion as well as reflection. In cooperative learning activities, the role of faculty member shifts from disseminating information to facilitating reflection on experience, helping physicians learn how to examine and improve their practice rather than telling physicians what is new.[8]

Applying Learning Types to Small and Large Groups

It has been suggested that independent learning—including that of the most common type of CME offerings, the formal lecture—is effective in achieving only three types of cognitive outcomes: individualistic skills, simple mechanical skills, and factual information.[7] Competitive strategies are useful in improving speed and quantity of work on simple drill activities and in competitive skills.

Most cognitive outcomes, including the following higher-order thinking processes, are most effectively taught using cooperative strategies in small groups: retention; application and transfer of factual information, concepts, and principles; mastery of concepts and principles; problem-solving; creative ability, including divergent and risk-taking thinking; productive controversy; awareness and utilization of one's capabilities; and reflection.

In light of these learning types, consider the types of educational problems addressed in medical education. Physicians rarely deal with only factual information or simple mechanical skills; instead, they regularly employ complex, higher-order thinking skills such as problem-solving, decision-making, and judgment. One model of decision-making illustrates the complexity of educational problems in medical education. Here, for example, the management of a complex patient with several comorbidities requires that a physician:

- recognize stimuli (patient symptoms, signs, conditions, etc), especially in a "noisy" environment,
- know the language of the stimuli,
- have in mind an algorithm for diagnosis and treatment for various conditions,
- have in mind relevant concepts and principles,
- restructure the problem situation,
- generate and think through alternative solutions and implications,
- make and act on a decision,
- see through the action, and
- self-correct one's actions.

Two of these skills can be adequately addressed in a lecture format: the presentation of general medical diagnosis and presentation of management algorithms, concepts and principles, new findings, etc.

Without cooperative learning strategies, physicians miss opportunities to apply and refine higher-order thinking processes to the problems they encounter in the practice of medicine, including recognition of symptoms, sorting out of symptoms, using patient data to restructure the patient's problem, generating alternative solutions, thinking through alternatives and implications, seeing through the action, and self-correcting one's actions. In choosing a group instructional strategy, the desired instructional outcomes must be identified. Once these are identified, they can be matched to the appropriate instructional strategy.

Figure 9-1 presents a matrix that may be useful to CME professionals in analyzing educational problems and planning CME activities designed to effectively address these issues.

In our scenario at the beginning of this chapter, Dr Jones wishes to develop a course for primary care physicians to communicate research facts and concepts. Communication of multiple facts on new advances in neurology may, however, have little impact on the participants' practice of medicine, although it may set the stage for such change. A CPD professional might suggest to Dr Jones that the

FIGURE 9-1

Choosing Group Instructional Strategies

Type of Educational Outcomes	Large Group	Small Group
Understand facts, concepts	×	
Understand algorithms for diagnosis, treatment	×	
Understand new research findings	×	×
Retain and master facts, concepts, principles		
Identify symptoms in "noisy" environment		×
Diagnose and manage using mentally available algorithms		×
Restructure problem		×
Generate alternative solutions		×
Think through alternative solutions		×
Make decisions		×
Act on decisions		×
Self-correct actions		×

Source: Adapted from Romiszowski AJ. *Designing Instructional Systems.* New York, NY: Nichols Publishing; 1999.

course include a lecture to transmit recent research results to a large audience, followed by breakout sessions of small, case-discussion groups. The purpose of small-group sessions would be to increase interactivity and the potential for participants to retain facts and apply them to problem-solving tasks related to their own patients.

WHY PROBLEM-BASED LEARNING?

In problem-based learning (PBL), learners study cases in small groups under the direction of a tutor. PBL arises from several learning principles from educational psychology. First, PBL activates prior knowledge in learners, providing a knowledge framework further elaborated through small-group problem analysis. Second, learners construct problem-oriented "semantic networks" that include cues from the context of professionally relevant problems. In these ways, PBL fosters professional curiosity.[9]

Is PBL Effective?

PBL, a form of discovery learning, has become a means of organizing undergraduate and graduate medical education curricula; although it has enormous potential for CME, it has not yet become the standard in CPD.[10] Few research studies have been conducted to compare the effectiveness of lecture- and problem-based formats. In a nonrandomized trial, Greenberg and Jewett found greater improvements in knowledge and performance as a result of the use of problem-based formats compared to traditional formats.[11] Comparing PBL in small-group instruction to large-group instruction in a randomized, controlled trial, however, Heale and colleagues found no significant differences in physician performance following these educational interventions, though they indicate that a one-day format may be too brief an intervention on which to make these comparisons.[12]

In a more recent study of 87 family physicians, PBL in the management of headache was associated with greater knowledge acquisition and improvement in clinical reasoning skills than a lecture-based approach. The problem-based approach was also preferred by the family physicians studied.[13] Meyer has reported ongoing efforts to apply PBL to the improvement of educational outcomes of traditionally didactic grand rounds programs; this application to grand rounds may strengthen the format by allowing immediate application of critical and creative thinking skills to real-world clinical problems. Anecdotal reports from participants and faculty have assigned value to this process.[14]

Incorporate PBL into CPD

In facilitating the development of CPD group activities, problems or cases may be incorporated into group learning by using audience-response technologies in large groups or by breaking large groups into smaller groups for problem-solving exercises.

The incorporation of problems into group learning immediately engages physicians in the use of problem-solving skills that will be more likely to transfer to patients in a real-world setting.

LARGE-GROUP INSTRUCTIONAL STRATEGIES

Why Is This Format so Common?

There are many reasons behind the commonplace nature of the lecture in the CPD of physicians. They are the easiest strategies to arrange and implement. They are familiar to physicians, require less space and fewer human resources,[15] and can convey a large amount of information in a condensed period of time.[16] For these and other reasons to be discussed later, large-group live instruction remains the predominant mode of instruction.[17] In 1998, 25,000 live CME courses and 18,000 regularly scheduled rounds and conferences were certified by accredited professionals of CME in the United States.[1]

Is It Effective?

As Romiszowski's categorization of group instruction suggests, the effectiveness of lectures in disseminating factual information has been demonstrated in short-term as well as longer-term knowledge retention.[15,18,19] However, as early as the 1970s, evidence has suggested that traditional programming has not been effective in facilitating changes in physician performance and changes in patient health outcomes.[20–23] Since that time, many well-designed research studies have only increased the evidence that traditional didactic teaching is not the most effective method for influencing physician performance or patient health outcomes.[24–29] Many studies have demonstrated that CME conferences have little impact on improving professional practice or on improving patient health outcomes. Didactic CME courses have also had weak effects on guideline adoption.[28]

Most recently, Davis and colleagues summarized the results of 14 randomized, controlled trials of physician education conducted between 1993 and January 1999, concluding, from this review at least, that didactic teaching sessions do not appear to be effective in changing physician performance.[28] There is evidence, however, that interactivity and sequencing of events (eg, two sessions held one month apart) increases learning effectiveness. In addition, data from this study suggest that adding adequate needs assessments prior to the course and/or adding enabling materials, such as patient education materials or flow charts, to the material distributed during the course can improve course outcomes.[28] Romiszowski's model can be used to explain this ineffectiveness; he predicts that formal courses based on independent learning will be most successful in demonstrating changes in performance of individualistic skills, simple mechanical skills, and factual information.[7]

Expository Large-group Instruction

Expository lectures are preplanned. They are controlled by a preset time limit. In a one-way expository lecture, the responsibility for the transfer of information remains with the instructor. Learners have little, if anything, to say about what is communicated or how it is communicated. Key characteristics of an effective expository lecture are the visibility of slides; the clarity of the presentation; the relevance of the material to the audience; and the speaker's presentation style, ability to engage the audience, and animation.[30] Many CME organizations have engaged in faculty development to improve these qualities.

Enhancing Large-group Instruction

Incorporating Practice and Feedback

Peloso and Stakiw note that the ability to change practice is enhanced if the information presented is supported by published evidence, if the changes are endorsed by opinion leaders, and if there is opportunity for practice and feedback.[31] An expository lecture becomes a two-way system when the instructor asks for feedback to verify that his or her message was correctly received. Based on this feedback, the instructor may modify the presentation to ensure that learners have understood what was said. The learners do not add new content to the lesson but serve as a check on reception and interpretation.[7]

Response systems make it possible for faculty to ask questions of the audience and to see their responses immediately. The simplest and most cost-effective approach is the use of a set of colored cards given to each audience member. When a question is asked, audience participants are asked to hold up the colored card that represents their answers to the question. Computerized audience-response systems are used for the same purpose, to elicit immediate responses from audience participants. A keypad is given to each member of the audience; participants are asked to touch the numbers on the keypad that represent their responses to the questions asked by faculty.

In a recent study of the use of audience-response systems in medical lectures, 85% of respondents felt that the system facilitated teaching clinical reasoning as well as medical facts. In addition, respondents felt the system helped identify learner weaknesses.[30] Gagnon and Thivierge[32] developed an instrument to evaluate the impact of keypad technology on a group of 255 respondents. They found that the technology was most beneficial in facilitating interaction and participation, self-evaluation, and immediate feedback. The technology had less impact on meeting learning needs, on learning itself, and on the practice of medicine. Cost, availability, lack of faculty development, and lack of personnel available to run the system are barriers to the more widespread use of this computerized technology.

Adding Discovery Learning

Although discovery learning strategies are most often used in small-group learning settings, they can be applied effectively to larger groups, even though all learners may not be equally involved in the discovery process. Within medical education, problem-based or case-based learning best describes the discovery learning process. In reflective lecturing, one-way exposition of a problem or case is made by the instructor. The instructor tries to simulate problem-solving by presenting the problem, posing questions, leaving pauses for reflection, and acting out the steps of discovering the solution.[7]

In medical education, faculty present patient problems in a variety of ways. Historically, in grand rounds case presentations, the patient was actually brought into the lecture hall for discussion. Although it is more common for cases to be presented using live patients on ward rounds, the opportunity exists for using live patients in group learning formats. In medical schools, faculty have access to standardized patients (individuals trained to act like a patient with a certain condition) who are used in undergraduate medical education to present cases. Faculty also present cases using videotaped (or less commonly, audiotaped) presentations. In courses such as advance cardiac life support, sophisticated mannequins are used to represent patients. Virtual reality is a complex, computerized environment for case presentations, used most frequently in teaching procedures. The simplest and least expensive case presentations are paper handouts, which give participants a narrative presentation of the patient.

A typical case format presentation for a reflective or one-way lecture includes the following: a recounting of a patient's demographic information; chief complaint; history of present illness; other medical history; family personal and social history; review of systems, physical findings, and laboratory tests; and diagnostic impression, differential diagnosis, and management plan. The patient is presented to a large group with little opportunity for experienced clinicians to demonstrate diagnostic reasoning.[16]

Ways to Improve Lectures

Ways to improve lectures include:

- facilitating improvement of faculty presentation skills (stressing interactivity);
- asking faculty to use cases, problems, clinical vignettes in presentations;
- asking faculty to model problem-solving in thinking through a clinical problem;
- using audience-response technology to engage learners;
- breaking large groups into smaller groups for discussions; and
- adding enabling materials such as patient education materials and flow charts to course handouts.

An alternative to the typical case presentation is the "chunked format."[16,33] Two presenters facilitate discussion—one acts as the presenter and the other as facilitator. Instead of presenting the total case, the presenting physicians present "chunks," or small collections, of data as they became available to the physician managing the case. After each piece of information is presented, an experienced clinician facilitates discussion of the case in thinking aloud through the problem. The facilitator does not participate in the discussion until the end of the case. Cases are chosen for their potential to facilitate decision-making skills.[16]

Large-group Distance Learning

In distance education, learners are linked by media to the resources of an educational institution. More recently, Dillon defined distance education more broadly, indicating that learners and learning resources may be separated by time or distance, or both.[34]

A range of telecommunications technologies offers linkages between learners and learning resources. For decades, physicians have had access to technologies such as teleconference and satellite broadcasts that required them to go to a certain location at a certain time to access group learning experiences. Earlier distance learning activities provided independent learning opportunities, using traditional lecture strategies with minimal interaction during a brief question-and-answer period at the conclusion of a lecture. Current technologies mediated by the Internet offer more continuous access to information technology as well as professional education. Learning can be accomplished from the work site, which may decrease the delay between learning and transfer of knowledge to the workplace.

More continuous access, however, does not guarantee the use of appropriate learning strategies within the medium. As technologies increase learner options, learner confusion may also increase.[34] Clearly, one role of the CPD professional may be to help guide the learner within this environment, discussed in greater detail in Chapter 11.

Small-group Instructional Strategies

Why Small-group Learning?
Many of the limitations of large-group instruction can be overcome simply by reducing group size. Small-group methods foster collaborative rather than independent learning and are most applicable to groups of 10 or less. Small-group instruction offers the opportunity for increased interaction among faculty and learners, which is a key to addressing the transfer of facts and concepts into practice, problem solving, and reflection. Peloso and Stakiw suggest several key elements: A learner-directed agenda; use of trusted opinion leaders as group facilitators; opportunity for practice and feedback; and information from various sources including peer discussion and

patient questions. These elements are readily applicable to small-group learning.[31]

Is It Effective?

In the summary of trials measuring the effectiveness of rounds and conferences, interactive sessions and mixed sessions (using both interactive and didactic techniques) demonstrated more evidence of enhanced participant activity than those sessions that were strictly didactic.[28] Small groups offer a range of instructional possibilities. Typical small-group instructional strategies will be discussed first, followed by some special techniques, such as the development of communities of practice, as examples of innovation in small-group instruction.

Discovery Learning in Small Groups

The term *small-group learning* is usually applied to groups with fewer than 10 members. Frequently, as groups become larger than 10, the instructional methodology automatically reverts to some type of expository strategy. In groups of 10 or less, however, discovery learning strategies dominate.

A typical pattern for formal courses is the combination of large-group lectures and breakout small-group sessions, usually labeled as open-group discussion. The topic is defined by the instructor or leader of the session who acts as a facilitator. Learning occurs through interactions within the group discussion. A seminar format is often used for rounds and conferences, appealing to both residents and physicians in practice. In a seminar, one of the learners (often a resident) has previously prepared a case to be presented to a group. A discussion of the findings follows and is usually facilitated by a faculty member. In this type of small-group session, more responsibility for the content is delegated to at least one of the learners.

Peloso and Stakiw describe their three-year experience with more than 25 sessions of a small-group format in which discussion of clinical problems among general practitioners was facilitated by an expert specialist. They suggest the benefits are twofold: the relevance of the cases to clinical practice and the opportunity to ascertain the standard of care of peers.[31]

The Workshop as an Approach to CPD

A workshop is another frequently used small- to mid-sized group format. The term *workshop* has come to refer to a variety of formats but has the intent of a practical application focus. The instructor may present concepts and principles or procedures. Learners are then expected to apply this to a real task under supervision. One form of workshop is that of demonstration, in which cases are used to generate discussion, analysis, and a demonstration of cognitive skills. Cases provide material for open-ended analysis and are intended to give the learners simulated practice in decision-making. Cases are most effective when they simulate real-life incompleteness and uncertainty and are not simplified to make solutions obvious.[7]

Workshops may also include the use of standardized patients. Standardized patients used for objective structure clinical examinations (OSCEs) have been used for years to assess and teach medical students and residents a variety of clinical competencies. Standardized patients are used infrequently in CME, except occasionally in the evaluation of CPD programs.[25]

O'Brien and colleagues, however, described the use of standardized patients during a 7.5-hour formal small-group session designed to improve community practitioners' clinical skills in cardiology. Participants rotated through a nine-station OSCE. Following the OSCE experience, faculty members reviewed and discussed each case with participants. Learners were encouraged to identify and discuss issues raised by the case. Reports of individual and group performance were presented to participants following the discussion. Although recruitment for the program was difficult, informal evaluations demonstrated that participants felt their communication skills and knowledge about cardiology issues had improved.[35]

Case-based instruction is also used for modeling and provoking discussion, eg, when medical ethics are at issue. Role-playing is another small-group instructional strategy occasionally used in the design of CME, eg, in courses centered on limiting potential malpractice liability or increasing/improving patient–physician communication.

Workshops may also allow hands-on demonstrations of procedures such as use of flexible sigmoidoscopy or laproscopic surgery in an animal model. Psychomotor skills can be learned effectively by demonstrations from experts followed by practice. In medical education, simulations are more carefully developed opportunities for workshop practice, usually of psychomotor skills involved in such tasks as surgical procedures. The following simulations are intended to reproduce the essential elements of a real-life situation and provide the learner practice without risks to real patients:

- Live patients
- Standardized patients
- Videotaped patients
- Audiotaped patients
- Mannequins
- Computerized cases

- Virtual reality
- Role plays
- Paper scenarios

In some areas such as surgery and cardiopulmonary resuscitation, virtual-reality methods provide elaborate simulations for learners. The costs of software, equipment, and personnel are limiting factors in the use of elaborate simulations. Instructional games other than simulations are rarely used in medical education but are potentially powerful small-group learning strategies.

Communities of Practice

Within business organizations, one form of interactive group method, designed to improve knowledge sharing and learning, is known as communities of practice. Communities of practice are being recognized as a means of radically galvanizing knowledge sharing and learning in the process of change.[36] Communities of practice are informal, self-selected groups of individuals with shared expertise and a passion for a similar enterprise. Members may meet face to face frequently or periodically or may be connected electronically by e-mail or other means, but the group only continues as long as there is interest in maintaining it. Communities of practice foster new and creative approaches to problems and, as they generate new knowledge, they reinforce and renew themselves. Because they are informal and form spontaneously, they are not especially easy to build or sustain. Bringing individuals together and providing an infrastructure, however, can support the formation and continuation of communities of practice. Communities of practice are characterized by their abilities to solve problems, develop professional skills, and transfer best practices.[36]

Evidence of the application of communities of practice to CME is sparse. Three examples, however, may serve as models for CPD professionals who wish to bring individuals together into communities of practices and provide an infrastructure to support their continuation.

1. Problem-based, Small-group Learning

Premi and colleagues have described a novel practice and problem-based approach in Canada. They have developed an extensive network of small learning groups in which primary care practitioners organized themselves into learning groups of five to nine physicians and met in local communities for one and one-half hours twice monthly. A group member was chosen as a learning facilitator who was trained to facilitate the group. Specific case histories and case commentary were provided.[8]

2. Collaborative Office Rounds

Collaborative office rounds have been developed as a format for small discussion groups, which meet regularly over a sustained period of time to improve early identification and intervention with mental disorders in children. These rounds are case-based but vary in their approach. One approach focuses on interesting and challenging cases presented by participants; a second defines topics and asks participants to bring cases related to them. The groups are jointly led by pediatricians and child psychologists. Preliminary evaluations of this process have demonstrated stability within the groups and regular attendance by participants, as well as endorsements of the process by participants.[37]

3. CPD Provider-facilitated Group Learning

An additional example of a physician community of practice is demonstrated by a CPD provider bringing practitioners together to form such a group and providing an infrastructure for its development. Primary care practitioners in Alabama were interviewed to determine key issues surrounding the higher prevalence of cardiovascular disease in the "Stroke Belt." Physician frustrations centered on lack of patient adherence to prescribed medical regimens, including lifestyle changes. Physicians were then recruited to participate in a series of case-based audioconferences conducted at noon by speakerphone in their offices. Cases were designed to increase physicians' knowledge and use of effective adherence-enhancing strategies in the management of hypercholesterolemic patients. Following the series of audioconferences, physicians were furnished with a reminder chart that briefly summarized several key adherence-enhancing strategies. A rigorous evaluation of this process was conducted using a nested-cohort, prospective, randomized, controlled trial design and unannounced standardized patients, as well as physiologic and survey instruments on actual patients. Results revealed increases in physician adherence-enhancing strategies, a significant improvement in patient understanding of hypercholesterolemia, and an increase in self-reports of fat intake. In addition, male patients enrolled in the study showed a significant reduction in total serum cholesterol levels nine months after the intervention.[38]

Technologic Advances

Advances in technology have offered new methods of facilitating the formation of communities of practice including asynchronous learning networks, ie, learning networks created for the purpose of linking, for a limited period of time, learners and faculty who may not be in geographic proximity. These learning networks essentially combine Web-based case problems or course content with a bulletin board or chat feature, which allows faculty and participants to contribute comments to a discussion. Networks are organized over specific time periods, varying from one week to as long as a semester or more. They are labeled "asynchronous" because both participants and faculty can log on and access the course and discussion at any time, so that the discussion is not conducted in a synchronous fashion. Both participant physicians in practice and faculty may access the course when it is most convenient.

Although asynchronous learning networks have been used effectively by other educational groups, including higher education, veterinarians, and engineers, as a means of radically changing how information is accessed and translated to practice, CPD professionals have yet to promote or evaluate learning networks for their potential with physicians in practice. These issues are explored in greater detail in Chapter 11.

An initial pilot study of feasibility among primary care physicians did not demonstrate effective outcomes among groups of physicians who did not typically use the Internet as a means of relating to colleagues or of obtaining CME.[38] A more recent trial of more than 300 pediatricians forming an asynchronous learning network to solve pediatric asthma case problems was highly successful in meeting participant and faculty expectations. The majority of those participating used the Internet daily, most often for literature searching. They were most likely to access the course at night or on weekends. In evaluating the course, most felt that information on the case should be presented once a week rather than three times a week, which was proposed for the pilot course.[39]

Much work remains to be done to assess the effectiveness of Web-based technologies in this area.

Multiple and Combination Group Instructional Strategies

Multiple Longitudinal Interventions

For the purposes of this discussion, multiple interventions are those that occur in more than one session over a longitudinal period of time. Many patterns fit the description of multiple interventions, including events that occur periodically over a longitudinal period of time (such as courses that meet every week for several months), a course that meets for a day or two and is followed up by additional educational sessions later, or variations of these patterns. Educational methods that are multiple in their format have been demonstrated to be more effective than those that are single episodic events.[28]

Combination Methods

Combination strategies blend more than one type of intervention, eg, combining a two-day course with reminder charts for physicians to use in their offices, courses coupled with patient-mediated strategies, and educational materials. Both large- and small-group instructional strategies have been combined with other methods in attempts to increase the effect of the intervention on facilitating changes in physician performance as well as on patient health outcomes. Of the 99 randomized controlled trials reviewed by Davis et al, 39 used three or more educational strategies, with 79% showing positive effects, compared to 60% effectiveness when one educational intervention was used.[25] Combined methods also appear to have more impact on the adoption of clinical practice guidelines.[24]

Summary: Applying Evidence to Practice

Large-group continuing education activities are the backbone of the CPD of physicians. The expectations of faculty, learners, and funders guarantee their survival.

However, several factors have the potential to significantly impact the planning of formal educational activities. Physicians are willing to devote less time and income to travel to formal events. Health care costs, medical errors in managed health care, and the increased focus on measurement of outcomes and return on investment will continue to challenge CPD professionals to demonstrate improved physician performance as a result of continuing education. Although large-group instruction may be effective in predisposing physicians toward making changes in their practices, rigorous evidence from randomized controlled educational trials does not support the use of large-group didactic sessions as an effective single educational strategy to promote changes in physician performance and in patient health outcomes.[25,27,28]

When group learning is planned, CME professionals may increase the chances of improving physician performance by improving the quality of large-group instruction through:

- faculty development to improve presentation and facilitation skills;
- integration of problems or case examples into large-group discussion;
- use of technologies and techniques that foster dialogue and interaction in large-group discussions;
- addition of small-group breakout discussions; and
- combination of large-group activities with other interventions, including audit and feedback, reminder systems, patient-mediated interventions, and office system improvements.

When group learning is planned, small-group discussions may also be added as breakouts from large-group sessions. Interactive small-group sessions will be more effective than large-group didactic sessions in facilitating changes in the following types of physician thought processes: retention, application, and transfer of factual information, concepts, principles; problem-solving; divergent and risk-taking thinking; productive controversy; awareness and utilization of one's capabilities; and reflection.[7]

Combination approaches are more effective in facilitating changes in physician performance and in patient health status than single, episodic large-group sessions. Planners should consider designing or recommending to faculty the combination of large-group sessions with one of the following more effective interventions: small-group interactive sessions, audit and feedback, patient-mediated interventions, reminder systems and other office system improvements, and outreach visits.

CPD professionals often develop educational activities reactively at the request of various physician course directors and faculty, just as in the scenario that starts this chapter. However, in designing, developing, and implementing such activities, planners have the opportunity to enhance the reach and effectiveness of group learning methods by advising faculty on the design of educational activities, by seeking funding for more innovative approaches to CPD, and by being proactive, eg, initiating the development of educational activities. If CPD professionals, funders, and faculty begin to use the evidence summarized in this chapter and elsewhere and apply their skills in new ways to develop effective educational activities, both physicians and patients will benefit.

REFERENCES—CHAPTER 9

1. Kopelow M. Unpublished data, Accreditation Council for Continuing Medical Education, 1999.

2. Erickson D. Less time, less money, less travel: Eighth annual physician preference survey. *Med Meetings.* January 1, 2001;28:32–38.

3. Moore DE, Bennett N, Knox A, Kristofco R. Participation in formal CME: Factors affecting decision-making. In: Davis D, Fox R, eds. *The Physician as Learner: Linking Research to Practice.* Chicago, Ill: American Medical Association; 1994.

4. Cividin TM, Ottoson JM. Linking reasons for continuing professional education participation with post-program application. *J Contin Educ Health Prof.* 1997;17:46–55.

5. Putnam RW, Campbell MD. Competence. In: Fox RD, Mazmanian PE, Putnam RW. *Changing and Learning in the Lives of Physicians.* New York, NY: Praeger Publishers; 1989.

6. Romiszowski AJ. *Producing Instructional Systems.* New York, NY: Nichols Publishing; 1984.

7. Romiszowski AJ. *Designing Instructional Systems.* New York, NY: Nichols Publishing; 1999.

8. Premi J. Individualized continuing medical education. In: Davis D, Fox R, eds. *The Physician as Learner: Linking Research to Practice.* Chicago, Ill: American Medical Association; 1994.

9. Schmidt HG. Foundations of problem-based learning: some explanatory notes. *Med Educ.* 1993;27:422–432.

10. Kantrowitz MP. Problem-based learning in continuous medical education: Some critical issues. *J Contin Educ Health Prof.* 1991;11:11–18.

11. Greenberg LW, Jewett LS. The impact of two teaching techniques on physicians' knowledge and performance. *J Med Educ.* 1985;60:390–396.

12. Heale J, Davis D, Norman G, Woodward C, Neufeld V, Dodd P. A randomized controlled trial assessing the impact of problem-based versus didactic teaching methods in CME. Conference on Res in Med Educ. Washington, DC: *Assoc Am Med Coll.* 1988;37:72–77.

13. Doucet MD, Purdy RA, Kaufman DM, Langille DB. Comparison of problem-based learning and lecture format in continuing medical education on headache diagnosis and management. *Med Educ.* 1998;32:590–596.

14. Meyer AI. Problem-based learning in grand rounds: an effective alternative to didactic lectures. Conference Proceeding. Congress 2000: The CME Summit: Practices, Opportunities and Priorities for the New Millennium, April 12–16, 2000, Universal City, California.

15. Romm FJ, Dignan M, Herman JN. Teaching clinical epidemiology; a controlled trial of two methods. *Am J Prev Med.* 1989;5:50–51.

16. Brose JA. Case presentation as a teaching tool: making a good thing better. *J Am Osteopath Assoc.* 1992; 92:376–378.

17. Miller GE. Continuing medical education for physicians. *J Contin Educ Health Prof.* 1994;14:61–62.

18. Silverberg J, Taylor-Vaisey A, Szalai JP, Tipping J. Lectures, interactive learning, and knowledge retention in continuing medical education. *J Contin Educ Health Prof.* 1995; 15:231–234.

19. Martenson D, Myklebust R, Stalisberg H. Implementing problem-based learning within a lecture-dominated curriculum; Results and process. *Teach Learn Med.* 1992;4:233–237.

20. Bertram DA, Thompson MC, Giordano D, Perla J, Rosenthal TC. Implementation of an inpatient case management program in rural hospitals. *J Rural Health.* 1995;12:54–66.

21. Dixen J. Evaluation criteria in studies of continuing education in the health professions: a critical review and a suggested strategy. *Eval Health Professions.* 1978;1:47–65.

22. Stross JK, Harlan WR. The impact of mandatory continuing medical education. *JAMA.* 1978;239:2663–2666.

23. Haynes RB, Davis DA, McKibbon A, Tugwell P. A critical appraisal of the efficacy of continuing medical education. *JAMA.* 1984;251:61–64.

24. Davis DA, Taylor-Vaisey A. Translating guidelines into practice. *Can Med Assoc J.* 1997;157:408–416.

25. Davis DA, Tomson MA, Oxman AD. A systematic review of the effectiveness of continuing medical education. *JAMA.* 1995;274:700–705.

26. Davis P, Russell AS, Skeith KJ. The use of standardized patients in the performance of a needs assessment and development of a CME intervention in rheumatology for primary care physicians. *J Rheum.* 1997;37:1995–1999.

27. Bero LA, Grilli R, Grimshaw JM, Harvey E, Oxman AD, Thomson MA. Closing the gap between research and practice: an overview of systematic reviews of interventions to promote the implementation of research findings. The Cochrane Effective Practice and Organization of Care Review Group. *BMJ.* 1998;317:465–468.

28. Thomson O'Brien MA, Freemantle N, Oxman AD, Wolf F, Davis DA, Herrin J. Continuing education meetings and workshops: effects on professional practice and health care outcomes. *Cochrane Database Syst Rev.* 2001.

29. Oxman AD, Thomson MA, Davis DA, Haynes RB. No magic bullets: a systematic review of 102 trials of interventions to improve professional practice. *CMAJ.* 1995;153:1423–1431.

30. Copeland HL, Stoler JK, Hewson MG, Longworth DL. Making the continuing medical education lecture effective. *J Contin Educ Health Prof.* 1998;18:227–234.

31. Peloso PM, Stakiw KJ. Small-group format for continuing medical education: a report from the field. *J Contin Educ Health Prof.* 2000;20:27–32.

32. Gagnon RJ, Thivierge R. Evaluating touch pad technology. *J Contin Educ Health Prof.* 1997;20–26.

33. Kassirer JP, Kopelman RI. Clinical problem solving at grand rounds. *Hosp Pract.* 1990;51:54–59.

34. Dillon CL. Distance education research and continuing professional education: Reframing questions for the emerging information infrastructure. *J Contin Educ Health Prof.* 1996;16:5–13.

35. O'Brien MK, Feldman D, Alban T, Donoghue G, Sirkin J, Novack DH. An innovative CME program in cardiology for primary care practitioners. *Acad Med.* 1996;71:894–897.

36.   Wenger EC, Snyder WM. Communities of practice: the organizational frontier. *Harvard Business Review.* Jan 2000:139–145.

37.   Fishman ME, Kessel W, Heppel DE, Brannon ME, Papai JJ, Bryun SD, Nora AH, Hutchins VL. Collaborative office rounds: continuing education in the psychosocial/developmental aspects of child health. *Pediatrics.* 1997;99:1–5.

38.   Casebeer LL, Gotterer G, Stokes D, Grad R, Kristofco R, Fulwinkle G. Comparing the effectiveness of a CME pediatric asthma asynchronous learning network, Web course and monograph. 2000. Conference Proceeding. Congress 2000: The CME Summit: Practices, Opportunities and Priorities for the New Millennium, April 12–16, 2000, Universal City, California.

39.   Casebeer LL, Grad R, Kristofco R. Internet CME lessons from the past and visions of the future. Unpublished paper; 2001.

chapter 10

Continuing Professional Development in the Learning Organization

Nancy L. Bennett, PhD; Robert Fox, EdD

Mr Fisher, the CEO of Lakeside Community Hospital, found an interesting report in Monday's interoffice mail comparing the length of stay of all hospitals in the state. When he compared the report to statistics from his hospital, he was surprised to learn that the length of stay for pulmonary patients in the pulmonary department was significantly higher than the reported average. The first step on his agenda was to meet with the department chair, Dr Cortier, who said that the length of stay was the same as it had been for the last five years and he remains very satisfied with the quality of care that the physicians are delivering. Still troubled, Mr Fisher requested that the physicians in pulmonary care participate in a task force to evaluate strategies to decrease length of stay without compromising patient care. Frowning, Dr Cortier asserted that he saw no need for physicians to change their current practices and his department was too busy to participate in any more meetings. They were at an impasse on the issue, one aware of a problem the other sought to avoid. But the hospital was underperforming and, at least for now, unable to change its behavior.

INTRODUCTION

The popular image of the delivery of health care has been transformed from the individual care offered over the years by a trusted primary care physician to a system of practitioners, medical and otherwise, providing care within the framework of an organization's policies, procedures, and regulations. It has evolved to specialized teams operating within an organization of specialized units, all working together to solve patients' problems. Health care organizations are knowledge-driven organizations of health care providers and administrators working interactively and collectively on specific problems to bring all resources to the problems at hand. Each member of the organization contributes his or her discreet knowledge and skill to a larger whole. Now, improved care means more than a relationship between patient and physician; it includes integration of the whole organization in a new kind of way, one that applies collective competence to health problems and goals. In order to provide improved care, the organization depends upon its ability to learn from within and without, as colleagues teach each other and as the organization learns from interacting with its environment. This means that when we act together as an organization, we must correctly identify problems, specify the need for new and different competencies, and create the ability to capture and move knowledge from inside and outside the organization to address the problems we face. This ability to manage the knowledge needs and resources in a way that expands the organization's competence and performance is the heart of organizational learning.[1-3]

For example, when first diagnosed with diabetes, Mrs Jones received a treatment plan from her physician, plus a series of visits with her dietitian and ongoing follow-up with her designated nurse. All of these professionals act on behalf of Mrs Jones, collectively and independently, but in concert within the resources, processes, and values of her managed care organization (MCO). The system will prompt other units in her MCO to automatically send reminders about ongoing laboratory tests and make available human, electronic, and material resources that respond to questions as they arise for Mrs Jones. All of this began behind the scenes when the MCO used its statistics about complications of diabetes for women over 65, coupled with guidelines developed by a team of in-house physicians to design this organizational approach to care based on new science, national recommendations, in-house experience, and the shared wisdom of professionals based on their experiences. The organization's behavior toward its patients reflects a collective competence built, not only from the individual competencies of its members but also from the interactive and synergistic effects of shared competencies. The combination of competencies generates new abilities not present until the organization functions as a competent entity in its own right. The knowledge and skill the organization exhibited was acquired from its personnel and from peer institutions and organizations; in addition, it was adapted as they acquired new competence from within and without. The organization learned from its formal and informal processes, as well as from its ability to reflect on experience and integrate solutions into standard processes and organizational behaviors.

The potential power of an organization is far greater than the sum of its parts when the power of individual thought and experience builds together for the purpose of innovative solutions to difficult problems. Assuming that one of the primary purposes for a health care organization is to continually learn better ways to provide care, then providing that care depends on the ability of individuals in the group to combine their knowledge in a way that extends their capacities and enhances their performance. They must be able to:

- work together seamlessly to identify familiar problems and solve them,
- recognize and appreciate different aspects of a problem that contribute to a more effective solution, and
- recognize new problems and construct ways to address them.

Although there is wide agreement that organizations must learn, act, and self-correct collectively in ways that enhance organizational effectiveness, there is very little data to demonstrate ways to use the models that attempt to explain organizational learning. It is a topic of discussion supported by logic and anecdotal experience rather than by large-scale systematic study. Consequently, it must be considered with an eye toward how organizational learning might occur rather than a firm grasp of how it does occur.

This chapter focuses on relationships within an organization. Individuals bring skills and knowledge to the organization that, in turn, provide a structure with policies, resources, and values. That interaction provides ways for both individuals and the organization to learn. We have selected three ideas from the broad literature to describe some of the facets of these relationships in a learning organization. These conceptually based explanations of how organizations learn are:

- *Learning from experience*: Learning effective solutions is based on the organization's experience dealing with unusual problems in a way that allows the problems and their solutions to be routine. In those positive results lies the key to allowing the organization to learn and to fulfill its mission.[4]
- *Learning within communities of practice in an organization*: The interactions and problem-solving efforts of colleagues learning in communities of practice within the organization provide an informal avenue to changes in the organization's performance while honoring its values and resources.[5]
- *The processes used for adoption of new practices*: A learning organization constantly faces the difficult problem of continuing with tried-and-true solutions versus incorporating new ideas and change into the day-to-day approaches to work. The literature on adoption of innovations and accounting for disruptive change suggests serious impacts on health care organizations.[6,7]

For most of the twentieth century, physicians practiced relatively autonomously, controlling the quality of their own work and delegating responsibility for the management of hospitals and other health care organizations to administrators and other health care professionals. With emerging pressures to control costs while improving quality and access, administrators and other members of the health care team have become more involved in new ways to think about practice patterns. At the same time, physicians have become more involved in running hospitals and clinics. Some of those shifts have resulted in shared goals for better health care, and some have not. Enhanced performance is based not only on the work of individuals but also on the whole collectivity of personnel in terms of how they reflect the values, resources, and processes of the organization. When individuals learn, they bring potential back to an organization; when an organization learns, it creates lasting change that communicates new competence and performance to all of its members. Learning and change go forward together in learning organizations.

LEARNING FROM EXPERIENCE

Mr Fisher, the hospital CEO, looked at the impasse in pulmonary medicine. He reflected on an early experience 12 years ago with a similar problem in cardiology. Hearing about strategies from his colleagues to reduce the rate of second myocardial infarctions (MIs), he pushed Dr Bishop, the head of cardiology, to expand and reform the cardiac rehabilitation unit. This included redistributing tasks and competencies to staff inside and outside of the unit. Other units involved in cardiac care, such as the intensive care unit, emergency medicine, behavioral medicine, and the diabetes center, were given new roles. Originally, Dr Bishop felt that unless he had a full-time physician to staff a center, the risks of distributing responsibilities were too high. Not only was the organization's problem difficult to identify and describe, the solutions lead to far-reaching consequences within the cardiac center, the hospital at large, and the way the professions trained and oriented their work. The various education units, such as continuing medical education (CME) and continuing nursing education (CNE), might have been effective partners in supporting training for this change, but they were bound to their own professional clients and not experienced at sharing problems or solutions across disciplines. The Quality Assurance Committee was also uncomfortable with making a change based on trust that they would act rationally in adopting new performance when faced with evidence suggesting potential negative outcomes.

An essential criterion for determining if a learning organization will thrive is whether, as an organization, it will learn from its experiences. Learning from experience has been addressed in earlier chapters as a way of understanding how clinicians change their competence and performance based on the kinds of cases they encounter. That process can be broken down into several important aspects summarized in a set of principles emerging from the theory of reflective practice, as originally articulated by Schön.[4] These principles, as described in a general way by Parboosingh et al. (Chapter 8) and Campbell and Gondocz (Chapter 5), can be restated to fit the learning from experience that characterizes organizations.

Organizations have a total fund of knowledge that they acquire from their personnel, who, in turn, acquire it from continuing education and self-directed learning. This formal body of knowledge is often bound to scientific evidence but may also reflect standard practices and historical precedents. Each health care organization adapts this body of knowledge in a variety of ways, including learning from experience in fulfilling its multiple goals and by supporting continuing professional education activities for its personnel.

Organizations identify their problems according to the solutions at their disposal. If they do not have solutions, they redefine the problem to fit the solutions they do have. For example, lack of financial support for a new cardiac rehabilitation center in the annual giving campaign is a problem of marketing, not of changing ways that the public defines the role of institutions in daily life. The first is a problem the organization set up to solve with its marketing competencies; the second is a problem that the organization has no solution for, so it is invisible until the solution becomes known. A learning organization may learn this new solution, for example, by mimicking peer institutions or by hiring new kinds of personnel with new solutions.

An organization's fund of knowledge is adequate for most problems; however, when its members face a problem that is unique, full of conflict, or ambiguous, they experience a disruption that moves out of its zone of competence. This zone of messy and difficult reflection and experimentation to solve problems was labeled a swamp by Schön.[4]

Moving from what one knows, to the unknown, back to the known, involves three processes: reflection-in-action, experimentation, and reflection-on-action. Organizations often face problems that require them to respond immediately, even if they do not have a clear definition of the problem. Initial response to infection with HIV or cases of anthrax are examples. Reflection-in-action[4] is the stage where the organization tries to sort out the nature of its problems. In health care organizations, this may mean that the hospital CEO has to act before he understands the best course of action. This is often a period of information and knowledge collection and assembly so that a better strategy for action may evolve. An organization's ability to assemble knowledge from within and without about problems in order to reduce ambiguity, conflict over alternatives, or coping with unique situations is often a critical element in a formula for success. Failure to learn at this point predicts an ultimate failure to solve the problem.

Experimentation[4] points to testing and evaluating a response to the difficulties of the organization. In our example about the cardiac rehabilitation unit, this stage may follow systematic and unsystematic efforts to collect information and knowledge about the problem in an effort to reduce ambiguity related to how to reorganize cardiology in a way that will improve outcomes. In experimentation, consultation for a limited number of new cases by behavioral medicine staff in the emergency room may be incorporated into organizational procedures. This kind of experiment may be a function of the experience of peer institutions or the opinion of experts in the center for behavioral medicine.

The last stage is reflection-on-action.[4] In this stage, the organization may use a variety of processes to judge the effects of the experiment. In our case, how much did it change the rate of MIs? Were there any negative outcomes? How much did the new process cost? How can it be refined to increase its effects while reducing time, money, and energy expended? And, how can it be incorporated into the strategic planning and budgeting process? Some of these questions are addressed as the new knowledge and competence is incorporated into the fund of knowledge and competence of the total organization. As this process of learning from experience draws to an end, the performance of the organization and of its individual workers may change in ways that accommodate some of the most important problems facing the new unit.

The focus for continuing professional development (CPD) professionals is to facilitate change that will endure. Changes and learning embraced by organizations in this way are institutionalized so that they provide support and reinforcement vertically and horizontally in the organization's patterns of behavior. CPD can become a critical part of this process, but only if that continued learning is vertically and laterally integrated into the change processes of health care organizations. However, this kind of learning from experience may not be the only way that organizational learning occurs or the only avenue to new roles for CPD. Learning groups or communities of practice may support the organization's goals through less-structured mechanisms with the goal of finding innovative solutions.[5,8]

LEARNING INFORMALLY IN COMMUNITIES OF PRACTICE

Dr Armstrong has been a general surgeon for 20 years and is informally known throughout his hospital for very low rates of postoperative complications. No one ever paid much attention to this until the hospital was found to have abnormally high rates of postoperative complications in a report card issued by CMS. The operating room director set up a meeting with Dr Armstrong to learn about what he does differently than the other surgeons and what types of strategies might be employed to decrease complications in the surgery department. The administrator suggested that a lecture on surgical technique would be appropriate. However, Dr Armstrong, in speaking with the Dr Jordan in the CPD department, questions whether this will be effective, because it is not clear why there is variation among the surgeons. Dr Armstrong is also quite clear that subtle distinctions in the kinds of problems presented during surgery are not conveyed well in lectures.

A responsive organization has put policies, procedures, and resources in place that draw from the work of its members in a systematic way so that experience is a building block for new policies, procedures, and resource allocation. That system is built on the values of the organization. Supporting the learning of individuals in acquiring and utilizing more knowledge needed to meet the institution's goals can result in improved practice or in no change at all. Dr Armstrong thought about and developed a way to work with the colleagues on his team for better outcomes.

Although examining assumptions about patient management strategies and how they play out in work was essential for the surgeons, there were also informal interactions that were critical to framing the problems about postoperative bleeding problems. Informal approaches are often very efficient and effective in bypassing a lack of flexibility or nimbleness at adopting new ways of doing business in an organization. Lack of flexibility on the part of an organization may be the result of efforts to standardize care, leadership that is not in touch with current changes in practice, disinterested physicians, lack of staff, or a number of other factors. But, within the organization, groups of individuals may find innovative ways to think about a problem, or unusual solutions, and ways to work around the rules while still supporting institutional goals. Informal conversations to share ways that people frame a problem or ways to think about innovative approaches to solutions can be very effective in making an organization flexible.

The missing piece for this problem was in the translation of those efforts for a broader group. As a follow-up, Dr Armstrong suggested that he ask his colleagues if he could assist on some of their surgeries to observe a range of techniques and think about the differences he has incorporated into his own work. He noted that looking for assumptions about what will improve outcomes might be a helpful way to talk about it. He also suggested that the general surgeons regularly get together for breakfast to compare their approaches to specific techniques and patient management problems. Six of the 10 surgeons decided to work out a way to compare notes. After three months, the rate of postoperative bleeding began to decline as a result of changes in operative technique, standardization of the type of suture material being used, increasing vigilance about discontinuation of anticoagulants prior to surgery, and changes in monitoring of patients by the nursing staff in the immediate postoperative period—all issues that were brought to light over breakfast conversations. The surgeons in this group were very excited, not only about their improved patient outcomes but also their enhanced collegiality and enthusiasm for their professional interaction. The strategy suggests that colleagues collectively working together may find solutions that individuals do not—and that the process may be outside of the formal structure.

To find meaning from what is learned, individuals use their own groups or communities to provide a context. Shared values, common uses of language, and ways of doing or practicing are based on being part of a community that derives shape and substance for the implementation of ideas.

Wenger's ideas[5] about communities of practice describe a kind of social community that is particularly helpful to understanding one kind of informal learning in a learning organization. Wenger[8] defines a community of practice as an informal group of people who get together to share expertise and passion for a specific problem or area. One image is the "watercooler group" that hangs out together in what might appear to be casual conversation. In reality, they trade ideas about unique ways to get things done. People are often a part of many communities of practice pointing to specific interests. A group thrives on the development of knowledge and on solving problems by sharing past experiences and innovative new approaches. The requirements for a community of practice are not rigid—they may meet regularly or not, in person or not, and may have a specific agenda or not. But, they add value to an organization by their effectiveness in suggesting creative strategies, solving problems quickly, facilitating the transfer of best practices, developing specialized skills, starting new kinds of services, and helping institutions develop talent. Rather than delivering a product or accomplishing a specific assignment, such as a new way to manage hypertension, a community of practice looks to develop capabilities of those who participate. A physician and nurse with a special interest in ensuring that specific populations improve their management of hypertension to avoid cardiac problems may join with a social worker and secretary to think about novel ways to help patients monitor their disease. They look for ways to build an understanding or a new way to frame the problem and they share possible solutions. If data show that patients are not compliant with a treatment plan, the group may talk with colleagues for suggestions for phone follow-up or mailed reminders. When a community of practice creates new knowledge, it renews the group. In the operating room, Dr Armstrong helped to mold a new kind of contact among some of his peers to frame problems and create a new kind of interaction around solving those problems. The success in making progress provided the group with the energy and incentive to continue their informal contact.

Because communities of practice are informal, they are fragile due to lack of support. Providing an official sponsor and designation for the community is one way to strengthen it. Rather than being prescriptive about the group's agenda and demanding selected kinds of products, providing resources and coordination support the continued health of the group. Understanding the value of the group demands nontraditional measures. Leaders must listen to the stories of the group to have a sense of the interplay between knowledge, solutions, and activities. Dr Jordan, in the CPD unit, supports communities of practice by providing space, encouragement, enthusiasm, responsiveness, and a conduit for outcomes to the CEO. Although Dr Jordan does not do the kind of planning that might occur with a formal CPD program, the skills needed to foster this kind of learning are equally important.

ORGANIZATIONAL INNOVATIONS

Bayside Hospital will be surveyed by the Joint Commission for Accreditation of Healthcare Organizations next year and is concerned about its compliance with the requirements for pain management. Some of the nurses have heard about an approach known as patient-controlled analgesia (PCA), which allows the patient to adjust the amount of pain medication after surgery. This concept is presented at the medical staff meeting, and the majority of physicians are adamant that it should not be introduced at the hospital because patients may get too much medication or might become dependent on narcotics. They serve a population with higher-than-average problems around substance abuse and feel that their current approaches to postoperative pain management are appropriate for their population and budget constraints. Dr Connors, who recently came from another institution, has experience with the technique and volunteered to conduct a pilot project with his patients on one unit. A 3-month study revealed that Dr Connor's patients who use PCA are discharged earlier and their total dose of narcotics is less than that of similar patients. Six months later, three-quarters of all surgeons on the staff are ordering PCA for their patients.

The idea that pain can and should be monitored by the patient demands that all the members of the organization think about the underlying values related to whether only the "professionals" are taking care of a patient or whether patients are part of the team. When a new idea is introduced, the first look is to see how it will improve what is currently being done. A second look, however, can envision whether the goals in practice are the right ones. That kind of double-look learning is essential in thinking about changes in health care.[9,10] Creating a health care team that includes the patient is just one of the major changes now in process.

Even with the support of double-look learning, the level of change in health care is almost overwhelming. Even before a new system is in place, new demands for changes are heard. The quality of "evidence" varies dramatically for making decisions. One way to help an organization manage the future is by understanding something about how innovations are adopted and how disruptive change impacts a learning organization.

Rogers's work[6] describing how innovations are adopted provides two important ideas for how to think about making effective changes by a learning organization. First, individuals adopt new things at different rates. The rate is predicated by how a person sees the world and the relative advantages and disadvantages of the specific innovation. Do I need to learn a new technique? Is my office staff supportive? Will we need to buy new equipment or change our record-keeping system? Will I get better results? These may be a few of the questions a physician asks when first deciding about a new way to manage a patient problem. Among any group of people there will be differing rates for adopting an innovation. There are also stages of preparedness in adopting an innovation, with different supporting resources. In the beginning, information is gathered, an individual is persuaded that the innovation is helpful, the innovation is put in place, and, finally, the innovation is integrated into standard practice. There may be support or barriers at any of those stages that will influence whether the change will be incorporated.

Beyond a learning organization knowing how to look at its work in several ways, and knowing that adoption of changes takes time and varies among members of the organization, one striking business pattern stands out. That pattern is the failure of successful companies to stay at the top of their business. For years, best care was thought to take place in the hospital—that is, until managed care organizations provided ways to keep patients at home with new kinds of services. Today, new care patterns, especially in ambulatory care, are emerging to challenge traditional MCOs. That pattern of disruptive change has been described by Christensen.[11–14]

According to Christensen,[12] a critical piece of advice has always been to stay close to the customer. Health care organizations asked patients what they needed; many patients felt they needed full-time nursing care found in the hospital. But evidence about healing patterns, coupled with cost constraints, encouraged and forced many patients to try managed care as another option. The heart of the problem is in the concept of staying close to one's customers or learners in the traditional view of needs assessment to provide something that is more effective and efficient. By listening closely to customers or learners, a company cannot develop products with attributes that are not historically valued. At the same time, if a company is to be successful, it must have customers who demand a response to perceived needs. For MCOs, that meant getting patients up and active quickly to preserve overall good health, thus providing more support for home care while decreasing high costs.

The activities of an organization result from resources, processes, and values.[12] When problems must be addressed, the automatic response tends to be a request for resources. Either funds must be provided to study the question, or the lack of money damages a pilot project. If an organization is to foster the development of disruptive change or a rigorous new way of thinking about a problem, part of its business plan should dictate that the organization's development be sheltered from mainstream ideas so that comparisons with current needs do not cause it to fail. It also demands that leaders support the development of projects that will disrupt the current way of doing business. The new product may change in what it values or in the resources that are needed. New processes may be essential. Although health care institutions are not measured solely on profits, financially failing organizations cannot attract professionals and provide quality care. The same idea fits well with learning provided by academic institutions: new ideas delivered in new ways may need support to avoid negative comparisons with traditional learning.

A disruption such as a new way to manage pain will be more apt to succeed if the organization values input from all members of the team and if it values change. If the processes for change are so cumbersome that new ideas are lost in complicated processes or the leadership makes clear that the informal opinion is to maintain the status quo, the organization will not learn from its members. In our case, if Dr Connor had not championed the new technique, if he could not find support for using the technique with his own patients, or if the nurses were dismissed as less knowledgeable about pain, the experiment could not have moved forward.

A NEW KIND OF CPD PROFESSIONAL

CPD that is effective deals with the formal and informal structure of the organization; takes into account the resources, processes, and values that are available; and is respectful of the culture when thinking about how to frame and solve problems. The purpose of learning by individuals is to support the continued learning of the organization so as to respond more effectively to the challenges it faces. Individuals can create lasting change by contributing to the responsiveness of the organization. None of the conceptual work is independent of the team that makes an organization work. Information from the outside and the inside must converge on the problem.

The new kind of educator in CPD has expertise in how adults learn and stages of their professional development, as well as organizational behaviors.[15,16] There is a skillful blend of matching the learning needs of individuals with the needs of teams and of the whole organization. Incorporating our understanding of the learning organization into a job description for the CPD professional offers some intriguing possibilities. Rather than thinking about planning a one-hour lecture to reflect a change in the protocol for diabetes, the CPD educator may become part of a team that looks at the development of treatment protocols and their integration into practice with physicians, nurses, pharmacists, therapists, financial experts, and managers. Rather than planning a self-study reading package on critical new literature in genetic counseling around newborn care, the educator may work on that project in the context of working with other units in order to create overlapping learning for the social work staff, nurses, lab technologists, and managers. The aim of that effort might be to design learning activities that will support a new view of the decision tree for genetic testing in newborns. Instead of inviting academicians to present grand rounds, an educator may work with one of the staff to provide a discussion of problem cases drawn from inside the hospital.

The new competencies required for those in CPD that reflect the areas we have discussed in this chapter can be divided into three sections. First, learning from experience demands that those in CPD:

- help an organization to establish systems that are sensitive to unusual problems and circumstances so that new responses are continually being built;

- develop internal and external monitors and contacts to encourage participation in the provision of new ideas, concepts, and knowledge relevant to that organization; and

- build strategies to expand a standard portfolio of traditional CME programming to include options that build organizational learning, such as innovative self-directed and group learning.

Second, to encourage informal learning, those in CPD must:

- understand informal learning options and recognize new ways to encourage groups to address problems. They must provide resources and support for informal groups by knowing who they are and how support can be provided. A community of practice is one example;

- reflect the values of the organization in learning opportunities by identifying problems across the organization and by working outside of the CME office; and

- link units of the organization in new ways that foster new teams that can build new ideas.

And, third, the adoption of new processes and values can be supported by:

- providing productive dissonance to recognize problems and time to foster change through strategies that provide ongoing learning and feedback;
- sheltering innovations in ways that allow them to grow until their contribution to the organization can be assessed; and
- implementing double-look practices to expand the kinds of problems that the organization will be able to recognize and address.

Removing barriers for new communities of practice, creating informal structures to support cross-discipline communication, and instituting reflective practices that support double-look learning are some of the necessary functions of the knowledge worker in CPD who facilitate organizational learning. But, the early state of research and practice in this area limits the extent to which this role can be prescribed. Those who believe they have experienced learning organizations base most of what is offered on the logical extension of either existing theories from other areas of research on learning or logical deductions.

More than anything, this area needs qualitative and quantitative research to elaborate on the explanations offered so far and to verify the relationships that are proposed in those theories. Without this body of research, discussion suggests that the phenomenon exists and offers attempts at explaining it. Discussion should not propose elaborate systems for actually facilitating organizational learning.

This chapter has offered three components of organizational learning, some reflections on how these explanations may work in organizational learning, and some suggestions as to what that might mean for the CPD of physicians and the organizations that offer health care. Although it is clear that organizations do learn to perform in different ways based on changing competencies needed to solve problems of care and problems of the delivery of care, exactly how this learning works requires closer scrutiny. However, to ignore it because the literature is too limited and poorly developed, at least for now, would be an error. Facilitating organizational learning will be part of the role of those who work in the CPD of physicians. It is not too early to include it in the paradigm of CPD.

REFERENCES—CHAPTER 10

1. Garvin D. Building a learning organization. *Harvard Business Review.* 1993;71:78–91.
2. Senge PM. The leader's new work: building learning organizations. *Sloan Management Review.* Fall 1990;7–23.

3. Argyris C. Teaching smart people how to learn. *Harvard Business Review*. May–June 1991:99–109.

4. Schön DA. *Educating the Reflective Practitioner: Toward a New Design for Teaching and Learning in the Profession*. San Francisco, Calif: Jossey-Bass Publishers; 1987.

5. Wenger, E. *Communities of Practice: Learning, Meaning and Identity*. Boston, Mass: Cambridge University Press; 1998.

6. Rogers EM. *Diffusion of Innovations*. 4th ed. New York, NY: Free Press; 1995.

7. Christensen, C. *The Innovators Dilemma*. Boston, Mass: Harvard Business School Press; 1997.

8. Wenger E, Snyder W. Communities of practice: the organizational frontier. *Harvard Business Review*. Jan–Feb 2000:139–145.

9. Frankford, DM, Patterson MS, Konrad TR. Transforming practice organizations to foster lifelong learning and commitment to medical professionalism. *Acad Med*. 2000;75:708–717.

10. Argyris C. Double loop learning in organizations. *Harvard Business Review*. 1977;55:115–125.

11. Bower J, Christensen C. Disruptive technologies: catching the wave. *Harvard Business Review*. Jan–Feb 1995:43–53.

12. Christensen C, Overdorf M. Meeting the challenge of disruptive change. *Harvard Business Review*. March–April 2000:66–76.

13. Christensen C. Armstrong E. Disruptive technologies: a credible threat to leading programs in continuing medical education? *J Contin Educ Health Prof*. 1998;18:69–80.

14. Christensen C, Bohner R, Kenagy J. Will disruptive innovations cure health care? *Harvard Business Review*. Sept–Oct 2000:102–112.

15. Barnes BE. Evaluation of learning in health care organizations. *J Contin Educ Health Prof*. 1999;19:227–233.

16. Confessore SJ. Building a learning organization: communities of practice, self-directed learning and continuing medical education. *J Contin Educ Health Prof*. 1997;19:5–11.

Using Technology in Continuing Professional Development

Barbara E. Barnes, MD; Charles P. Friedman, PhD

INTRODUCTION

Information and telecommunications technology (ITT) offers the opportunity to revolutionize the way we provide education. In view of the rapidly expanding volume of medical information and expectations for evidence-based decision-making, continuing professional development (CPD) professionals must be able to leverage the expanding capabilities of ITT to help physicians meet the demands of practicing in the twenty-first century.

For a number of years, computers have been used to improve traditional CPD venues. High-quality still pictures and multimedia facilitate the incorporation of clinical images into lectures and assist faculty in explaining issues. Through the use of audience-response systems, attendees can give feedback during a presentation, enabling faculty to tailor content to learner needs. Self-study materials can be made more interactive and interesting as the result of CD-ROMs and increasingly sophisticated computer programs.

However, even with these enhancements, traditional models of CPD are suboptimal in terms of effectiveness, efficiency, and convenience.[1] CPD has been constrained by time, place, and content because we have lacked adequate tools to link teachers and learners in disparate locations, manage information from a variety of sources, and simplify highly complex problems.[2] Traditional venues such as formal courses might be described as *discontinuous* professional development: a process that occurs apart from clinical

---

The authors express appreciation to Ann McKibbon, MLS, for her contributions to this chapter.

practice, requiring that physicians assess their own needs, find an appropriate CPD activity, and, if possible, apply the information to their practice.[3]

A variety of factors motivate CPD professionals to develop new educational models that overcome these limitations:[4]

- Physicians have less time to participate in CPD. Continuing education must be accessible, convenient, and affordable.

- Physicians need education that is relevant to the patient population they serve. Physicians require assistance in defining individual learning needs, seeking out the best learning venues, and measuring the outcomes of education on clinical performance.

- Society has become aware of variation in the quality of care delivered by practitioners and there is growing public concern about medical errors. In order to be relevant to the health care system, CPD professionals must demonstrate that their activities improve provider competence and health care outcomes.

- Medical knowledge is proliferating rapidly and it is increasingly difficult for physicians to keep up. Physicians need help in finding the information they need, ensuring that it is valid, and translating it to the care of their patients.

Advances in ITT make it possible for CPD professionals to use technology not just to improve existing models of education but also to transform the way physicians learn and change.[5] This chapter, through the use of a case study, will describe how the field of CPD can employ technology to help physicians manage medical information, gain greater access to CPD, practice clinical skills and problem-solving, and integrate education into their day-to-day clinical practice.

AN INTRODUCTION TO THE TECHNOLOGY

In order to understand how ITT can be applied to CPD, it is important to review a few key concepts related to the technology and its applications:

- *Hardware:* According to Moore's law, the capabilities of computer hardware double every 12 to 18 months.[6] Advances in memory and processing allow large quantities of data, including high-resolution images, to be stored and manipulated. The miniaturization of computing devices, including notebooks and handheld devices, permits individuals to carry information resources with them at all times, whether they are at the office, hospital, or home.

- *Software:* Increasingly sophisticated software allows users with minimal training to use the power of modern computers to solve everyday problems and perform a variety of tasks. "Course-ware" can provide a variety of functions to help educators develop computer-based learning activities, including authoring tools, testing modules, and communication vehicles, such as discussion lists and Web chat groups that allow persons with common interests to exchange ideas without meeting face to face.

- *The Internet:* The Internet links computers across the world through a set of internationally accepted communication standards that allow the exchange of information according to those standards. The World Wide Web is a network of sites created and maintained by individuals. The pages within them may contain text, images, or multimedia.[7] Web browsers such as Microsoft® Internet Explorer and Netscape® Navigator contain the basic software needed to find, retrieve, view, and send information over the Internet, obviating the need for specialized software on individual machines. In addition to providing access to information, the Internet serves as a vehicle for communication through the use of e-mail.

- *Transmission:* Bandwidth expresses the "thickness" of the electronic pipeline that allows data to be communicated from one location to another. Standard text may be easily transmitted over "plain old telephone services" (POTS) at 28 or 56 kilobits per second, whereas practical use of high-resolution images and broadcast-quality video may require transmission in the range of millions of bits per second. All else being equal, increases in bandwidth improve image quality, speed of transmission, and fidelity of motion. Data transmission may be accomplished through terrestrial lines, microwave links, or satellite.

- *Synchronicity:* Communication is synchronous when users from different locations interact at the same time. Examples include real-time chat lines, audio conferences, and video conferences. Asynchronous communications, such as e-mail or discussion lists, allow users to interact at their convenience, accommodating personal schedules and disparate time zones.

PROVIDING EDUCATION WHEN AND WHERE IT IS NEEDED

Alan Peterson has just returned home from a university hospital where he underwent liver transplantation. He is on four different antirejection medications. Dr Mary Baldwin, Alan's general internist, has not cared for a posttransplant patient since residency and she cannot find any pertinent information in the textbooks or pharmaceutical references kept in the office. She is pleased to learn that the transplant institute offers a Web portal containing full-text articles, textbook chapters, practice guidelines, drug information, evidence-based reviews, and patient education materials. Dr Baldwin can also obtain an application for her handheld computer containing prescribing information, dosing calculations, and major side effects of antirejection drugs. She is informed of a monthly video or audio continuing medical education (CME) conference offered by the university to help primary care physicians manage these complex patients. There is also a quarterly case conference discussion conducted as an on-line chat group. Dr Baldwin can earn CME credit for taking part in televideo patient consultations.

As the amount of medical knowledge expands, physicians have an increasingly difficult time remaining current, particularly in regard to situations that they encounter infrequently or in specialty areas that advance rapidly. The university might consider offering a presentation on management of the transplant patient in its internal medicine update course that Dr Baldwin routinely attends. However, by the time many of the participants actually see one of these cases, it is likely that they would have forgotten much of the information and that some of the recommendations would be out of date. Lacking the most current information, physicians' decisions are made according to a "best guess" about the optimal course of action.[8] Recent studies demonstrate that physicians' inability to integrate up-to-date evidence into clinical practice can lead to deviations from recommended guidelines as well as medical errors.[9] In order to deliver optimal care to her patients, Dr Baldwin needs to have resources available "just in time" to assist in decision-making.[10]

Traditionally, physicians have relied on textbooks or journals kept in their offices or local library to provide information they need. However, these resources quickly go out of date and it is not feasible for a physician practice or even a local hospital to retain hard copies of all books and journals that may be required as reference material. Public and proprietary electronic literature repositories accompanied by search tools, such as PubMed[11] and Ovid©,[12] allow physicians access to continuously updated databases of medical knowledge via the Internet, including abstracts, full-text journal articles, systematic reviews, and practice guidelines.

Access to knowledge resources is not a universal blessing, however. If Dr Baldwin searched the last three years of PubMed on the topic of liver transplantation, she would find more than 4400 references. Limiting this to only review articles would still yield more than 650 citations. An Internet search engine might find tens of thousands of Web sites on this topic, many of uncertain credibility. The usefulness of knowledge resources is dependent not only on their validity but also the work involved in accessing a relevant and navigable subset of the information they contain.[13] A variety of tools are available to help busy physicians deal with the expanse of medical literature.[14,15]

The Skolar[©] program, developed at Stanford University, is an advanced Web-based knowledge-management system that allows learners to rapidly search a variety of resources in order to efficiently answer clinical questions.[16] The information sources are carefully reviewed by experts to assure their usefulness and credibility. With such a system, users can select resources such as original research articles, systematic reviews, guidelines, and synopses to answer the questions that arise in clinical practice.[17] The results of each individual's queries are archived into an electronic log that contains the results of previous searches, providing a means of tracking educational activities. A project is underway to determine how use of the Skolar[©] program can be made eligible for category 1 CME credit.

Web portals offer a single point of access to an array of resources: "one-stop shopping" for information on a particular topic.[18] To create these portals, content experts and information specialists select credible resources relevant to the prospective target audience. Sources may include primary research reports, review articles, meta-analyses, synopses, custom-written didactic content, multimedia resources, practice guidelines, certified CME activities, patient education materials, and links to other Web sites, allowing the user to choose the items most relevant to his or her needs and interests. These Internet-based resources can be updated as appropriate to incorporate new research and current recommendations for care.

Searching the literature and accessing Web portals are examples of how physicians can retrieve, or "pull," information from knowledge repositories using ITT. However, practitioners may not be aware of their learning needs (ie, they may not know where to find the answers to their questions or have time to get the required information). The use of telecommunications technology, such as e-mail, allows educational resources to be sent, or "pushed," to physicians, either in the form of a text message, attachment, or link to a Web site from which further information may be obtained. This approach may be useful for educating physicians on a timely issue, such as Federal Drug Administration approval of a new device, recently discovered drug interaction, or outbreak of a communicable disease.

ITT can also support synchronous learning activities in which faculty and learners in different geographic locations are brought together at the same time. A wide range of modalities are available, permitting attendees to communicate through text, audio, or video, with the choice of venue being determined by the level of interactivity, cost, ability of attendees to conveniently access the program, and types of images being employed. For example, the demonstration of a surgical procedure may require the use of satellite or video conferencing with high bandwidth. On the other hand, a discussion of optimal diabetes treatment may be adequately conducted by means of telephone conference or e-mail chat group. Teleconsultations offer a unique opportunity for CPD, allowing experts and practitioners to discuss a clinical issue in the context of a particular patient.

The convergence of computing and communications devices into portable units, such as personal digital assistants (PDAs), allows physicians to easily retrieve information important to day-to-day patient care, such as drug dosages and interactions. From the office, hospital, or home, it is possible to send and receive e-mail as well as access information available over the Internet, allowing communication with consultants or patients and access to online library resources and practice guidelines. These communications devices provide a vehicle for receiving voice or electronic alerts about critical patient events, such as abnormal laboratory values or outbreaks of communicable diseases. Through the use of Web links or e-mail attachments, it is possible to include supporting educational materials with these notifications in order to give practitioners more information about the appropriate management of the patient's condition.

The use of electronic tools enables CPD to be liberated from the constraints of time, place, and content. Technology helps educators reach a diverse and disparate audience while conserving the time of both faculty and learners. Participants can be given a wide choice of educational modalities and knowledge resources, accommodating individual learning styles and the nature of the educational need that is being addressed. In contrast to traditional concepts of education that differentiate between self-directed venues driven by the learner (such as literature searches) and formal activities designed by the faculty (such as a lecture), ITT can support a variety of levels of interaction between practitioner and expert (Figure 11-1). For example, a Web portal permits physicians to select information relevant to their needs, knowing that experts have reviewed the resources to assure scientific merit and currency. Information "pushed" by e-mail allows content developers to provide timely information on important issues such as recently identified drug side effects or emerging epidemics that can be reviewed at the practitioner's convenience. Through the use of video conferencing, specialists and referring physicians can conduct case discussions, sharing information and collaboratively determining optimal management strategies for their patients. The availability of these new modalities allows CPD to occur when and where it is needed, with the potential to improve the quality of patient care, optimize learning, and enhance the productivity of both learners and teachers.

FIGURE 11-1

The Use of Different Technologies Supports Learning Activities with Varying Degrees of Learner and Faculty Involvement

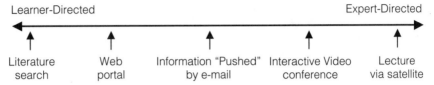

Learner-Directed   Expert-Directed

| Literature search | Web portal | Information "Pushed" by e-mail | Interactive Video conference | Lecture via satellite |

NEW MODELS OF EDUCATION: SIMULATION

Six months after his transplant, Mr Peterson's condition has deteriorated due to organ rejection. He requires intravenous medications and has received a new type of vascular access device that must be changed every eight weeks. Dr Baldwin's practice group has a number of patients with these devices. The university transplant team invites Dr Baldwin or one of her colleagues to spend a half day in their skills-simulation center to learn how to insert the device, saving Mr Peterson travel to the university hospital and affording the community physicians an opportunity to generate increased revenue by doing the procedure. The transplant group also offers to provide Dr Baldwin with a computer software program that will allow her to evaluate the risks and benefits of various experimental treatment options available to Mr Peterson.

Educators have long struggled to determine the optimal method for teaching clinical skills.[19] The "see one, do one, teach one" model has a number of limitations. Even under close supervision, it may not be safe to learn new procedures on patients. Animal laboratories are expensive and may not replicate the human condition. A variety of computer technologies, ranging from simple software programs to virtual reality, may be employed in order to develop "medical flight simulators." These systems allow physicians and trainees to learn in a near real-life situation while being observed and obtaining feedback.[20] Skills can be repeated under varied conditions until competency is achieved. Emergencies and complications can be simulated so learners can practice the management of unlikely but serious problems. Following training conducted with the simulator, tools such as video conferencing can permit experts to remotely observe the clinician performing the procedure on a patient (teleproctoring) to assure that competency has been achieved.

Anesthesia simulators allow learners to not only practice technical skills such as intubation and venous access but also manage a variety of clinical situations. Computer-based algorithms permit the effects of pharmaceutical and other interventions to be translated into physiological parameters (such as heart rate, respirations, and blood pressure), producing a very realistic learning environment.

Participants are able to demonstrate how they implement clinical algorithms (such as the American Heart Association guidelines for management of acute cardiac events) and can practice using different therapeutic strategies. Such simulation tools support not only individual learning but also provide a mechanism for evaluating how well clinicians function on a patient care team, such as in an operating room or emergency department.

Simulations can assist physicians in evaluating treatment options for complex clinical situations, particularly those for which there is insufficient evidence to mitigate for one particular treatment option or in which treatments carry a variety of risks and benefits.[21] These tools assist physicians in processing large amounts of information and allow them to practice complex decision-making in "high fidelity, low-risk" conditions.[22] By employing computers to generate a variety of clinical scenarios, participants can experiment with diagnostic and therapeutic options that would not be considered in practice because they are unfamiliar or potentially too hazardous.[23] Using sophisticated algorithms, various parameters can be altered in order to determine their effects on patient outcomes. For example, the university transplant team could evaluate the impact of different postoperative management strategies on length of stay, cost of inpatient care, and time until patients return to work. Such simulation tools are also valuable for informing patients about the benefits and risks of alternative treatment options. Of the experimental treatment alternatives available to Mr Peterson, one may be much more effective in eliminating organ rejection but may also carry a danger of permanent side effects that will affect his quality of life. Other choices may have a lower likelihood of assuring organ survival but may have a higher safety profile. Having this information clearly delineated supports collaborative decision-making between physicians and patients, allowing an informed choice of treatment options.[24] The use of such simulations can improve the care of the patient under consideration in addition to helping physicians improve their diagnostic reasoning and clinical management skills in the care of other, similar patients.[25]

THE INTEGRATED PRACTICE-LEARNING ENVIRONMENT

It is 2010 and Mr Peterson is now a long-term transplant survivor. Dr Baldwin has installed a state-of-the-art clinical information system and electronic health record that continuously assesses the quality of care she delivers, comparing her performance with peers as well as practice guidelines. If consistent patterns emerge, customized electronic learning modules are sent to her desktop. When a medication is prescribed outside of the standard dosage range or in combination with other drugs that might produce an interaction, Dr Baldwin is notified by means of her personal digital companion (combination pager, cell phone, and handheld computer). If she needs to obtain more information about these issues, she can immediately retrieve selected full-text articles by clicking on a Web link that accompanies the alert. The clinical information system tracks Dr Baldwin's practice patterns to assure that the CPD interventions have resulted in changes in her clinical performance. A log of all of her educational activities and resulting improvements in her clinical practice is maintained electronically. Dr Baldwin submits this information annually to her state licensing and specialty boards in order to demonstrate the maintenance of professional competency.

New models of CPD are currently available through the use of a variety of technological tools. However, the real power of ITT will be realized only when there is full integration of education and clinical care. By employing data contained in clinical information systems and electronic health records, physicians' learning needs will be determined based on clinical performance; educational resources will be delivered "just in time" to improve patient care; and the effectiveness of learning will be assessed on the basis of patient outcomes. "Smart systems" will simultaneously evaluate a variety of data sources, such as compliance with practice guidelines, adverse events, the cost of care, and patient satisfaction. These systems will use this information to assemble and deliver learning resources to the appropriate target audience, be it an individual, practice group, or multidisciplinary team. A variety of learning modalities may be incorporated, including feedback, reminders, and electronic methods of academic detailing. Physicians will be able to "mine" the clinical databases to gather information about their patient population and compare their practices with those of other doctors. Through the use of integrated information and telecommunications systems, physicians will have unlimited access to educational resources, patient care data, and colleagues across the world.

Such a model of CPD will be organized not on the basis of episodic learning activities but in terms of ongoing clinical improvement processes specific to each practitioner and care team. The demarcation between learning and practice will be eliminated, with physicians functioning in a seamless environment of multifaceted improvement interventions, including courses and grand rounds, consultations and feedback from colleagues, alerts about critical events, and prompts for ordering preventive services and lab tests required for monitoring therapy.[26] Education will be appropriate to a physician's scope of practice and performance, with objective data being used to assess outcomes. As described in Chapter 5, electronic learning portfolios can be used to document the linkage between performance gaps, educational interventions, and subsequent practice patterns.

The integrated practice-learning environment is a strategy to address many of the concerns about physician practice in the modern health care environment, including ongoing demonstration of competency, reduction of medical errors, and evidence-based decision-making. However, the model as described is beyond what can currently be achieved. Although components exist in some institutions, fulfilling the complete vision will require a significant commitment to integrated information architecture as well as additional technological innovations; enhanced competencies of both educators and learners to use technology and information resources; and critical research on new models of education. Moving CPD to this next level involves a variety of opportunities and challenges.

THE ROLE OF CPD PROFESSIONALS IN THE DEVELOPMENT OF TECHNOLOGICALLY ENABLED LEARNING ACTIVITIES

The appeal and availability of advanced ITT generate considerable enthusiasm in the CPD community to find uses for these new modalities. Such eagerness creates a natural propensity to put the technology first, generating questions such as, Can the Internet be used as a method for delivering continuing education? It is critical that CPD professionals differentiate projects designed to explore the feasibility of using technology in education from the development of learning activities that happen to employ ITT. Educators must always begin with questions such as, What is the best way for primary care physicians to learn about the management of a patient after liver transplantation?, with the choice of the venue being determined by the needs of the target audience rather than the availability of the technology. Although the university may be proud of its capability to provide live Web casts, this might not be the optimal mechanism for educating referring physicians. Dr Baldwin might prefer audiotapes that she can use while driving to the office or printed information that she can review while waiting to pick up her children at school. The goal of using ITT in CPD is not to do things differently but to do them in the way that best meets the needs of learners and the patients for whom they provide care.

In order to use ITT effectively, CPD professionals must assure that technical development is driven by a systematic process of instructional design. In addition to the steps of routine educational planning process, the use of technology introduces several other considerations:

■ *Assessment of the target audience in regard to the use of technology:* Following identification of an educational need, it is critical to determine the interests of the potential target audience in using new instructional modalities and the ability of these recipients to access and employ the venues under consideration.

Factors that need to be considered include availability of required hardware and software, access to bandwidth, and technical literacy. The type of program developed for a university faculty may be very different from that intended for rural physicians. The academic medical center's high-speed network and state-of-the-art computers might allow high-quality still images and video to be incorporated into learning activities and, through the organization's purchase of licensing agreements, faculty may have access to a large number of online library resources. Rural practitioners unaffiliated with the university may be limited to publicly available journals. Their use of modems through telephone lines and hardware with limited memory and processing capabilities may necessitate the provision of content in text form with limited graphics.

- *Delineation of educational requirements and specifications:* In order to define technical specifications, level of professional and staff expertise required for development, and potential project cost, CPD professionals must clearly define the learning model that is being employed and level of evaluation required.[27] Issues to be considered included the characteristics of learner–faculty interaction, requirements for multimedia and images, and necessity for testing and certification. For example, if the goal of the activity is to provide mandatory safety training, a highly self-directed model may be appropriate with content in text format and post-test designed to assess knowledge. On the other hand, the presentation of complex issues might necessitate some degree of discussion between faculty and learners. Skills training might require the use of simulation, observation by an expert, and development of a mechanism for competency assessment.

- *Determining the composition of the design team and evaluation of current capabilities:* CPD professionals and technical experts (such as programmers, multimedia technicians, IT architects, and telecommunications staff) must work closely to assure alignment of educational goals with ITT capabilities. Other members of this team will include content experts and perhaps library and information specialists. A systematic evaluation must be conducted to determine the benefits and challenges of using various modalities, taking into account factors such as cost; existing organizational capabilities; and the ability of the institution to develop, deploy, and support the technology.

- *Assessing the need to train faculty and end users in the use of technology:* Faculty may require training in authoring Web-based activities, presentation skills, or use of multimedia. The selection of software and hardware should take into account the existing skills of the proposed target audience, with the development of a training plan, if needed. Prior to full implementation, accommodation should be made for pilot testing to further assess the ability of learners to participate in the activity as well as the reliability of hardware and software.

- *Development of a plan for evaluation and project sustainability:* Activity evaluation should assess factors associated with ITT such as ease of use, appropriateness of the technology to the learning activity, and adequacy of technical support. In addition, consideration must be given to how hardware and software will be maintained, content will be updated, and users will be supported.

In order to accomplish these goals, CPD professionals must forge partnerships with professionals from other disciplines, including technical experts and library and information specialists.[28,29] The use of ITT in education may lead to the formation of new kinds of professionals such as "informationists" who can assist educators and clinicians in bridging the body of medical evidence and clinical practice.[30] Although it is not necessary for CPD professionals to be highly skilled technical experts, they need to understand the principles of medical computing and information management in order to be able to determine the capabilities and limitations of using ITT in the development of lifelong learning activities.

CHALLENGES IN USING ITT IN CPD

The success of technologically assisted education will be determined by a variety of factors. First, physicians must embrace the new methods of CPD. A recent study indicated that 89% of physicians use the Internet, spending an average of eight hours per week online.[31] While 78% of practitioners read electronic journal articles, only 45% report using the Web for completion of CME activities. According to the annual report of the Accreditation Council of Continuing Medical Education in 2000, only 3.57% of all physicians participating in certified CME activities chose an Internet venue.[32]

The core competencies promulgated by the Accreditation Council for Graduate Medical Education and endorsed by the American Board of Medical Specialties state that physicians must be able to "use information technology to manage information, access online medical information, and support their own education" as well as to "locate, appraise, and assimilate evidence from scientific studies related to their patients' health problems."[33] In order to help physicians achieve this level of technical and information literacy, CPD professionals will need to join with colleagues responsible for the undergraduate and graduate curricula to:

- define the knowledge, skills, and attitudes required to function in a technically enlightened environment;

- determine how these competencies can most effectively be taught; and
- establish the best time within the medical education continuum to develop and refine these skills.[34,35]

Increased access to computers and the Internet is needed in clinical settings. Information systems were initially introduced into hospitals and offices to support billing and administrative functions. The importance of physician interaction with clinical information systems is now being recognized, but many, if not most, of the inpatient and outpatient care settings lack sufficient hardware, software, and connectivity to support the practice-learning environment described in the scenarios above. Potential educational applications must be taken into consideration during the design and development of clinical information systems and electronic health records. CPD professionals should accordingly find ways to participate in organizational ITT planning efforts. Institutions funded by the National Library of Medicine's IAIMS (Integrated Advanced Information Management Systems) program[36] have a unique opportunity to explore ways to integrate education with clinical care.

CPD professionals who use electronic clinical data for needs assessment and evaluation will have to remain current on regulations related to data privacy and security.[37] At a time when ITT has increasing capability to analyze patient care information, there are rising concerns about confidentiality, integrity, and access to this data.[38] Technology for de-identification of clinical information and maintenance of security will become an essential component in efforts to integrate CPD and medical practice.

CPD must find ways to fund the new models of education. The incentives of equipment vendors and telecommunications carriers who capitalize development efforts may lie in use of the highest-end technology and maximum bandwidth, not necessarily the most cost-effective strategy for educating physicians. CPD providers must remain mindful that educational activities will be evaluated on their ability to improve physicians' knowledge, skill, competence, and performance, rather than the performance of the ITT being used. Accordingly, funding for new ways to deliver CPD should include support for rigorous evaluation procedures. Although some critical assessments of ITT in CPD have begun to appear in the literature,[39–41] many questions remain, particularly in regard to barriers to employing technology and the cost-benefit of new educational models. A comprehensive research agenda must address optimal methods to improve technical and information literacy and required competencies for CPD professionals in the technologically capable educational environment.[42]

A MANDATE FOR CPD

Increments to human material power are not paced by increments in the wisdom to use that power. . . . We are driving faster without necessarily steering better.[43]

Achieving the vision of a digital health care environment affords a promise of seamlessly integrating learning and clinical practice. It is critical that CPD professionals assume a central role in transforming the way physicians work and learn. The new vision will be accomplished through the application of sound educational theory and practice to technological deployment and will require the acquisition of new competencies by educators, faculty, and learners, as well as the forging of partnerships among a variety of disciplines. The field of CPD will progress only if new ways of delivering education are critically evaluated in the context of the literature and theory of how physicians learn and change.

Advances in technical capability will certainly stimulate changes in the way we provide education. The responsibility for demonstrating that these innovations are truly improving the health of our patients and communities rests on the field of CPD.

REFERENCES—CHAPTER 11

1. Davis DA, Thompson O'Brien MA, Freemantle N, Wolf FM, Mazmanian P, Taylor-Vaisey A. Impact of formal continuing medical education: do conferences, workshops, rounds, and other traditional continuing education activities change physician behavior or health care outcomes? *JAMA*. 1999;282:867–874.

2. Friedman, C. The marvelous medical education machine or how medical education can be 'unstuck' in time. *Med Teacher*. 2000;22:496–502.

3. Barnes BE. Creating the practice-learning environment: using information technology to support a new model of continuing medical education. *Acad Med*. 1998;73:278–281.

4. Bennett N, Davis DA, Easterling WE, Friedman P, Green JS, Koeppen BM, Mazmanian PE, Waxman HS. Continuing medical education: A new vision of the professional development of physicians. *Acad Med*. 2000;73:1167–1172.

5. Gibson CC. When disruptive approaches meet disruptive technologies: learning at a distance. *J Contin Educ Health Prof*. 2000;20:69–75.

6. Khanna R, Kwan J, Lamin J, White I. More on Moore's Law. www.eco.utexas.edu/undergraduate/Forum/ML/ppframe.htm

7. Wyatt JC. Knowledge and the Internet. *J Royal Society Med*. 2000;93:565–570.

8. Gorman PN, Helfand M. Information seeking in primary care: how physicians choose which clinical questions to pursue and which to leave unanswered. *Med Decis Making.* 1995;15:113–119.

9. Institute of Medicine. *Crossing the Quality Chasm: A New Health System for the 21st Century.* Washington, DC: National Academy Press; 2001.

10. Chueh H, Barnett GO. "Just-in-time" clinical information. *Acad Med.* 1997;72:512–517.

11. www.ncbi.nlm.nih.gov/entrez/query.fcgi

12. www.ovid.com

13. Smith R. What clinical information do doctors need? *BMJ.* 1996;313:1062–1068.

14. Williamson JW, German PS, Weiss R, Skinner EA, Bowes F. Health science information management and continuing education of physicians. *Ann Intern Med.* 1989;110:151–160.

15. Morrison I. The future of physicians' time. *Ann Intern Med.* 2000;132:80–84.

16. Dev P, Tsai MC, Strasberg H, Rindfleisch TC, Melmon KL. SHINE: helping tame the wilds of CME. *MD Computing.* 2001;17:15–18.

17. Haynes RB. Of studies, syntheses, synopses, and systems: the "4S" evolution of services for finding current best evidence. *ACP J Club 2001*; March/April:A11–A13.

18. Examples include: MD Consult www.mdconsult.com and Medscape www.medscape.com.

19. Issenberg SB, McGaghie WC, Hart IR, Mayer JW, Felner JM, Petrusa ER, Waugh RA, Brown DD, Safford RR, Gessner IH, Gordon, DL, Ewy GA. Simulation technology for health care professional skills training and assessment. *JAMA.* 1999;282:861–866.

20. Akay M, Marsh A. *Information Technologies in Medicine: Medical Simulation and Education.* New York, NY: John Wiley & Sons; 2001.

21. Plsek P. Redesigning health care with insights from the science of complex adaptive systems. In. Institute of Medicine. *Crossing the Quality Chasm: A New Health System for the 21st Century.* Washington, DC: National Academy Press; 2001.

22. Guest CB, Regehr G, Tiberius RG. The life long challenge of expertise. *Med Educ.* 2001;35:78–88.

23. Dörner D. *The Logic of Failure: Recognizing and Avoiding Errors in Complex Situations.* Reading, Mass: Addison-Wesley; 1996.

24. Barry MJ. Health decision aids to facilitate shared decision making in office practice. *Ann Inter Med.* 2002;136:127–135.

25. Friedman CP, Elstein AS, Wolf FM, Murphy GC, Franz TM, Heckerling PS, Fine PL, Miller TM, Abraham V. Enhancement of

clinicians' diagnostic reasoning by computer-based consultation: a multisite study of 2 systems. *JAMA*. 1999;282:1851–1856.

26.   Negreponte N. *Being Digital*. New York, NY: Vintage Books; 1995.

27.   Sonwalkar N. The sharp edge of the cube: pedagogically driven instructional design for online education. *Syllabus*. 2001;15:12–16.

28.   Schacher LF. Clinical librarianship: its value in medical care. *Ann Intern Med*. 2001;134:717–720.

29.   www.sacme.org/Research/default.htm#pbm

30.   Davidoff F, Florance V. The informationist: a new health profession. *Ann Intern Med*. 2000;132:996–998.

31.   Taylor H, Leitman R. The increasing impact of ehealth on physician behavior. *Health Care News (Harris Interactive)*. 2001;1:1–14.

32.   www.accme.org/incoming/2000_annual_data_tables.pdf

33.   www.acgme.org/outcome/comp/compFull.asp

34.   Candy PC. Preventing "information overdose": developing information-literate practitioners. *J Contin Educ Health Prof*. 2000;20:228–237.

35.   Frisse M. Re-imagining the medical informatics curriculum. *Acad Med*. 1997;72:36–40.

36.   www.nlm.nih.gov/pubs/factsheets/iaims.html

37.   Gostin LO. National health information privacy: regulations under the health insurance portability and accountability act. *JAMA*. 2001;285:3015–3021.

38.   Jennett P, Watanabe M, Igras E, Premkumar K, Hall W. Telemedicine and security. Confidentiality, integrity, and availability: a Canadian perspective. *Studies in Health Technology & Informatics*. 1996;29:286–298.

39.   Jennett PA, Hunter BJ, Husack JP. Telelearning in health: a Canadian perspective. *Telemed J*. 1998;4:237–247.

40.   Yuh JL, Abbott AV, Ontai S. Pilot study of a rating system for educational web sites. *Acad Med*. 2000;75:290.

41.   Bell DS, Fonarow GC, Hays RD, Mangione CM. Self-study from web-based and printed guideline materials: a randomized, controlled trial among resident physicians. *Ann Intern Med*. 2000;132:938–946.

42.   President's Information Technology Advisory Committee. Using information technology to transform the way we learn. 2001. www.itrd.gov/pubs/pitac/pitac-tl-9feb01.pdf

43.   Grudin R. *The Grace of Great Things: Creativity and Innovation*. New York, NY: Ticknor & Fields; 1990.

chapter 12

Feedback and Reminders: Tools for Change in the Practice Setting

Nancy L. Bennett, PhD; Robert D. Fox, EdD; Dave Davis, MD

The pile of papers spills off Dr Atkins' desk—too many ads, continuing medical education (CME) course brochures, and articles to be read. The push to see more patients is draining and frustrating and, given the time pressures, he worries about the little ways he's forgetting to follow up, especially on some of the preventive care and "life" issues with patients that he thinks are a good investment of time. Pushing the papers aside, one CME brochure on ways to use feedback and reminder systems to help with loose ends and details catches his attention. He considers the possibilities.

His colleague, Dr Westlake, is the director of quality assurance at their HMO. Sighing, she reviews a report of instances where the health care providers in her organization are not complying with an array of policies and guidelines, especially in primary prevention. She notes some underuse phenomena (eg, low levels of mammograms for women over 50, no flu shots for those over 65 years), some related to overuse (too many third-generation cephalosporins for routine infections), and a distressingly long list of medical errors. She requests a meeting with the director of CME, guessing that doctors do not always know the relevant protocols and need to learn about these areas of their practice. Deep down, she suspects the problem is either more complicated than a "need to know" or much simpler. In either case, the usual list of current educational activities does not seem to be the answer.

INTRODUCTION

Sometimes medical news seems more focused on the problems—diminishing levels of clinical knowledge, incompleteness, retention of poor practices, and out-of-date material, as well as access and application problems. How can we help clinicians have the best information when and where they need it? The good news is that medicine has a rich history of clinicians demanding the latest and best information, and experts and educators responding with opportunities to learn about advances in science and clinical care. Although physicians expect to continue learning throughout their careers in order to provide high-quality care, the traditional educational system has not been as demanding about expectations for continually assessing or improving that performance and its contributions to a patient's care.

We know there are problems in transferring new knowledge and skill from the classroom to the hospital or office and in having the right information at the right time. The traditional variety of continuing medical education (CME) activities has not been sufficiently satisfying in that role. Faced with gaps in practice and the realization that knowledge management is difficult for each individual, what can we do? One approach is to provide opportunities in the practice setting so that physicians receive information related to specific clinical problems as they need it.

Reminder and feedback systems create point-of-care interactions, not only as effective ways to assist physicians to use what they have learned but also to organize their behavior and reinforce new knowledge or skills in the context of care. They prompt clinicians to review more of what they know and to use new ways of practicing. However, reminder and feedback systems are not all the same and they are neither equally useful nor effective in every setting or situation. To take their place in the list of strategies for facilitating learning and change in clinical care, we must examine and think through their advantages and limitations.

DEFINITIONS

In fulfilling the need for strategies to extend the clinician's capacity to have information provided at the point of care, to judge his/her performance against peers, and to process the large number of variables presented by each patient, health managers, educators, researchers, and others have created information-delivery systems. This chapter focuses on reminders and feedback systems that show promise as techniques to extend the ways we can effectively support change in patient care.

The literature defines and differentiates each system as follows: *Reminder systems* provide practitioners with specific clinical information matched to specific criteria about a patient at the time of a patient visit. Oxman and colleagues[1] define reminders as consisting of any intervention, manual or computerized, that prompts the health care provider to perform a clinical action.

Reminder systems provide one-way communication from an expert source to an individual physician. This might be in the form of a recommendation regarding the need for a specific test, exam, or procedure, generally at the time of a patient visit or encounter. The chief complaint may be entirely separate from the subject of the reminder. For example, although patients come in to primary care practices for episodic visits, a reminder system might identify who is most at risk for influenza (eg, diabetics, seniors) and therefore would most benefit from a flu shot. Or the reminder might identify when, in the course routine diabetic care, is diet consultation most useful in the primary treatment for diabetes.

Feedback systems provide a clinician with information about his or her own performance in specific clinical areas, generally compared to other individuals, groups, practices, or standards. Oxman et al.[1] define a feedback system as "any summary of clinical performance of health care over a specified period, with or without recommendations for clinical action. This information may have been obtained from medical records, computerized databases, patients, or by observation." A feedback system might look to answer questions such as, How does Dr Bartlett's performance in preventive care compare with that of her peers? What is the ratio of lumpectomy versus modified radical mastectomy in group A compared to group B?

Reminders and feedback systems are similar in two ways: they are based on summarizing objective rather than subjective health care practices and they are intended to persuade or suggest rather than regulate. Generally, the clinician is free to accept or reject the clinical direction pointed to by the reminder or feedback. As such, they are not intended to dictate care but to raise points of patient management and questions for the physician to consider. (See Table 12-1.)

There are also differences between the two systems. For the most part, reminders are delivered at the time of a patient visit. On the other hand, although most often delivered in the office, ward, or other practice setting, feedback is less immediate and does not require the precise timing or location of a reminder. It can occur at any time after a visit or clinician-patient encounter—immediately or several weeks to months later. Further, the use of the standard or

TABLE 12-1

Reminders and Feedback—Common Characteristics

Reminders and feedback have two characteristics in common:

■ They're driven by someone other than the learner, based on objective rather than subjective needs.

■ They possess few, if any, regulatory, coercive strategies or incentives: the clinician is free to choose or refute the clinical directive pointed to by the reminder or feedback.

point of comparison for the reminder or feedback system differs between the two. Whenever possible, reminder systems are set against a background of evidence-based guidelines or practices. Feedback systems, although often based on guidelines, generally compare clinician to peer group, group to group, or clinician to standard. Reminder systems allow general standards, protocols, or norms to be applied in a specific encounter. Feedback permits a specific series of encounters to be generalized to groups, again applied against external standards, guidelines, and protocols.

DEVELOPING REMINDER AND FEEDBACK SYSTEMS

Key Players in Development

There are a variety of actors in the development of reminder systems, each of whom may use an array of information sources and distribution techniques. The process of creating reminder systems ranges widely, from straightforward attempts to put rational actions in front of practitioners (eg, a group agreeing that smoking-cessation programs are a "good thing" and instituting a simple prompt system) to complex processes involving the assessment of incidence and prevalence of clinical problems, performance reform, assessment of barriers, and evaluation of rate and extent of change.

An example of the latter might be Dr Westlake's decision in the scenario outlined above. The system might implement a major preventive health initiative, using prompts for mammograms and pap smears at each visit for eligible female patients and flu shots on a seasonal basis for every elderly patient or others at risk.

There are other promoters of these practice-based systems. Many reminder systems begin with a physician team member who wants to remember information or actions learned from a recognized expert source, eg, a senior colleague or a teacher in a CME course. Champions for such change often emerge from the quality assurance or improvement committee, managers of health care organizations, clinics and hospitals, and, increasingly, continuing professional development (CPD) professionals.

Using Feedback and Reminders to Meet Standards of Care

How do physicians and others establish standards in the development of feedback and reminders? Sometimes this initiative comes from the simple agreement that a particular clinical article formulates the right approach to a problem. However, faced with a plethora of literature, individual physicians, physician groups, and health care team members may customize a practice system that merges information from a professional society, government standards, literature, and/or institutional standards into a more personalized system that accounts for community standards and specific patient panels.

In any discussion of reminders and feedback, clinical practice guidelines (CPGs) form an important concept. Inasmuch as they provide the basis for many feedback and reminder systems, using the Institute of Medicine's initial work, we define them here as "systematically developed statements about specific clinical problems intended to be used as decision aids for both patients and practitioners."[2] Although arguments beyond the scope of this book ensue regularly about CPGs as "cookbook" medicine and the degree to which "evidence" (versus opinion) is applied in the making of the guideline, they are clearly one of the major forces behind decisions driving the development of reminders and feedback.

REMINDER SYSTEMS

A 58-year-old man comes in to his internist for a yearly physical. He is mildly hypertensive, moderately overweight, and concerned about his risk for a heart attack. He offers that his father died of a stroke at 55. Two kinds of reminders are clipped to his chart.

First, a simple prompt in the form of a sticker is attached to the patient record by the office receptionist indicating, "smoker; try counseling about quitting." Second, a more complex reminder takes the form of a checklist of screening and preventive health care strategies for men over age 50 based on national guidelines. That reminder is automatically generated by the office system because of the age of the patient. The link between excess weight, smoking, and hypertension is flagged for the latest patient information handouts.

Types of Reminders

Reminders appear in a variety of forms. They may be directed to health care professionals or to patients. These reminders are categorized by their method of transmission: print, team-member, computerized, public, and patient reminders.

Reminders in Print

Printed prompts clipped to a chart or patient record are the simplest form of reminder. These might include a note about a standard of care (eg, checking potassium when a patient is taking potassium-losing diuretics), suggestions about follow-up for an abnormal laboratory test, or a screening reminder specific to a particular population or type of problem briefly summarized or referenced. Wilson and colleagues, in their study of smoking cessation,[3] used prompts placed by receptionists on charts to encourage physicians to ask about smoking and to provide counseling about quitting.

Reminders Delivered by Team Members

Messages delivered by nurses, social workers, therapists, staff, or other team members form the second method. They may remind the physician (or others on the team) about a test or make recommendations for an intervention or a follow-up procedure. Foley and colleagues improved clinical compliance with recommendations about mammography by using a nurse-initiated system of clinician and patient reminders.[4] Further, Rhew and colleagues demonstrate that nurse-initiated vaccine protocols raised rates substantially more than physician or patient reminder systems in preventing certain types of pneumonia.[5]

Reminders Delivered by Electronic or Computerized Means

A third form of reminder makes use of electronic data and computer-based systems about patients and processes, described in more detail in Chapter 11. Balas[6] described a variety of electronic forms in the primary care setting including physician prompts, algorithm-generated decision-support systems, and interactive patient education or instruction.

Provider Prompt/Reminders. Two examples of noncomputerized prompts are provided by the vignette at the beginning of this section; delivering these at the time of a visit, in a computerized office setting, is relatively easy to imagine. Such computerized prompts appear to be useful in disease prevention, reminding primary care physicians to screen for cholesterol, hypertension, cancer, or other disorders. Further, they also appear to help in the management of complex chronic problems such as diabetes, flagging those at risk for complications such as amputation.[7] Finally, unlike paper formats, these systems can require physicians to respond to computer-generated prompts—an apparently successful maneuver.[8]

Decision-support Systems. A variety of authors report on the use of computerized support systems useful in diagnosis, case management, and treatment—each providing reminders in the form of electronically mediated algorithms, protocols, or flow charts. Johnson and colleagues[9] reviewed controlled trials of such systems, finding positive effects on physician performance in the following areas: three of four studies in computer-assisted dosing, one of five studies of computer-aided diagnosis, four of six studies in preventive care, and seven of nine studies of computer-aided quality assurance for medical care. These data are suggestive of a powerful effect for this more complex reminder system in disease management in most of these areas. Even more elaborate "expert systems" have also been described, eg, in pediatrics. Johnson and Feldman describe the usefulness, both real and potential, of Meditel, Iliad, Quick Medical Reference, and Dxplain™.[10] A study about approaches to acute abdominal pain confirms that using computer-aided decision support improved diagnostic and decision-making performance.[11]

Interactive Treatment, Patient Education.   Some computer systems target the patient, not only for the purposes of health promotion or understanding disease but also as an attempt to encourage appropriate physician or other health provider behavior. Examples can be found in lifestyle modification, the results of which may be forwarded to the physician, prompting questions and action.

Portable Technologies.   Increasingly, many physicians use handheld devices, such as palm pilots, on which they have downloaded reminders in the form of short algorithms, formulas, or treatment protocols. These innovative technologies, when electronically linked to the Internet, can also deliver reminders to clinicians throughout their workday, on hospital rounds, during home visits, or in the offices, replacing and augmenting older forms of information delivery by page, beeper, phone, or email.[12]

Reminders as Public Messages

Messages directed to the public encourage adults and teens to bring new kinds of questions to their physicians and to be empowered in their own care. First, public health messages, recommendations from government agencies, and other sources occur in schools, at work sites, on TV, and in newspapers and magazines. Examples include smoking cessation ads and domestic abuse messages. Second, some messages from the pharmaceutical industry form an emerging type of reminder system, providing the patient with specific questions about treatment options (among many other areas) for allergies and acid reflux problems. Third, there are many examples of joint efforts. For example, specialty societies, disease-specific groups (eg, the American Diabetes Association), and others such as government or industry may work together to reduce the incidence or to spot the early signs of such entities as Alzheimer's disease, diabetes, heart disease, and mental illness.

Reminders to Patients

In contrast to widespread public media campaigns, several forms of more targeted patient reminders are available. There are many types—phone calls from staff members to patients, post cards and other mailed reminders, waiting room posters, and flyers are common examples. Saywell and other investigators[13] tested the cost-effectiveness of five patient-focused interventions geared to increase mammography for breast cancer screening. Three of the methods (in-person, telephone plus letter, and in-person plus letter) had significantly better compliance rates compared with the control, physician letter, or telephone alone. However, when considering costs, only one emerged. In this study, telephone plus letter was the most cost-effective strategy.

Another study by Lythgoe[14] details the success of phoned patient reminders for immunizations, cancer screening, and other preventive measures. As in the case of physician reminders, computerization of office records can play a sizable role. Further, computer telephony integration technology shows promise: it automates wellness and recall messages. This technology can be personalized and can remind patients of preventive or other health measures.

Reminders Coupled with Other Methods.   Reminders can be used with any of the other educational methods and strategies outlined in this chapter and elsewhere throughout the book.

Casebeer and her colleagues[15] in Alabama determined the effectiveness of case-based, interactive audio conferences and chart reminders in increasing physicians' adherence-enhancing skills and improving cholesterol levels. In a prospective randomized controlled trial (RCT) of 28 community physicians and more than 200 outpatients with high cholesterol, physician learning was measured by unannounced standardized patients, and patients' health by serum cholesterol levels, weight, knowledge of hypercholesterolemia, self-reported dietary habits, and health status. The authors found significant differences in the intervention group's patients' knowledge of cholesterol management, reductions in their self-reported dietary intake of fats, and a decrease in the serum cholesterol level of men in the intervention group nine months after the intervention. They conclude that combining standard audio conferences with chart reminders shows promise in increasing physicians' adherence-enhancing strategies, but note that the "problem of enhancing adherence remains complex."

FEEDBACK

Ashish Bageria is a 35-year-old general practitioner practicing in inner city Chicago. He's reviewing his month-end summary of preventive practices and notes that— judged against his peers—his rate of anticoagulation for atrial fibrillation in patients over 65 is very low, below that of all his colleagues, in fact. He puzzles over this, thinking, first, that he is sure his rate is much higher and, second, that *his* patients are different than others', perhaps much older, more frail, and more prone to falls, perhaps cognitively less able to take daily medications on a regular basis.

Halfway around the world, Jeannette VanVoerd studies feedback on her performance over the last six months in diabetes management. An Australian general internist practicing in a large ambulatory care clinic, Jeannette notices with some pleasure that her patients' glycosolated hemoglobin (HbA1C) levels, averaged over the period, are within a highly acceptable range, compared to the national diabetic care standards. But she wonders about those cases in which she knows there is poor compliance with diet and other measures, and thinks that her group should be developing their own local standards.

A feedback system represents specific communication about physicians' actual practices in managing patients, other practitioners' performance, and/or a set of standards for optimal care. Such systems help a physician measure his or her practice compared to that of others and to an outside source of expertise. They raise and help answer questions such as these:

- How often did you record blood pressure measurements for your patients in July?
- What are the recommended standards?
- How does your performance compare to that of your peers or team members or to other groups?
- Do you use more complex, expensive antibiotics more often than a comparable group of physicians in another setting?
- Do you refer more patients to specialists than the standards set by your employer?

Specific criteria are used to review the performance data of a particular physician or group of physicians and are then compared to national or local standards, institutional mandates, or practices of other physicians in a group. Here are some examples:

- A primary care physician receives a note comparing her rate of diagnosis of depression with others in her group over the past three months;
- General internal medicine team members review graphs outlining how frequently they screen for hypertension, document smoking status, or order HbA1c tests on their diabetic patients;
- Obstetricians interpret comparative data outlining how frequently they perform certain procedures (eg, Cesarean sections, Pap smears) on their patients compared to other groups or to themselves, within groups.

Feedback is explained in terms of its importance to the learning process, the time of delivery, its sources, and its targets.

Learning Depends on Feedback

When practicing a new procedure or applying a new concept, learners need and value tests, assessments, and feedback in order to learn. Optimal learning uses feedback, early and often. Without specific, direct information about a work pattern, an individual must guess whether he or she is "in compliance" with best practices, a notoriously difficult task. Although any group of physicians may have good reasons for noncompliance with established patterns for some or all of their patients, feedback systems provide a way to help physicians look at their work in very specific, concrete ways. Agreement from physicians that the comparative standards are practical, useful, and demonstrate good medicine is essential. Feedback works best when there are agreed upon standards that fit the patient panel for the individual or group involved.

Feedback may be part of a learning experience. In one study, the authors provided primary care physicians with video feedback of real and role-played psychiatric consultations.[16] In another, a brief training program on skills, attitudes, and knowledge about problem drinking was followed by individual tutorials and feedback; participants scored significantly higher on measures of counseling skills, among other items.[17] In a third study, simulated patients provided immediate systematic feedback to physician learners about their approach to breast cancer screening. With background information, instruction, and brief feedback, improvements were significant.[18]

Outside of these resources that are dependent on other people, most feedback is the result of audit or other systematic review of the data in patient care provided by charts, utilization data, surveys of patients, and other sources. This type of feedback is explored in greater detail in Section II of the book.

Timing of Feedback

Feedback to a clinician may summarize his or her performance data over a period as short as a week or over much longer periods. Once summarized, these data may be provided to the physician, a week, month, or several months later. Although study effects vary, most believe that the more immediate the feedback, the better. For example, results of last month's Pap smear procedures (or barriers to performing them) are more present in the physician's mind, more able to be recalled, and thus (at least in theory) more apt to produce change in physician performance.

Sources of Feedback

Three major sources, individually or in combination, provide the basis for establishing a feedback system. They are discussed in the following paragraphs.

First, and most commonly, uninterpreted data is generated from clinical records, using such sources as chart audit, prescribing summaries, records of lab tests, utilization, and other information sources. Second, using survey methods, individuals or groups of patients may provide feedback to a physician, team members, or clinic about communication, interpersonal skills, or perceptions of quality of care. Hospital satisfaction questionnaires are a common example. Third, group discussion by peers, consultants, or team members may be directed to changing practices by agreement within a group. Such a process, reported by Fidler and her colleagues in Alberta, Canada, generates change and learning on the part of most physicians.[19] When physicians received feedback from peers, referring physicians, coworkers, and patients, 83% reported having contemplated a change and 66% reported having initiated a change for at least one aspect of practice. Finally, when respected clinical leaders help establish the process of feedback, dissemination of local and national utilization data, guidelines, and outcome studies are more powerful.[20,21]

Target of the Feedback

Individual Feedback

Directing data to individual clinicians appears in numerous studies, with good results noted in many of these trials and across a wide range of clinical topics.

First, positive performance changes have been noted in acute and ambulatory medical management of patients, in such diverse subjects as the time to initiate thrombolytic (clot-busting) treatment[22] and diabetic care[23] in diverse settings. Eagle and colleagues demonstrated that practice guidelines were more effective in reducing intensive care unit and hospital utilization with feedback.[24] In the primary care setting, group practices enhanced their effectiveness in using guidelines by means of an ambulatory care medical audit system.[25]

Second, test ordering is a popular subject of audit and feedback, as a few examples demonstrate. Feedback about lab test ordering and their costs decreased requests for tests among physicians,[26] and among physicians, nurses, and physician assistants in thyroid testing.[27] In a further study, when physicians received a monthly overview comparing individual use of laboratory tests with a group of peers, individuals indicated they valued the information as a way to think about their own practices.[28]

Third, in the area of preventive care, intensive medical record review with individualized feedback to primary care residents produced high levels of compliance with practice guidelines for preventive care.[29] In addition, Holmboe and colleagues, using medical record audit and individualized feedback on prevention guidelines, produced exceptionally high levels of compliance with preventive care practices among internal medicine residents.[30] Finally, representing specialist practice, anesthesiologists' performance changed in regard to preventive measures with individual feedback and enhanced education.[31]

Not all areas of medical care, however, may lend themselves to feedback; less promising outcomes were found in some studies. One of these, by Socolar and colleagues, sought to improve physician documentation and knowledge of child sexual abuse, tailoring feedback to physicians with directed educational materials. The intervention failed to improve most aspects of documentation and knowledge.[32] This study, and others, may reflect our poor understanding of management for some complex problems and the role of feedback in that process.

Group Feedback

There are several examples of feedback delivered to groups of practitioners. For example, Norton and his colleagues employed simple annual feedback to a group of family physicians during a one-hour discussion to improve Pap smear rates.[33] Similarly, Billi implemented a cost feedback intervention to alter group behavior in general medicine services, demonstrating a decreased length of stay and decrease in costs.[34] Finally, Freeborn et al. used bimonthly feedback about group practices for use of X-rays of the lumbar spine.[35] This study's failure to decrease these rates may raise questions about practice setting and patient expectations as powerful forces, in this case not overcome by the feedback process.

EVIDENCE FOR EFFECTIVENESS: DO REMINDERS AND FEEDBACK WORK?

Individual studies provide an interesting view of the use of reminder and feedback systems. Systematic reviews of the literature are another source of interpretation, which provides a somewhat broader look. And, negative studies round out the picture by their help describing some of the barriers to change.

Reminders

Physician Reminders

A 1995 review of randomized controlled trials of interventions to change physician performance indicated that, along with multiphasic interventions and perhaps patient-mediated strategies, only physician reminders showed promise of being an effective single change agent.[36] Here, reminders to physicians effected change in 22 of 26 studies.

Further, more specific reviews analyze the effect on reminder systems, highlighting the effect of a variety of parameters. For example, a meta-analysis of 16 randomized controlled trials of such systems supports the view that, in the ambulatory care setting, computer-based reminders improved most (though not all) preventive practices.[37] Improvements were noted in immunization, mammography, colorectal cancer screening, and cardiovascular risk reduction, but not, for example, in cervical cancer screening or other preventive measures. As we have seen earlier in this chapter, practice setting, physician characteristics, and patient demographics also influence the effectiveness of reminders. Yarnall et al, in a family practice setting, described the implementation and subsequent use of a computerized health maintenance tracking system in a large, urban North Carolina community health center with low-income African-Americans.[38] At each office visit, clinicians received a computerized encounter form indicating needed screening tests, counseling, and immunizations for each randomly selected study patient. However, even with prompting, clinicians only addressed health maintenance with this population of patients about half of the time.[38]

Patient Reminders

Wagner uses a meta-analysis of the effectiveness of mailed patient reminders on mammography screening to provide an answer to the question of the effectiveness of patient prompts. In 16 published articles, women who received reminders were approximately 50% more likely to get a mammogram. Further, personalized letters were found to be more effective than generic reminders.[39]

However, not all studies of patient reminders produce positive results, indicating the effect of patient age, insurance plans, and other variables need consideration in the development of any patient reminder system.[40] Clayton evaluated the effectiveness of an annual public health strategy in a managed care setting. In that study, patients 65 and older who had previously received influenza immunization were randomized to an intervention group (a mailed postcard reminder) or a control group (no postcard).[40] There were no differences in vaccination rates between the groups.

Feedback

O'Brien and her colleagues reviewed the effects of audit and feedback on professional practice and health care outcomes.[41] Overall, these reviewers found 37 studies that matched their criteria. They targeted outcomes in diagnostic test ordering, prescribing practices, preventive care, and general medical management. The relative percentage changes ranged from −16% to 152%. Eight of 13 trials in which audit and feedback were used alone changed physician behavior. Similarly, in 15 studies in which feedback was combined with educational materials or meetings, 10 showed positive changes. When audit and feedback were used as one strategy of many, 6 of 11 studies showed such a positive outcome.

Other citations about the difficulty of changing physician behavior for specific practices are also readily available. The effectiveness (and the ineffectiveness) of some trials using feedback methods speaks to a variety of issues. First, the changes required may be too difficult to address in a single study, or a single patient visit, or in many busy practice settings. The treatment of depression in the elderly, for example, is a complex problem; enhancing diagnostic skills by feedback is only one piece of a large management puzzle. Second, feedback systems may not be part of the culture of interaction for a given group of physicians. In many offices, hospitals, ambulatory care clinics, and other settings, peer interactions and many other factors influence the methods and patterns of learning. Third, clinical settings may not be using feedback with other supportive mechanisms for change. If a physician wants to follow new guidelines, but equipment, paper methods, and staff support are missing, such changes may not be possible. Fourth, and finally, the physician's perception of the feedback (does he agree with it? does she truly believe that her practice and patient population are different? is he prepared to act on it?) speaks to intraprovider issues, explored elsewhere in this book.

FROM EVIDENCE TO CPD: USING NONTRADITIONAL TOOLS TO EFFECT CHANGE

Educators, clinicians, CME providers, quality-assurance managers, and others share the attempt to turn the flood of educational and CPD literature, studies, surveys, and theories into usable, workable techniques. The following outlines several steps in the process of implementing such information using audit, feedback, and reminders.

Step 1: Choose what to change: establish evidence for action and gaps in performance or care. We might also call this step, "choose your battles," or "you can't solve all problems all the time." In the face of this advice, and in a situation in which a large number of clinical areas require attention, the CPD provider needs to select areas of need in practice among groups of physicians in health care teams, in hospitals, or in managed care organizations that fit at least two criteria. First, there is clear evidence that the proposed clinical change will benefit patient outcomes. Second, there is evidence that a gap exists in practice or outcomes at the intended level.

Step 2: Lay the groundwork: establish buy-in on the part of clini-cians. There's pretty clear evidence—from the clinical world, stud-ies on guideline implementation, and the educator's perspective in adult education (two sides of the house represented in this book)—that ownership of the need for change, the evidence behind that need (both medical evidence and the evidence about the size and extent of the gap), and the type and frequency of educational inter-ventions are important.

With that in mind, securing buy-in is a clear and necessary sec-ond step, a process that reviews barriers to change, clinician and team motivation, and other success-dependent factors. The jury's out on exactly how to do this, but we propose considering some of the following strategies, including focus groups, interactive educa-tional meetings, consensus conferences, and Delphi methods, to name a few. These meetings also provide a necessary first step in allowing all physicians and team members an educational "level playing field," in which they are exposed to shared information at the same time.

Step 3: Decide what to do. There are two parts to this apparently simple statement.

> *A: Consider the theoretical basis on which reminders and feed-back work.* It is useful to think about the essential components of the models of change outlined elsewhere in this book. In part, this helps to clarify how and why these strategies work for the CPD professional. In addition, they help to explain the strat-egy to others who will be affected by it.
>
> *B: Choose the strategy.* Consider some questions, such as the nature of the change required, the size of the gap, the barriers to change, the clinical topic areas, and the provider of feed-back, among other variables. Figure 12-1 provides a checklist that may be helpful in this regard.

Step 4: Implement the strategy. Those who wish to foster change must decide how these change strategies will work, using their own experience, the evidence and theory presented in this chapter, and an understanding of facilitating professional development and best practices. Although knowing when to use feedback is neither clear nor simple, all learning systems consider feedback to be essential for success. One way to approach this dilemma of when and how to use feedback and reminder systems is to develop a rich defini-tion for these systems, using examples of systems in place or tested elsewhere, and to suggest ways to think about their roles in an in-tegrated learning system.

Step 5: Evaluate the outcomes. Use practice data and the perfor-mance gap outlined in Step 1 to determine whether the intervention has made a difference.

FIGURE 12-1

Choosing the Strategy: Using Feedback and Reminders

Feedback Systems			
Timing:	Immediate	Delayed	Ongoing
Data Source:			
Chart audit			
Utilization review			
Peer/outside group			
Patients			
Expert opinion/external body			
Delivery Method:			
Colleague			
Supervisor/chair/director			
Educational influential/opinion leader			
Employer			
Professional associate/outside expert			
Reminder Systems			
Method:	Paper	Electronic	Combined
Target:	Physician Team	Patients	Combined
Type:	Simple	Complex (algorithms)	Decision-support
Use of Collateral Methods			
Educational meetings, sessions, workshops			
Educational materials—print, computerized, audiovisual			
Opinion leaders			

TABLE 12-2

Using Feedback and Reminders to Change Practice Performance

Step 1: Decide what to change: use practice guidelines, other clinical evidence, and establish gaps in care

Step 2: Lay the groundwork: establish buy-in among clinicians

Step 3: Decide what to do:
    a) Use theory
    b) Choose reminders, feedback both +/− other methods

Step 4: Establish the intervention

Step 5: Measure the outcome by re-measuring the gap

See Table 12-2 for steps to use feedback and reminders to change practice performance.

CONCLUSION

This chapter has explored reminders and feedback as useful additions to the large and growing armamentarium of the CPD professional. Their ability to be grafted onto the practice setting, and their differences from traditional educational activities, help in situations of information overload and data overload, like those outlined by Drs Atkins and Westlake at the chapter's outset. Further, both reminders and feedback provide direct, point-of-care measurable learning systems. Evidence suggests that these can be effective, especially in preventive care and the management of specific medical issues.

Despite their overall effectiveness and growing use, as shown in the examples, many questions remain unanswered. We do not yet have a widespread understanding of and standards for disclosure of specific behaviors found in feedback systems. Further, we have little information about feedback to both patients and health providers. Should patients have information about the number of times their physicians prescribe certain classes of drugs or make selected diagnoses? Is it helpful to know how many times a physician has done a procedure and the complication rate?

In addition, our understanding of individual behavior within a system calls for at least three sorts of inquiry. First, we need to examine more closely the role of the learner/health practitioner when faced with reminders and feedback. Second, we need to understand the system itself, not only the particulars of the reminder or feedback but also the larger practice setting in which these play out. Managed care and fee-for-service provide widely different variables. Third, we need a better understanding of what kinds and formats of information to use in reminder and feedback systems, in addition to clearer pictures of how that information can be used most productively. These are provided by quality assurance professionals like Dr Westlake, by practitioners such as Ashish Bagheria and Jeannette VanVoerd, and by CPD professionals like ourselves. The rich and complex questions appeal to investigators and practitioners in their ability to clarify and apply these ideas in practice.

REFERENCES—CHAPTER 12

1. Oxman AD, Thomson MA, Davis DA, Haynes RB. No magic bullets: a systematic review of 102 trials of interventions to improve professional practice. *Can Med Assoc J.* 1996;153:1423–1431.

2. Institute of Medicine. *Clinical Practice Guidelines: Directions for a New Program.* Field MJ, Lohr KN, eds. Washington, DC: National Academy Press; 1990.

3. Wilson DM, Taylor DW, Gilbert JR, Best JA, Lindsay EA, Wilms DG, Singer J. A randomized trial of a family physician intervention for smoking cessation. *JAMA.* 1988;260:1570–1574.

4. Foley EC, D'Amico F, Merenstein JH. Improving mammography recommendation: a nurse-initiated intervention. *J Am Board Fam Pract.* 1990;3:87–92.

5. Rhew DC, Glassman PA, Goetz MB. Improving pneumococcal vaccine rates. Nurse protocols versus clinical reminders. *J Gen Intern Med.* 1999;14:351–356.

6. Balas EA, Autin SM, Mitchell JA, et al. The clinical value of computerized information services—a review of 98 randomized controlled trials. *Arch Fam Med.* 1996;5:271–278.

7. Khoury A, Landers P, Roth M, et al. Computer-supported identification and intervention for diabetic patients at risk for amputation. *MD Compu.* 1998;15:307–310.

8. Litzelman DK, Dittus RS, Miller ME, Tierney WM. Requiring physicians to respond to computerized reminders improves their compliance with preventive care protocols. *J Gen Intern Med.* 1993;8:311–317.

9. Johnson ME, Langton KB, Haynes RB, Mathieu A. Effects of computer-based clinical decision support systems and patient outcome. A critical appraisal of research. *Am Intern Med.* 1994;120:135–142.

10. Johnson KB, Feldman MJ: Medical informatics and pediatrics. Decision-support systems. *Arch Ped Adolsc Med.* 1995;149:1371–1380.

11. De Dombal FT, Dallas V, McAdam WA: Can computer aided teaching packages improve clinical care in patients with acute abdominal pain? *BMJ.* 1991;302:1495–1497.

12. Wagner MM, Eisenstadt SA, Hogan WR, Pankaskie MC. Preferences of interns and residents for e-mail, paging, or traditional methods for the delivery of different types of clinical information. *Proc AMIA Symp.* 1998;140–144.

13. Saywell RMJ, Champion VL, Skinner CS, McQuillen D, Martin D, Maraj M. Cost-effectiveness comparison of five interventions to increase mammography screening. *Prev Med.* 1999; 29:374–382.

14. Lythgoe MS. Computerized telephone reminder system facilitates wellness and prevention. *J Med Pract Manage.* 1999;14:204–208.

15. Casebeer LL, Klapow JC, Centro RM, et al. The intervention to increase physicians' use of adherence-enhancing strategies in managing hypercholesterolemic patients. *Acad Med.* 1999;74:1332–1339.

16. Gask L. Small group interactive techniques utilizing videofeedback. *Int J Psychiatry Med.* 1998;28:97–113.

17. Ockene JK, Wheeler EV, Adams A, Hurley TG, Hebert J. Provider training for patient-centered alcohol counseling in a primary care setting. *Arch Intern Med.* 1997;157:2334–2341.

18. Costanza ME, Greene HL, McManus D, Hoople NE, Barth R. Can practicing physicians improve their counseling and physical examination skills in breast cancer screening? A feasibility study. *J Cancer Educ.* 1995;10:14–21.

19. Fidler H, Lockyer JM, Towes J, Violato C. Changing physicians' practices: the effect of individual feedback. *Acad Med.* 1999;74:702–714.

20. Soumerai SB, McLaughlin TJ, Gurwitz JH, Guadagnoli E, Hauptman PJ, Borbas C, Morris N, McLaughlin B, Gao X, Willison DJ, Asinger R, Gobel F. Effect of local medical opinion leaders on quality of care for acute myocardial infarction; a randomized controlled trial. *JAMA.* 1998;279:1358–1363.

21. Conway AC, Keller RB, Wennberg DE. Partnering with physicians to achieve quality improvement. *Jt Comm Qual Improv.* 1995;21:619–626.

22. Cummings P. Improving the time to thrombolytic therapy for myocardial infarction by using a quality assurance audit. *Ann Emerg Med.* 1992;21:1107–1110.

23. Lobach DF. Electronically distributed, computer-generated, individualized feedback enhances the use of computerized practice guideline. *Proc AMIA Annu Fall Symp.* 1996;493–497.

24. Eagle KA, Mulley AG, Skates SJ. Length of stay in the intensive care unit: effects of practice guidelines and feedback. *JAMA.* 1990;264:992–997.

25. Palmer RH, Hargraves JL. Quality improvement among primary care practitioners: an overall appraisal of results of the ambulatory care medical audit demonstration project. *Med Care.* 1996;34:SS102–SS113.

26. Gama R, Nightingale PG, Broughton PM, et al. Modifying the request behavior of clinicians. *J Clin Pathol.* 1992;45:248–249.

27. Schectman JM, Elinsky EG, Pawlson LG. Effect of education and feedback on thyroid function testing strategies of primary care clinicians. *Arch Intern Med.* 1991;151:2163–2166.

28. Winkens RA, Pop P, Bugter-Maessen AM, et al. Radomized controlled trial of routine individual feedback to improve rationality and reduce numbers of test requests. *Lancet.* 1995;345:498–502.

29. Nasmith L, Boillat M, Rubenstein H, Diagle N, Goldstein H, Franco ED. Faculty advisor program for family medicine residents. *Can Fam Physician.* 1997;43:1257–1263.

30. Holmboe ES, Scranton R, Sumption K, Hawkins R. Effects of medical record audit and feedback on residents' compliance with preventive health care guidelines. *Acad Med.* 1998;73:901–903.

31. Cohen MM, Rose DK, Yee DA. Changing anesthesiologists' practice patterns: can it be done? *Anesthesiology.* 1996;85:260–269.

32. Socolar RR, Raine B, Chen-Mok M, et al. Intervention to improve physician documentation and knowledge of child sexual abuse: a randomized controlled trial. *Pediatrics.* 1998;101:817–824.

33. Norton PG, Shaw PA, Murray MA. Quality improvement in family practice. Program for Papsmears. *Can Fam Physician.* 1997;43:503–508.

34. Billi JE. The effects of a low-cost intervention program on hospital cost. *J Gen Intern Med.* 1992;7:411–417.

35. Freeborn DK, Shye D, Mullooly JP, Eraker S, Romeo J. Primary care physicians' use of lumbar spine imaging tests: effects of guidelines and practice pattern feedback. *J Gen Intern Med.* 1997;12:619–625.

36. Davis DA, Thomson MA, Oxman AD, Haynes RB. Changing physician performance. A systematic review of the effect of continuing medical education strategies. *JAMA.* 1995;274:700–705.

37. Shea S, DuMouchel W, Bahamonde L. A meta-analysis of 16 randomized controlled trials to evaluate computer-based reminder systems in preventive care in the ambulatory setting. *JAMA.* 1996;3:339–409.

38. Yarnall KS, Rimer BK, Hynes D, et al. Computerized prompts for cancer screening in a community health center. *J Am Board Fam Pract.* 1998;11:96–104.

39. Wagner TH. The effectiveness of mailed patient reminders on mammography screening: as meta-analysis. *Am J Prev Med.* 1998;14:64–70.

40. Clayton AE, McNutt LA, Homestead HL, et al. Public health in managed care: a randomized controlled trial of the effectiveness of postcard reminders. *Am J Public Health.* 1999;89:1235–1237.

41. O'Brien G, Lazebnik R. Telephone call reminders and attendance in an adolescent clinic. *Pediatrics.* 1998;101:E6.

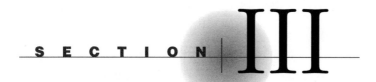

Deciding About Effectiveness

Primary editor: Robert Fox, EdD

A Clinical Thematic: Deciding What Was Done and How Well It Was Done

Dave Davis, MD; Robert Fox, EdD;
Barbara E. Barnes, MD; Karen Costie, RN

Two months have passed since Dr Ted Brucken first saw Marjory Hall for symptoms related to diabetes. It took weekly visits following her initial complaint before Marjory was fully diagnosed and her treatment plan was in place. She is now on medication and her blood sugar is under good control. She continues to lose weight, but this is because of the changes she has made in her eating habits. An appointment with a local ophthalmologist has uncovered mild diabetic retinopathy, but her lowered blood sugar has improved her vision so that Marjory can now better see her computer screen at work. Her energy level has returned to a level that she thinks is good; she has not missed a day of work in over a month. She admits that the anxiety over her social situation can sometimes be overwhelming; being the sole caregiver for her young granddaughter made her realize that she must do all she can to maintain good health.

Reflecting back on that time, Ted recalled how unhappy he was at the way that he handled Marjory and her concerns. He felt that he should have been more aware of the risk for Marjory; the warning signs had all been there in one way or another for a few years. He certainly didn't pick up on the high level of fear and anxiety that expressed itself in his office on her second visit to him. He knew that he should be thanking Marjory for being the catalyst in his new plan for his own professional development.

As he drives home from the office, he remembers the stack of unread journals on his desk. He remembers feeling a little disconnected from his Monday night "quality circle" at the Mountainside Medical Group. The members of the group seemed to have a better handle on the latest literature and advancements than Ted. And he remembers how concerned he was when he realized that mandatory board recertification was less than two years away and that he didn't have a plan to help him prepare.

Members of the "quality circle" and their suggestions helped to provide some direction for his own education related to diabetes. Taking the first step, Ted went to the American Diabetic Association (ADA) Web site and found the practice guidelines. As he read them, he realized that he really knew more than he thought he did; there were only two or three of the recommendations that he thought he might need to learn more about. It came as a relief for him to discover that he was not as far away from current practice as he thought he was. The ADA also offered an online self-assessment exercise that helped him to narrow his focus of learning even more. Now, knowing that he had only several issues to research, he felt that he could find the materials and resources he needed. His plan involved scanning the table of contents of all the journals stacked on his desk and looking specifically for articles related to the management of diabetes. His search yielded three articles, all relevant to his learning needs, written in peer-reviewed journals. He could manage to read three articles while having lunch.

He was concerned over the cost of medication for Marjory, since she covers this bill out of her own pocket. The articles covered the newer, more expensive hypoglycemic (sugar-lowering) agents, but Ted felt these were not necessary for Marjory. Making rounds on his patients in the Rainier County General Hospital, Ted bumps into an old friend from medical school, now an endocrinologist. Ted asks for some advice on effective, low-cost pharmacological treatment options for Marjory. His friend also suggests that, given the widespread nature of this disease in the local community, Ted might attend a mini-symposium on type 2 diabetes to be held in the hospital auditorium next week. The symposium has a track for health professionals and for patients and family members. Ted agrees it is a good idea and plans to attend.

Ted found a diabetic flow chart in one of the articles he was reading. How could this help him? One of his colleagues in the "quality circle" used a similar flow chart. Comparing the items on both sheets, Ted developed his own, adding specific items he had learned from his recent readings. This would stand not only as a reminder to check the status of Marjory's diabetes but also as a measure of the progress of her disease and its management. He determines to put this diabetic checklist in the front of all of his diabetic patients' charts where he could use it at the point of care.

Finally, he returned to the "quality circle" to update the group on Marjory and her clinical status and to share his own new knowledge and flow chart with them. He reported to the group that he had been unaware of the community resources available for patients and that a phone call to a local diabetes education center helped steer him in the right direction for a group that would educate, motivate, and encourage Marjory to succeed. She was now part of a monthly support group. This group helped Marjory deal with her newly diagnosed diabetes and also gave her a social outlet where, in fact, she had made a few new friends.

DISCUSSION

The Impact of CPD

It is interesting that there are so many outcomes in this scenario—each positive, but each different. This section is designed to help the continuing professional development (CPD) professional search for and identify the variety of outcomes that indicate the value, nature, and extent of the processes and products of CPD activities. The case describes how some outcomes are part of an ongoing process of development in which Ted is engaged. They are merely milestones, or stepping-stones, to the next need, the next project, and the next outcome, all in a flow of development that represents the heart of professionalism.

Likewise, the outcomes for the patient are many and varied—part of the continuous process of management of her chronic illness in the context of her complicated life. Finally, the system of health care changes as Ted learns new ways of performing his role and assisting Marjory to better health.

The Patient

Patient outcomes can present in many ways, and in this particular case the patient experienced mostly positive outcomes. Improved clinical parameters, increased level of function, and reduced anxiety are all outcomes of the interventions employed by both the patient and physician, working in collaboration to improve health. The patient is the direct recipient of a concerted effort on Ted's part to raise his knowledge and skill and alter his attitude related to her illness. In fact, this new learning has been incorporated into the management of Ted's other diabetic patients.

The Physician

Although Ted is pleased with the outcomes related to this particular case, he is not happy that he found himself lacking the knowledge about diabetes he needed to have in order to practice with confidence and to match his own personal standard of a high level of competence. This experience has led him to become more focused in his own professional development.

Ted has developed a method of learning that he hopes will change several things. By identifying his actual learning needs, he has saved valuable time. He may follow this approach with each new gap that he uncovers. In this way, the mountain of journals and the fear that his patients may not be optimally cared for are reduced. He may make a diagnosis in one visit instead of two and may have found a treatment plan that benefits the patient and the insurance company in terms of cost-effectiveness.

Perhaps most importantly, Ted has learned that the gap between where he was and where he needed to be in his knowledge of detection, diagnosis, and treatment of diabetes was not large or insurmountable. In fact, it only took a few hours to learn what he needed to know. Ted now has a plan that helps him identify areas of his practice that fall short of his own desire for competence. He systematically chooses the materials and resources, such as literature, self-assessments, colleagues, and his "quality circle" group, to help answer the questions he has related to his own specific learning needs. This method of streamlining knowledge gaps has shown Ted that once you can be specific about your own learning needs, the time, effort, and resources needed to learn will be directed efficiently and effectively toward that goal. In fact, Ted has learned more about how to learn, an important outcome in his overall development.

The System of Care Delivery

The system of care delivery is a complex one. The stakeholders range from the patient and his or her physician, the immediate practice environment, including practice groups or hospital and health networks, third-party payers, and the community itself. Each, some more than others, has felt the impact of the changes in Ted's performance related to diabetes care—the introduction of flow charts is only one example at his local clinic level. In addition, Ted has been able to share new knowledge with his "quality circle" peers, changing the usual practices of several parts of the health care system.

The Health of the Public

By expanding his reach to include colleagues and other health professionals involved in the care of the diabetic patient, Ted can learn more about diagnosing and managing diabetes in his community. He recognizes that participating in population-based educational strategies, such as the mini-symposium, will assist in the process of sharing and learning in a community of practice. Ted's engagement in his own CPD will also benefit his colleagues in the "quality circle," as well as patients in his practice. By introducing new screening strategies recommended by one of the guidelines, diabetes may be detected before organ damage occurs and perhaps before the cost of treatment is an issue for the patient, physician, and supporting health system. Taken together, the dissemination of the processes and outcomes that result from Ted's odyssey of learning have led to ripples throughout the population of the community as new knowledge, skills, and ways of practicing are disseminated, formally and informally, throughout the community.

The CPD of Physicians

This section offers three chapters, each addressing important aspects of the ways that CPD provides and educators may search out and describe the outcomes of efforts to facilitate learning and development of physicians. In Chapter 13, Don Moore describes the different levels of outcomes that may result from attempts to facilitate learning and change. He expands the earlier models of evaluation of CPD to include new elements such as population health in the conceptual models and practical plans of CPD providers.

Penny Jennett and her coauthors offer in Chapter 14 an expansive array of practical tips and guidelines for the many methods and techniques associated with the evaluation of CPD efforts. The approach is to synthesize and apply knowledge of evaluation methods that is fugitive to the education of many CPD professionals. The extensive use of tables and figures adds to this authoritative reference for daily application. It expands perspective and builds a toolbox for describing and explaining the changes offered by Moore.

Finally, in Chapter 15, Paul Mazmanian also expands perspectives on evaluation by describing ways the new approaches may be used to identify outcomes and evaluate both evaluations and evidence. His perspective speaks to the need for new ways to think about this process. He offers a firm philosophical foundation that may enable practitioners to sort out the relative merits of different approaches to discovery, description, and explanation of processes and products of efforts to facilitate learning and change. He also introduces readers to the important distinctions and uses for qualitative and quantitative approaches to research and evaluation. Overall, this chapter focuses on the horizons of evaluation—the outcomes of CPD activity.

chapter 13

A Framework for Outcomes Evaluation in the Continuing Professional Development of Physicians*

Donald E. Moore, Jr, PhD

INTRODUCTION

It has become increasingly important for continuing medical education (CME) practitioners to assess and document the effectiveness of CME activities that they offer to physicians. What was once a research issue that concerned a small cadre of investigators has now become an operational issue for all CME practitioners. This challenge is being driven by increasing concerns about the quality and cost of health care,[1,2] due, in part, to the wide variability in physician practice that does not appear to be based on research-derived evidence.[3] Under these conditions, leaders in the medical profession, health care administrators, and state regulatory officials are concerned that physicians and the health care system may not be performing at optimal levels and have begun to establish mechanisms to monitor and ensure the maintenance of physician competence.[4]

CME has long played a central role in the maintenance of physician competence, although its precise role has remained obscure because of the lack of adequate measurement techniques or

---

* An earlier version of the material presented in this chapter can be found in: Moore DE, Jr. Needs assessment in the new health care environment: combining discrepancy analysis and outcomes to create more effective CME. *J Cont Educ Health Prof.* 1998;18.3:133–141. An expanded version with links to resources entitled *Evaluating Educational Outcomes Workbook* is available at www.acme-assn.org.

strategies. In fact, there have been complaints for many years, not only about the lack of effectiveness of CME[5–9] but the inadequacy of the evaluation mechanisms that have been used to measure CME effectiveness.[10–12]

Over the last 15 years, there has been important work that has challenged the assertion that CME is not effective. The work of Fox and his colleagues[13] demonstrated that physicians make changes in their personal and professional lives and rely heavily on CME in their change strategies. Slotnick[14] has elaborated the multiple-stage description of physician learning, originally developed by Geertsma and coworkers,[15] and suggests that effective CME should build on the questions physicians develop based on problems encountered in practice. Davis and his colleagues examined randomized controlled trials where CME was involved and showed that when CME was planned and implemented correctly, ie, incorporating needs assessment and multiple learning activities that focused on the identified need, physician behavior changed.[16–21] Central to the analysis of Davis and his colleagues was the work of Dixon who described four levels of evaluation in continuing education for the health professions: satisfaction, learning, performance, and health status.[22]

Dixon's conceptualization of four levels of evaluation was similar to other evaluation models popular in the human resource development field at the time. In 1959, Kirkpatrick[23] devised a four-level evaluation model that was in widespread use in business and industry in the 1970s when Dixon published her work. In the 1980s, Walsh[24] suggested a similar model and added attendance as a level before satisfaction, creating a five-level model. In the 1990s, about the same time that this multilevel evaluation model became known through the work of Davis' group, trainers in the human resource field began to adapt the Kirkpatrick model to contemporary conditions by suggesting that the model should consider return on investment (ROI) for training or benefits–cost analysis.[25] Finally, some in the health professions want to expand the model further by adding a level that would examine population health status.[26,27]

The combination of important research on physician learning and change and CME planning, as well as the adaptation of the multilevel evaluation model developed by Kirkpatrick to health care by Dixon and Davis and his colleagues, provides an opportunity to propose an approach to evaluating CME that consists of six levels: attendance, satisfaction, learning, performance, patient health status, and population health status.

At the same time, it appeared to many in the field of CME that the focus of the activities at each level in this emerging approach to evaluation was outcomes. Outcomes had become very important in health care,[28–34] it seemed only natural that outcomes should be important in CME as well. An *outcome* is defined as "the result or

TABLE 13-1

Levels of an Outcomes-based CME Evaluation Model

Level	Outcome	Definition
1	Participation	The number of physicians and others who registered and attended.
2	Satisfaction	The degree to which the expectations of the participants about the setting and delivery of the CME activity were met.
3	Learning	Changes in the knowledge, skills, and/or attitudes of the participants; the development of competence.
4	Performance	Changes in practice performance as a result of the application of what was learned.
5	Patient health	Changes in the health status of patients due to changes in practice behavior.
6	Population health	Changes in the health status of a population of patients due to changes in practice behavior.

effect of an event or the consequences of an action." And in CME, an outcome would be defined as the result or consequence of a CME event or events. Table 13-1 depicts how this definition is applied to the six-level approach to evaluation in CME.

EVALUATING "THE VALUE" OF
CONTINUING MEDICAL EDUCATION

In CME, evaluation of a CME activity is typically conducted by individuals who are responsible for planning and organizing that CME activity. In most cases, CME is evaluated by asking participants in a CME activity to respond to questions on an evaluation "form" that address issues of interest to a variety of stakeholders, including planners, the course director, speakers, and administrators who provide funding support. Currently, these questions focus more on administrative and customer satisfaction issues and do not provide information that address the concerns of leaders in the medical profession, health care administrators, and state regulatory officials about physician performance.

To provide this information, CME evaluation should focus on identifying, measuring, and describing the value provided by CME that leads to enhanced physician performance, improved health care quality, and reduced costs. In one way or another, most educators who write about evaluation define it as a "process of determining value." And most also state that an important first step in evaluation is defining "value."[35–36] The approach described in this chapter will define "value" in terms of "outcomes."

Evaluation of a CME activity could be planned at one or more of the six levels outlined earlier, depending on the purposes of the evaluation and the information needs of CME planners, the course director, speakers, or other stakeholders. At each level where evaluation occurs, data are collected to assess the effectiveness of the educational activity in meeting its goals defined in terms of that level.

Level 1: Participation

Evaluation at level 1 provides information about attendance and determines if attendance goals were met. Attendance issues are usually important issues for the course director, planning committee members, speakers, and administrators. Typically, attendance data are psychologically gratifying; course directors and planning committee members feel that an auditorium filled to capacity is testimony that the CME activity is successful. Information about participation can be obtained as a summary report from registration records with relative ease. Including characteristics of participants in a report will permit CME planners and others to obtain answers for questions beyond raw numbers, eg, Did members of the target audience participate? What percentage of the target audience participated? On the surface, there may seem to be "loftier" questions than those about attendance to ask; appropriately detailed questions about attendance can help CME planners understand what kind of coverage of the target audience occurred and whether a CME activity designed to address the educational needs of a particular group of physicians must be repeated because sufficient numbers of that group of physicians did not attend. Typically, attendance is described in terms of contact hours, which are computed by multiplying the number of credit hours by the number of participants.

Level 2: Satisfaction

Satisfaction surveys are ubiquitous in CME. Denigrated as "happiness indexes" by many, these surveys can nonetheless provide important information for CME planners if the right questions are asked. Satisfaction surveys for CME participants are very much like patient satisfaction surveys in hospitals, clinics, and physician's offices. Questions on well-designed satisfaction surveys ask participants in CME activities if their expectations regarding the setting and delivery of the CME activity were met. These are important issues for CME planners to consider; Malcolm Knowles[37] has suggested that a satisfactory educational setting is a prerequisite for learning. Questions might ask about expectations about location, scheduling, meeting rooms, food and beverage, mailing of the brochure, the style of the speakers, and relevance of content to work. Much of this work is done by meeting planners in CME settings and is crucial for effective CME. The effectiveness at this level is typically measured by participant responses using a five-point Likert scale. A goal is set as a score on the Likert scale; if the actual score meets or exceeds the goal, the arrangements are considered successful.

Level 3: Learning

Learning is divided into three major domains: knowledge, skills, and attitudes. After satisfaction surveys, assessment of changes in knowledge is the next most common evaluation technique, usually a test of multiple-choice and/or true–false questions. Clinical knowledge usually includes epidemiology, etiology, pathophysiology, signs and symptoms, diagnostic tests, treatment strategies, and effect on patients. Clinical skills could include psychomotor skills such as surgical or laparoscopic technique, decision-making skills like interpretation of test results and developing a management plan, interpersonal skills such as interviewing and communicating with patients, and working with and communicating with other members of the health care team. Assessment of learning clinical skills usually occurs by observation in the educational setting. Attitudes are a combination of beliefs and feelings that cause people to act in a certain way. Physicians may have certain attitudes toward hospital administration that may cause them to adopt or reject a clinical pathway. Physicians may also have developed attitudes toward certain patients, eg, those who do not take care of themselves or are chronically noncompliant, that make it difficult for them to provide the best possible care. Or they may develop attitudes that motivate them to go out of their way to help patients who ask intelligent questions about their conditions. Attitudes are typically assessed with questionnaires that use the semantic differential.

Combining new knowledge, skills, and attitudes in a given area and integrating this with a physician's existing knowledge, skills, and attitudes enables a physician to enhance his or her competence in a given area. When a physician is said to be competent, it means that he or she has the knowledge, skills, and attitudes to perform as expected.[38,39] Evaluation of competence occurs in the educational setting and typically involves observation of the physician managing a patient with a given disorder. Developing knowledge, skills, and/or attitudes is important, but the ultimate goal for a CME activity is to improve the competence of physicians to manage patients. Best practices usually define the competencies of physicians. Unfortunately, most CME activities do not provide the educational experiences to help physicians develop competencies. Knowledge, skills, and attitudes in clinical areas have dominated CME activities until just recently. Now it is recognized that physicians need other skills to function effectively in the modern health care environment. Consequently, physicians are beginning to learn knowledge, skills, and attitudes and to develop competence in areas such as communications, leadership, and quality management.

Level 4: Performance

In a level 4 evaluation, the focus is on the professional behavior of physicians in the work setting. Specifically, physician behavior is examined to determine if competencies that were developed as a result of participating in a CME activity are being implemented in practice. Typically, indicators are identified that serve as evidence that physicians are performing competently. For example, a course on diabetes management might have indicated that measuring hemoglobin A1c is an important part of best practice. Evaluation of physician performance after such a course would include monitoring physician measurement of hemoglobin A1C, an indicator for competence. Monitoring of this type usually occurs by abstracting charts, but observation of practice or use of simulated patients are other methods that could be used. Because it is often difficult or expensive to monitor indicators, "proxies" are used. Length of stay and returns to the operating room are two examples of proxies; administrative databases are excellent sources of proxies.

Level 5: Patient Health Status

Patient health status has been studied extensively in recent years. Improved patient health is the ultimate goal of health care and physician practice and is the focus of quality-improvement efforts throughout the country. The goal of CME is to provide physicians with educational activities that will help them develop the competencies they need to provide the very best possible care to their patients so as to improve their patients' health status. Many variables come into play between the time a physician develops improved competence in a CME activity and the time the health status of his or her patient improves, and there may be interest in ascertaining the impact. There are several ways to measure the health status of patients. Subjective measures include the Standard Form 12 and Standard Form 36 and condition-specific tYpes developed as part of the Medical Outcomes Study.[30,40,41] Objective measures include condition-specific lab tests and observation of a functional test.

Level 6: Population Health Status

Population health has been an increasing concern in the new health care environment. Use of epidemiological data can help CME planners understand if their programming has any impact on the health of the population in their catchment area. Again, many variables come into play between the time a physician develops improved competence in a CME activity and the time the health status of his or her patient improves, and there may be interest in ascertaining the impact. Morbidity and mortality rates and incidence and prevalence data may be compared before and after a CME activity.

IMPLEMENTING AN OUTCOMES-BASED CME EVALUATION PLAN

Evaluation should begin as soon as planning for a CME activity starts and should be imbedded in the planning process. An outcomes-based evaluation plan, consisting of six steps,[42] is suggested:

1) Involve all of those who are affected.
2) Specify evaluation questions.
3) Determine data-collection strategy.
4) Collect the data.
5) Analyze the data.
6) Report the data to all who are affected.

1. Who Should be Involved in Developing and Implementing an Evaluation Plan?

For most CME activities, individuals within the CME administrative unit assume responsibility for developing an evaluation strategy and have typically used a form that collects information about issues that reflect the meeting planning interests of the CME unit. But there are many other stakeholders in a CME activity, individuals who have interest in or are affected by the CME activity. Experts advocate a collaborative approach to planning CME activities, an approach that calls for broad-based involvement of learners, speakers, content experts, educational planners, and administrators, usually brought together on a planning committee. These individuals can contribute significantly to the development of evaluation questions and a data-collection strategy, drawing on their different backgrounds and role perspectives. The most obvious individual who should be involved in developing an evaluation strategy is the course director. He or she has stated and unstated goals for the CME activity that should be ascertained and incorporated into the evaluation strategy. Planning committee members should be involved for some of the same reasons. In fact, development of the evaluation strategy should be an important part of the early discussions of the planning committee.[43] These discussions may indeed

FIGURE 13-1

Gap Analysis in Framing Evaluation Questions

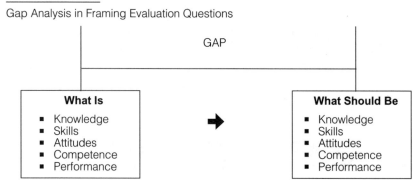

focus the planning efforts in a way that results in a more effective CME activity. Other stakeholders may include administrators responsible for the CME program or the area covered by the CME activity, members of the target audience, third-party payers, and regulatory officials.

2. What Questions Should be Answered by the Evaluation?

Evaluation questions will focus the evaluation activities. Each question should be stated in terms of outcomes, selecting one of the six levels of outcomes. In addition, each question should be amplified by a "what is" and "what should be" statement. Needs assessment can and should provide the data to describe "what is" (the entering behavior of the target audience) and "what should be" (behavior goal of the CME activity) (Figure 13-1).

For example, the course director for a CME activity in thrombolytic therapy may be concerned about the performance of physicians in the emergency department of his hospital (level 4) and wants to know if the CME activity will reduce the amount of time between onset of chest pain and administration of thrombolytic therapy. The current average time from door to medication is two hours (what is); best practice is one hour (what should be).

Some additional examples are provided below.

■ If the evaluation question asks about participation, the "what is" could be attendance at last year's course, and the "what should be" could be the desired attendance for this year's course.

■ If the evaluation question asks about participant satisfaction, the "what is" could be participant ratings of speakers from last year's course, and the "what should be" could be a target rating for this year's course.

■ If the evaluation question asks about participant learning, the "what is" could be the level of knowledge, skills, and attitudes before the CME activity, and the "what should be" could be an increased level of knowledge, skills, and attitudes.

- If the evaluation question asks about participant performance, the "what is" could be the performance level before the CME activity or series of CME activities, and the "what should be" could be some standards of achievable best practice.

- If the evaluation question asks about patient health status, the "what is" could be patient health status measured before the CME activity or series of CME activities, and the "what should be" could be some achievable level of health status, perhaps as described in the health status surveys.

- If the evaluation question asks about population health status, the "what is" could be population health status measured before the CME activity or series of CME activities, and the "what should be" could be some achievable level of health status, perhaps as outlined in a publication like *Healthy People 2010.*[44]

Combining the notions of discrepancy and six outcome levels appears to provide a more powerful framework for assessing CME effectiveness than has existed previously. In this approach, the CME planner contrasts "what is" and "what should be," establishes criteria for measurement based on the six outcomes levels, takes measurements, and makes judgments about the reduction of the discrepancy or gap that results from the educational activity.[45–47]

3. How Should Data be Collected?

Once the question(s) has been formulated, several important decisions have to be made to devise a data-collection strategy. These decisions consist of determining the types of data required, identifying sources for the data, and then selecting data-collection techniques. The data-collection strategy differs for each level of evaluation. And, it may be that the strategy for collecting data describing "what is" will be different from the strategy for collecting data describing "what should be."

Types of Data
Only data related to the evaluation question(s) should be collected. The type of data to be collected will be determined by the nature of the evaluation questions. For example, if the evaluation question asks about attendance, data related to participation should be collected. If the evaluation question asks about physician performance, data related to the behavior of physicians should be collected. In addition, data should be collected for both sides of the gap, ie, data should be collected about "what is" (current performance) as well as about "what should be" (standards, benchmarks, best practice).

Sources for Data

There are two primary sources of data: people and documents. The most common people source is the learner. Other people sources include experts in the field, peers of the learners, planning committee members, speakers, representatives of professional associations, hospital staff and administrators, pharmaceutical company and device manufacturer representatives, researchers, and patients. Individuals who have knowledge about or experience in the areas covered by the evaluation question(s) should be sought as sources of data.

A variety of documents can be used as sources of data for outcome evaluation studies. Patient records are the most obvious; administrative databases within health care organizations are becoming increasingly useful as techniques for data manipulation become more user-friendly. Hospital-based records, such as minutes of regularly convened committees, are also helpful. The professional literature is extremely valuable, especially for describing standards of practice. And there are an increasing number of reports from various government and nongovernment agencies that provide information that can be used in outcomes-evaluation studies. Four questions should be asked about sources of data:

1) Are the data accessible?
2) Does the source provide accurate and reliable data?
3) Does the source provide meaningful and relevant data?
4) Is the cost of obtaining the data reasonable?

Data-collection Techniques

There are a wide variety of data-collection techniques from which to choose. The nature of the evaluation question, the data required to answer it, and the sources of the data are all-important determinants of the data-collection technique. Techniques range from very simple and unsystematic to comprehensive and highly systematic. Unsystematic techniques include hunches, intuition, and "informed guesses." Slightly more formal techniques include the use of external consultants, informal networks of experts, or group meetings. More systematic techniques include analysis of reports by government or nongovernment agencies, tests and examinations, observation, or self-assessment. Currently, the most frequently used data-collection techniques are questionnaires and interviews, including focus groups.

In many cases, it is difficult for CME providers to gain access to data or develop instrumentation to collect objective, or "observed," data. In these cases, CME providers are encouraged to use approaches that will collect "self-report" data, rather than not collect any data. Self-report data are usually the opinions or perceptions of individuals and may reflect the personal biases of the reporter.

Objective data result from the systematic observation and recording of events and are collected according to procedures that prevent the introduction of personal bias. An example of objective data is a report by an unbiased observer of the performance of a physician in an area of interest, eg, the use of sterile technique in the operating room. An example of subjective data would be a self-report by surgeons about their use of sterile technique in the operating room. Studies have shown that the reliability and validity of self-report data compare favorably with objective data.[48] Although objective sources are certainly more desirable, the cost and inconvenience of using objective data sources in many CME evaluation projects may be prohibitive. Self-report data will not produce data and judgments that are scientifically rigorous, yet, the data that result from these approaches are still useful for administrative decision-making and outcomes-evaluation projects. Triangulation is a useful analysis technique when working with "subjective" or self-report data.[49] Table 13-2 shows that self-report and observed data can be collected at each level, except for level 1, which is attendance (only observed) and satisfaction (only self-report).

4. When Should the Data be Collected?

After decisions have been made about what data are needed to answer the evaluation question(s), where to get that data, and what techniques will be used to collect the data, timing of data collection is the next decision to be made. Framing your evaluation question with "what is" and "what should be" implies at least two different data-collection points: one before and one after the educational activity.[50] To answer the evaluation question, an initial assessment of "what is" must be taken. In some evaluation studies, the initial assessment occurs at the educational activity; in other cases, it can occur several weeks or months before the educational activity. To determine if "what should be" is accomplished, measurements can

TABLE 13-2

Self-Report and Observed Data in an Outcomes-based CME Evaluation Model

Level	Outcome	Subjective	Objective
1	Participation		X
2	Satisfaction	X	
3	Learning	X	X
4	Performance	X	X
5	Patient health	X	X
6	Population health	X	X

be made immediately after the educational activity (before the participants leave the educational activity) or several weeks or months after the educational activity is completed. Sometimes, a measurement is taken during the educational activity (formative evaluation) to determine if there is observable movement from "what is" to "what should be."[51] Finally, recent CME research suggests that "what should be" is more likely to be attained if physicians participate in multiple educational activities focused on "what should be."[52] Measurement can be taken before, during, and after these multiple CME activities.

5. How Should the Data be Analyzed?

At this step, you determine if the evaluation question has been answered. Again, use of gap analysis, as portrayed in Figure 13-2, will provide a more powerful framework for assessing CME effectiveness than has existed previously. Analysis methods can range from the statistics-based methods used by educational psychologists and social scientists to more ethnographic methods typically used by historians and anthropologists. Statisticians and research design consultants should be used when needed.

6. How Should the Data be Reported?

No matter what the size or scope of an evaluation project, it must always result in a written report. The detail and thoroughness will

FIGURE 13-2

Using Gap Analysis to Determine the Effectiveness of a CME Activity

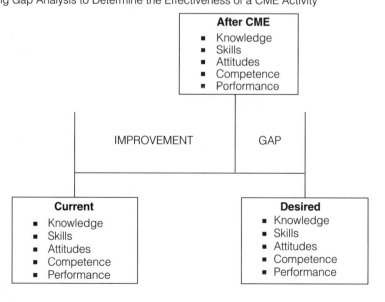

depend on the needs of the stakeholders and could range from sketchy notes sufficient to remind the CME planner to full reports needed by management to market health care services to a potential purchaser or justify funding for the CME department. In general, the report should follow the components of the plan.

BENEFITS, EFFECTIVENESS, AND COSTS IN CME EVALUATION

The CME enterprise is under an increasing number of pressures in all of its settings. One pressure centers around the resources provided to do the work of the CME enterprise. Individuals responsible for managing CME programs will increasingly be required to justify the level of resources provided to the CME program. In this environment, it is important for CME leadership to be able to demonstrate the benefits that accrued to their organization as the result of its investment of resources in the CME program. In other words, a benefit-cost analysis should be performed. Information about ROI will be useful for justifying the resources that have been provided to the CME enterprise and for making decisions about continuing, modifying, or terminating programming as well.

Phillips[53] added "return on investment" to the four-level evaluation model developed by Kirkpatrick. Phillips is correct in saying that cost analysis of an educational activity and the outcomes it produces is necessary. But this author feels that this analysis should occur at each outcome level, not only after the fourth level. The Kirkpatrick–Phillips model assumes that every educational activity will progress through four stages. In CME, application of the Kirkpatrick–Phillips model would mean that all CME would look like this: satisfaction with a CME activity leads to learning, which leads to improved performance, which leads to improved health status in patients, and then a benefit-cost analysis is done. The reality is that not all CME programming will progress through all four levels. And, the truth is that if the manager of a CME enterprise decides it can work only on performance or learning outcomes, he or she will still want to analyze the benefits in terms of the costs of its efforts. Figure 13-3 shows that benefit–cost analysis can occur at each level of outcomes.

In CME, benefit–cost analysis can provide answers to questions about the relationship between the cost of a CME activity or program and the benefit(s) that the educational activity or program provides. For example, did the educational activity, or program of activities, provide any added value to the CME enterprise or its parent organization? Or, were the benefits received by the CME enterprise or its parent organization worth the investment made in the educational activity or the program?

FIGURE   13-3

Cost–Benefit Analysis in an Outcomes-based CME Evaluation Model

Level of Evaluation		Benefit	Cost
1	Attendance		
2	Satisfaction		
3	Learning		
4	Performance		
5	Patient health status		
6	Population health status		

Typical ROI questions compare the funds expended to the funds received. For example, if the General Products Company (GPC) invested $10,000 on a project to produce a new product and revenue from sales of the new product was $13,000, all things being equal, it could be said that GPC received a 30% return on its investment, or profit, which would, in most cases, be considered very good. A similar question, did the CME enterprise make a profit?, cannot be answered as easily. Although there are some CME enterprises that do focus on making a profit, the predominant orientation of CME programs is toward social outcomes, rather than financial benefits.

A comprehensive benefit–cost analysis requires measurement or estimates of the benefits of a program, both tangible and intangible, and the costs of undertaking the program, both direct and indirect.[54] Once specified, the benefits and costs are translated into a common measure, usually but not necessarily, a monetary unit. The benefits and costs can then be compared, generally by computing benefit-to-cost ratio (the monetary value of the benefits divided by cost; any ratio above 1 being considered a good benefits-to-cost ratio) or net benefits (benefits minus the cost; a positive value is considered good).

Benefit-cost analysis is relatively easy to do for technical and industrial projects but difficult for many social programs where setting a monetary value on benefits may be impossible. For these reasons, cost-effectiveness studies can be used. This type of study requires quantifying both program costs and benefits, but only the costs are described in monetary terms. Cost-effectiveness analysis allows comparison of programs based on the magnitude of their effects related to costs. For example, it would be difficult to assign a monetary value to the compilation of ratings from an evaluation form for a CME program for which goals for CME outcomes are set at the satisfaction level. However, ratings and costs could be summarized for each CME activity, and judgments could be made about cost-effectiveness by comparing the ratings and costs for each activity. For example,

- Course A received a total rating of 4.5 and cost $10,000 to produce. Using the same evaluation form, course B also received a total rating of 4.5 but only cost $7,500 to produce. It would appear that course B was more cost-effective.

- Course C received a total rating of 4.7 and cost $15,000 to produce. Using the same evaluation form, course D received a total rating of 4.2 and also cost $15,000 to produce. It would appear that course C was more cost-effective.

- Course E received a total rating of 4.6 and cost $20,000 to produce. Using the same evaluation form, course F received a total rating of 4.4 and cost $16,000 to produce. The answer to the question about cost-effectiveness here centers around the question, Is the increase of 2 in the rating score worth the additional $4,000 in cost?

Benefit–cost and cost-effectiveness studies can be undertaken either during educational planning (using estimates about benefits) or after the course is completed. Retrospective analyses are more common because of the difficulty of estimating potential benefits.

There are several steps in performing benefit–cost and cost-effectiveness studies. The first step is to decide what accounting perspective will be used: individual, organizational, or societal. In this chapter, the perspective of the organization, the CME enterprise, has been chosen as an example. The next step is to specify and measure costs and benefits. Then monetary values of each are calculated and compared.

The organizational perspective takes the point of view primarily of the CME enterprise and secondarily of the parent organization. From the point of view of the CME enterprise, there may be several benefits that result from sponsoring a CME activity or series of activities. These benefits may be characterized broadly using the outcomes levels covered in the initial sections of this chapter, ie, satisfaction, learning, performance, and health status. In addition, there may be additional benefits such as a better image for the parent institution, increased referrals from physicians who participate in CME, and use of excess CME revenue to support other goals of the parent organization. Some of these benefits are more difficult to measure than others and are therefore difficult to quantify in financial terms. For some, effectiveness criteria could be developed and assigned. Then, a financial value could be attributed only to benefits resulting from improved performance, eg, the reduction in cost of providing a particular service or prescribing patterns for a certain condition after a series of CME activities designed to change that physician behavior.

The costs for the series of CME activities have three components: direct costs, indirect costs, and overhead. Direct costs are the actual costs of the educational activity and include, but are not limited to, honorarium and expenses for speakers, travel expenses incurred by staff supporting a CME activity on site, promotion and marketing, food and beverage service for the CME activity, audiovisual expenses, educational materials, and credit application and processing fees. Indirect costs are the resources required to support planning, organizing, and implementing a CME activity and include, but are not limited to, salary and benefits of staff, office supplies, telephone, office equipment, rent, postage and mailing for general correspondence, and professional development of staff. Overhead costs are the general costs of operating the organization that can be assigned to providing administrative support for the CME operation and include institutional personnel services, institutional financial services, institutional maintenance and repair services, institutional information services, institutional housekeeping services, and institutional governance.

In most CME enterprises, the costs of the CME activities may be offset by revenue. Revenue can be obtained from several sources: registration fees, commercial support, grants, exhibit fees, contracts, institutional funds, membership fees, volunteer time, and in-kind contributions.

The next step is to calculate the monetary value for the benefits and the costs and make judgments about the difference. Let's say that the costs of organizing and offering a series of CME activities on congestive heart failure were $16,450. There was $8,250 in revenue, reducing the cost to $8,200. The CME activities included presentation and discussion of feedback, distribution of pertinent articles, a formal CME course, discussion with a consultant in weekly video conferences, mailed local guidelines, and an order set on a computerized order-entry system.

The outcomes of this series of CME activities were that length of stay was reduced by 15% and use of ACE inhibitors was increased by 70%. The benefit of these outcomes, as determined by the hospital fiscal staff, was a 15% reduction in cost for managing patients with congestive heart failure, amounting to savings of approximately $4.5 million per year. The benefits of this series of CME activities clearly outweighed the costs; therefore, it can be said that there was significant ROI, ie, it was cost-effective to change the behavior of physicians through CME (Figure 13-4).[55]

Implementation of this approach in most CME settings may be difficult. Collection, compilation, and manipulation of financial data for educational activities are not a priority of most organizations. And many managers of CME enterprises will not be in a position to rework formal institutional accounts to obtain the information

FIGURE 13-4

Benefit–Cost Analysis in an Outcomes-based Approach to Evaluation in CME

Level of Evaluation	Was the CME activity effective?	What is the benefit?	What is the cost?	Was there a return on investment?
	Have the agreed upon outcomes been accomplished?	*What is the dollar value of the benefits created by the outcomes?*	*How much did it cost to offer the CME activity?*	*Were the benefits (in dollars) greater than the cost?*
Attendance				
Satisfaction				
Learning				
Performance				
Patient health status				
Population health status				

necessary to perform benefit-cost analysis. Typically, the accounting processes used by the parent organizations of most CME enterprises are not useful because they provide information about accounting issues, not programmatic issues.

A FRAMEWORK FOR EVALUATING THE OUTCOMES IN CME

The term *framework* has been chosen for the approach to evaluation that is being described here because the approach combines elements of many of the evaluation "models" that have been developed to assess educational and human services programs. In evaluation, the term *model* does not necessarily refer to a mathematical model that describes proven theory. Rather, a model in evaluation is a summary of the way a particular evaluator conceptualizes and describes the evaluation process. The model that bears an evaluator's name does not necessarily describe evaluation as it actually occurs; it describes how evaluation should be conducted according to the beliefs about evaluation and education that are held by the evaluator.[56]

The framework described in this chapter was developed to help CME practitioners answer the question, Does a CME activity, or a program of CME activities, change physician behavior in the area of focus of the CME activity? Corollary questions would be: Did the changed behavior lead to improved patient or population health status? and Was there a return on the investment of resources in developing and offering the CME activity? The framework, as it is currently constructed, does not answer questions about the CME activity itself. For example, it would not help the CME practitioner to answer questions about the design of the CME activity or the role of speakers in helping participants achieve their learning objectives. But, it may be useful in a recently proposed evaluation-based accreditation system in which CME providers would be accredited to offer CME activities at one of four levels based on the level of evaluation that was performed.[57]

At first glance, it appears that the framework resembles a model that has been called goal-achievement. In the goal-achievement model, the merit of a program is equated with its success in achieving a stated goal.[58] This model is based primarily on the work of Tyler, who developed an objectives-oriented model that was focused on school learning.[59] In Tyler's model, which has been used in all educational settings, defined objectives are compared with student performance in order to measure the extent to which the objectives have been achieved. The framework also draws on the discrepancy evaluation model, originally described by Provus,[60] but adapted for adult education by Knox[61] and described for CME by Fox.[62] The discrepancy model developed by Provus expanded on Tyler's model by focusing on measuring the difference, or discrepancy, between student performance and some agreed upon program standard. Knox redefined the approach by suggesting that student performance (in this case, adult students) be measured before the educational activity and that it be compared with a desired level of performance or standard, creating a "gap" that could guide the development of program activities (see Figure 13-1). Fox applied "discrepancy analysis" in CME, and Moore described the use of gap analysis in needs assessment for CME.[63] In this framework, the discrepancy can be described as a gap between "what is," a measurement taken before the educational activity, and "what should be," a standard. Evaluation in this framework measures how much of the gap is reduced after the CME activity. The effectiveness of an educational activity is determined by how much of the gap is reduced (see Figure 13-2).

In this framework, the discrepancy is the distance between two descriptions of outcomes, a description of "what is" and "what should be." As mentioned earlier, outcomes have become increasingly important in health care. In education, outcomes evaluation has become important as well. The relatively new model of outcome evaluation in education has been defined as activities designed primarily to measure the effects or results of an educational program, rather than their inputs or processes.[64,65] The

FIGURE   13-5

Underlying Theory of Continuing Medical Education

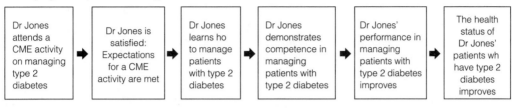

framework for outcomes evaluation proposed here assumes a logical progression from learning to improved performance to enhanced health status (Figure 13-5). As such, it draws on a logic model of evaluation, which describes a progression of traits or characteristics that have a developmental relationship.[66,67] For example, using the terms of the logic model, learning could be considered an initial outcome, performance an intermediate outcome, and change in health status the long-term, or ultimate, outcome.

The framework for evaluation of the continuing professional development (CPD) of physicians also draws on an emerging theory of how physicians learn and change. Simply, this emerging theory states that physicians learn and are more likely to change their behavior if the educational activity(ies) is focused on the behavior to be changed (needs assessment) and if multiple educational activities are offered—organized as predisposing, enabling, and reinforcing activities.[68–70] In this sense, the framework described here resembles the theory-based model of evaluation, which assumes that a program is based on explicit or implicit theories of change and about how and why the program will work. Although the current framework can answer the question, Did improved outcomes occur?, it cannot answer questions like, Did the CME activity cause the intended outcomes? and What elements of the underlying program theory contributed to achieving the outcomes?[71] The framework also appears to resemble the experimental model in which the behavior of one group after an intervention by one group is compared to the behavior of another group who did not receive the intervention.[72] In fact, the design of the proposed evaluation framework is more like a time series than an experiment because there is no control group.

Finally, the framework also contains elements of the cost-based evaluation models. There are three approaches in this model: cost feasibility, cost-effectiveness (integrating information about cost and effects to identify the option that most efficiently uses resources to accomplish outcomes), and cost–benefit analysis (collecting information to determine if the results of an intervention are "worth" the investment of resources).[73]

TABLE 13-3

CIPP model

	Context	Input	Process	Product
Objective	Define the institutional context, identify the target population, and assess their needs; identify opportunities for addressing those needs; diagnose problems underlying needs; judge whether proposed objectives are sufficiently responsive to the assessed need	Identify and assess system capacity and capabilities, alternative program strategies, procedural designs for implementing the strategies, budgets, and schedules	Identify or predict in the process defects in the procedural design or its implementation; provide information for decisions; record and judge procedural events and activities	Collect descriptions and judgments of outcomes and relate them to objectives and to context, input, and process information; interpret their worth and merit
Method	System analysis, survey; document review; hearings; interviews; diagnostic tests; Delphi technique	Inventorying and analyzing available human and material resources, solution strategies, and procedural designs for relevance, feasibility, and economy; literature search; visits to exemplary programs, advocate teams, and pilot trials	Monitoring the activity's potential procedural barriers and remaining alert to unanticipated ones; obtaining specified information for program decisions; describing the actual process, continually interacting with and observing the activities of the project staff	Defining operational and measuring outcome criteria; collecting judgments of outcomes from stakeholders; performing both qualitative and quantitative analysis
Relation to Decision-making and Change	Deciding on setting, goals and objectives; planning needed changes; providing a basis for judging outcomes	Selecting sources of support, solutions, strategies, and procedural designs; structuring change activities; providing a basis for judging implementation	Implementing and refining the program design, procedures, and process control; documenting the actual process for later use in interpreting outcomes	Deciding to continue, terminate, modify, or refocus a change activity; present a clear record of effects (intended and unintended, positive and negative)

DIRECTIONS FOR RESEARCH INTO CME EVALUATION

Although the framework for evaluation of the CPD of physicians draws on elements of many evaluation models, it has not been tested in a comprehensive way in any CME setting. This framework was developed to meet the needs of CME practitioners who are increasingly being asked to provide more sophisticated information about the outcomes of CME activities to a variety of stakeholders. Research is needed to determine if the proposed framework meets the needs of CME practitioners or if another approach should be developed.

The most important research question is, Does the framework provide reliable and valid information about the impact of CME on physician behavior? Once that question is answered satisfactorily, research efforts should focus on the factors that contribute to the success or lack of success of CME activities in improving physician performance.[74] Two evaluation models may provide approaches for identifying and examining the factors that contribute to a successful CME activity. First, the CIPP (context, input, process, product) approach, developed by Stufflebeam and his colleagues,[75] focuses on the interaction among context, inputs, process, and product (outcome) (Table 13-3). Second, use of the theory-based evaluation will clarify the causal relationships implicit in CME program development and identify factors contributing to successful program development.[76–79]

SUMMARY

A framework for evaluating the CPD of physicians is proposed in this chapter. It combines features of a number of evaluation models that have been developed in other education settings. There appears to be some promise for this framework to help CME practitioners answer questions about the impact and cost-benefit of CME. Answers to questions about what leads to successful CME programs await further research.

REFERENCES—CHAPTER 13

1. Committee on Quality of Health Care in America, Institute of Medicine. *To Err is Human: Building A Safer Health System.* Washington, DC: National Academy Press; 2000.

2. Committee on Quality of Health Care in America, Institute of Medicine. *Crossing the Quality Chasm: A New Health System for the 21st Century.* Washington, DC: National Academy Press; 2001.

3. Wennberg J, Gittlesohn A. Variations in medical care among small areas. *Scientific American.* 1982;246:120–134.

4. Policy on maintenance of certification adopted by the Assembly of the American Board of Medical Specialties on December 13, 2001.

5. Miller GE. Medical care, its social and organizational aspects: the continuing education of physicians. *N Eng J Med*. 1963;269.6:295–299.

6. Miller GE. Continuing education for what? *J Med Ed*. 1967;42:320–326.

7. Miller GE. Why continuing medical education? *Bull NY Acad Med*. 1975; 51.6:701–706.

8. Miller GE. The assessment of clinical skills, competence, and performance. *Acad Med*. 1990;65.9(Supplement):S63–S67.

9. Sibley JC, Sackett DL, Neufeld V, Gerrard B, Rudnick KV, Fraser W. A randomized controlled trial of continuing medical education. *N Engl J Med*. 1982;306:511–515.

10. Bertram DA, Brooks-Bertram PA. The evaluation of continuing medical education: a literature review. *Health Educ Monogr*. 1977;5:330–362.

11. Stein LS. The effectiveness of continuing medical education: eight research reports. *J Med Educ*. 1980;56:103–110.

12. Lloyd JS, Abrahamson S. Effectiveness of continuing medical education: a review of the evidence. *Eval Health Prof*. 1979;2:251–280.

13. Fox RD, Mazmanian PE, Putnam RW. *Changing and Learning in the Lives of Physicians*. New York, NY: Praeger Publishers;1989.

14. Slotnick HB. How doctors learn: physicians' self-directed learning episodes. *Acad Med*. 1999;74:1106–1117.

15. Geertsma RH, Parker RC, Whitbourne SK. How physicians view the process of change in their practice behavior. *J Med Educ*. 1982;57:10:752–761.

16. Haynes RB, Davis DA, McKibbon A, Tugwell P. A critical appraisal of the efficacy of continuing medical education. *JAMA*. 1984;251:61–64.

17. Davis DA, Haynes RB, Chambers L, Neufield VR, McKibbon A, Tugwell P. The impact of CME: a methodological review of the continuing medical education literature. *Eval Health Prof*. 1984;7:251–283.

18. Davis DA, Thomson MA, Oxman, AD, Haynes RB. Evidence for the effectiveness of CME: a review of 50 randomized controlled trials. *JAMA*. 1992;268:1111–1117.

19. Davis DA, Thomson MA, Oxman AD, Haynes RB. Changing physician performance: a systematic review of the effect of continuing medical education strategies. *JAMA*. 1995;274:700–705.

20. Davis DA, Taylor-Vaisey AL. Translating guidelines into practice: a systematic review of theoretic concepts, practical experience and research evidence in the adoption of clinical practice guidelines. *Can Med Assoc J*. 1997;157:408–416.

21. Davis DA. Does CME work? An analysis of the effect of educational activities on physician performance or health care outcomes. *Int J Psychiatry Med*. 1998;28.1:21–39.

22. Dixon J. Evaluation criteria in studies of continuing education in the health professions: a critical review and a suggested strategy. *Eval Health Prof*. 1978;1.2:47–65.

23. Kirkpatrick DL. *Evaluating Training Programs: The Four Levels*. San Francisco, Calif: Berrett-Koehler Publishers; 1998.

24. Walsh PL. Evaluating educational activities. In: Adelson R, Watkins FS, Caplan RM, eds. *Continuing Education for the Health Professional: Educational and Administrative Methods*. Rockville, Md: Aspen; 1985.

25. Phillips JJ. *Handbook of Training Evaluation and Measurement Methods*. Houston, Texas: Gulf Publishing; 1997.

26. US Department of Health and Human Services. *Healthy People 2010: Understanding and Improving Health*. 2nd ed. Washington, DC: US Government Printing Office, November 2000.

27. US Department of Health and Human Services. *Healthy People 2010. With Understanding and Improving Health and Objectives for Improving Health*. 2 vols. 2nd ed. Washington, DC: US Government Printing Office, November 2000.

28. Ellwood PM. Outcomes management: a technology of patient experience. *N Engl J Med*. 1988;318:1549–56.

29. Tarlov A, Ware JE, Greenfield S, Nelson EC, Perrin E, Zubkoff M. The medical outcomes study: an application of methods for monitoring the results of medical care. *JAMA*. 1989;262:925–930.

30. Stewart AL, Ware JE Jr. *Measuring Functioning and Well-being: The Medical Outcomes Study Approach*. Durham, NC: Duke University Press; 1992.

31. Greenfield S. The use of outcomes in medical practice applications of the Medical Outcomes Study. In: Couch JB, ed. *Health Care Quality Management for the 21st Century*. Tampa, Fla: American College of Physician Executives; 1991.

32. Ellwood PM, Huber MR, Couch JB. The future: clinical outcomes management. In: Couch JB , ed. *Health Care Quality Management for the 21st Century*. Tampa, Fla: American College of Physician Executives; 1991.

33. Williamson JW. Evaluating quality of patient care: a strategy relating outcome and process. *JAMA*. 1971;218:564–569.

34. Williamson JW, Moore DE Jr., Sanazaro PJ. Moving from "small qa" to "LARGE QA": an outcomes framework for improving quality management. *Eval Health Prof*. 1991;2:138–160.

35. Bennett NL. The voices of evaluation. *J Contin Educ Health Prof*. 1997;17.4:198–206.

36. Rossi PH, Freeman HE, Lipsey MW. *Evaluation: A Systematic Approach.* 6th ed. Thousand Oaks, Calif: Sage Publications; 1999.

37. Knowles MS. *The Modern Practice of Adult Education.* New York, NY: Association Press; 1970.

38. Neufeld VR, Norman GR. *Assessing Clinical Competence.* New York, NY: Springer; 1985.

39. Senior JR. *Toward the Measurement of Competence in Medicine.* Philadelphia, Pa: National Board of Medical Examiners; 1976.

40. Curtis LH, Phelps CE, McDermott MP, Rubin HR. The value of patient reported health status in predicting short-term outcomes after coronary artery bypass graft surgery. *Medical Care.* 2002;40:1090–1100.

41. Ware JE, Jr, Sherbourne CD. The MOS 36 Item Short Form Health Survey (SF-36): Conceptual framework and item selection. *Medical Care.* 1992;30:473–483.

42. Grotelueschen AD, Gooler DD, Knox AB, Kemmis S, Dowdy I, Brophy K. *An Evaluation Planner.* Champaign, Ill: Office for the Study of Professional Education, College of Education, University of Illinois; 1974.

43. Moore D. Needs assessment in the new health care environment: combining discrepancy analysis and outcomes to create more effective CME. *J Contin Educ Health Prof.* 1998;18:133–141.

44. US Department of Health and Human Services. *Healthy People 2010: Understanding and Improving Health.* 2nd ed. Washington, DC: US Government Printing Office, Nov 2000.

45. Provus M. Evaluation of ongoing programs in the public school system. National Society for the Study of Education (NSEE) 68th Yearbook, Part II, 1969, pp. 242–283; reproduced in Worthen BR and Sanders JR, eds. *Educational Evaluation: Theory and Practice.* Worthington, Ohio: Charles A. Jones Publishing Company; 1973, pp. 170–209.

46. Fox RD. Discrepancy analysis in continuing medical education. *Mobius.* 1983;3:37–44.

47. Moore D. Needs assessment in the new health care environment: combining discrepancy analysis and outcomes to create more effective CME. *J Contin Educ Health Prof.* 1998;18:133–141.

48. Curry L, Purkis IE. Validity of self-reports of behavior changes by participants after a CME course. *J Med Educ.* 1986;61.7:579–584.

49. Lockyer J. Needs assessment: Lessons learned. *J Contin Educ Health Prof.* 1998;18.3:190–192.

50. Fink A, Kosecoff J. *An Evaluation Primer.* Washington, DC: Capitol Publications; 1978.

51. Scriven M. The methodology of evaluation. In: Worthen BR, Sanders JR, eds. *Educational Evaluation: Theory and Practice.* Worthington, Ohio: Charles A. Jones Publishing Company; 1973.

52. Davis DA, Thomson MA, Oxman, AD, Haynes RB. Evidence for the effectiveness of CME: a review of 50 randomized controlled trials. *JAMA.* 1992; 268:1111–1117.

53. Phillips JJ. *Handbook of Training Evaluation and Measurement Methods.* Houston, TX: Gulf Publishing; 1997.

54. Thompson MS. *Benefit Cost Analysis for Program Evaluation.* Beverly Hills, Calif: Sage Publications; 1980.

55. Mason J, Freemantle N, Nazareth I, Eccles M, Haines A, Drummond M. When is it cost-effective to change the behavior of health professionals? *JAMA.* 2001;286.23:2988–2992.

56. Madaus GF, Kellaghan T. Models, methods, and definitions in evaluation. In: Stufflebeam DL, Madaus GF, Kellaghan T, eds. *Evaluation Models.* Revised edition. Boston, Mass: Kluwer; 2000.

57. Mazmanian PE, Mazmanian PM, Moore MA. Evaluation-based accreditation: Alternative approach to regulating continuing medical education providers. *J Contin Educ Health Prof.* 1996;16.2:112–116.

58. Madaus GF, Kellaghan T. Models, methods, and definitions in evaluation. In: Stufflebeam DL, Madaus GF, Kellaghan T, eds. *Evaluation Models.* Revised edition. Boston, Mass: Kluwer; 2000.

59. Tyler RW. *Basic Principles of Curriculum and Instruction.* Chicago, Ill: University of Chicago Press; 1949.

60. Provus M. Evaluation of ongoing programs in the public school system. National Society for the Study of Education (NSEE) 68th Yearbook, Part II, 1969, pp. 242–283; reproduced in Worthen BR and Sanders JR, eds. *Educational Evaluation: Theory and Practice.* Worthington, Ohio: Charles A. Jones Publishing Company; 1973.

61. Knox AB. Critical appraisal of the needs of adults for educational experiences as a basis for program development. Department of Adult Education, University of Nebraska, 1963. (ERIC Document 022 090, 1969).

62. Fox RD. Discrepancy analysis in continuing medical education. *Mobius.* 1983;3:37–44.

63. Moore D. Needs assessment in the new health care environment: combining discrepancy analysis and outcomes to create more effective CME. *J Contin Educ Health Prof.* 1998;18:133–141.

64. Kellaghan T, Madaus G. Outcome evaluation. In Stufflebeam DL, Madaus GF, Kellaghan T. *Evaluation Models.* Revised edition. Boston, Mass: Kluwer; 2000.

65. Grippin P, Peters S. *Learning Theory and Learning Outcomes: The Connection.* New York, N.Y: University Press of America; 1984.

66. Reed CS, Brown RE. Outcome-asset impact model: linking outcomes and assets. *Evaluation and Program Planning.* 2001;24:287–295.

67. Julian DA, Jones A, Deyo D. Open systems evaluation and the logic model: program planning and evaluation tools. *Evaluation and Program Planning.* 1995;18.4:333–341.

68. Fox RD, Mazmanian PE, Putnam RW. *Changing and Learning in the Lives of Physicians.* New York, NY: Praeger Publishers; 1989.

69. Davis DA, Thomson MA, Oxman AD, Haynes RB. Evidence for the effectiveness of CME: a review of 50 randomized controlled trials. *JAMA.* 1992; 268.9:1111–1117.

70. Green LW, Kreuter MW. *Health Promotion Planning: An Educational and Environmental Approach.* Mountain View, Calif: Mayfield Publishing Company; 1991.

71. Rogers PJ. Program theory: Not whether programs work but how they work. In: Stufflebeam DL, Madaus GF, Kellaghan T, eds. *Evaluation Models.* Revised edition. Boston, Mass: Kluwer; 2000.

72. Madaus GF, Kellaghan T. Models, metaphors, and definitions in evaluation. In: Stufflebeam DL, Madaus GF, Kellaghan T, eds. *Evaluation Models.* Revised edition. Boston, Mass: Kluwer; 2000.

73. Tsang MC. Cost analysis for improved educational policymaking and evaluation. In: Stufflebeam DL, Madaus GF, Kellaghan T, eds. *Evaluation Models.* Revised edition. Boston, Mass: Kluwer; 2000.

74. Wholey JS, Hatry HP, Newcomer KE. *Handbook of Practical Program Evaluation.* San Francisco, Calif: Jossey-Bass Publishers; 1994.

75. Stufflebeam DL, Foley WJ, Gephart WJ, Guba EG, Hammond RL, Merriman HO, Provus MM. *Educational Evaluation and Decision-making in Education.* Itasca, Ill: Peacock; 1971.

76. Rossi PH, Freeman HE, Lipsey MW. *Evaluation: A Systematic Approach.* 6th ed. Thousand Oaks, Calif: Sage Publications; 1999.

77. Bickman L. *Using Program Theory in Evaluation. New Directions in Program Evaluation.* San Francisco, Calif: Jossey-Bass Publishers; 1987.

78. Lipsey MW, Pollard JA. Driving towards more theory in program evaluation: more models to choose from. *Evaluation and Program Planning.* 1989;12:317–328.

79. Bickman L. The application of program theory to the evaluation of a managed mental health care system. *Evaluation and Program Planning.* 1996;19:111–119.

chapter 14

Methods, Tools, and Techniques of Evaluation*

Penny A. Jennett, PhD, Lynne B. Sinclair, BSc, MA; R. Van Harrison, PhD

You are a continuing medical education (CME) coordinator and have been asked to provide comments regarding the impact of a series of cardiology CME events (a cardiology program) scheduled to occur over the summer. You will be hiring a research assistant for the summer to select and design measurement tools that can be used to collect and monitor related data.

You have begun to think about the following questions:

- What will you be measuring?
- What evaluation tools would be most appropriate for this task?
- What are key references to which you could direct the student?
- What resources are available to help the student design, use, and test the appropriate tools?
- What guidance would you give the student regarding the strengths and limitations of various evaluation approaches and tools?

This chapter reviews some of the major principles and practices that influence your decisions in regard to each of the questions above. It also provides a ready resource for questions related to reports and articles that evaluate the process and products of continuing professional development (CPD). Key to the effective and efficient use of evaluation tools in continuing professional education is an understanding of evaluation terms, a clear knowledge of what is being evaluated with the associated evaluation questions, and an appreciation of available relevant approaches and tools.

*We gratefully acknowledge the valuable work of the research assistants and clerical staff of the Health Telemetrics Unit, who helped in the preparation of this chapter.

INTRODUCTION

When continuing professional educational events are evaluated, the evaluator(s) is systematically "determining the merit, worth, or value" of a particular activity,[1] empowering decision-makers to make needed changes,[1] and, at times, assessing the "meaning of something"[2] related to the program. Evaluation tools or instruments are selected to collect data through a monitoring and reporting process. Decision-makers review data and reports to make a judgment on the value of the activity. Reviews of evaluative feedback can occur at various times throughout the activity (formative evaluation) or can be conducted at its conclusion (summative evaluation). Self-, as well as peer, reviews, can be involved.[3]

As discussed in preceding chapters, several aspects of a continuing professional activity can be evaluated, including learning, the learning process, competence, performance, outcomes, programs, and cost–benefits. The same approaches and tools (Table 14-1) can be used to collect data across many of these domains. It is important, however, to understand the definitions, strengths, and limitations of your choices.

The first part of this chapter details five major categories of evaluation tools:

- *Survey tools* can measure perceived attitudes, beliefs, and reported behavior.
- *Knowledge tests* can measure factual knowledge, interview and clinical skills, problem-solving ability, and judgment.
- *Observations* can measure attitudes and beliefs, knowledge and skills, competence, and behavior.
- *Document review* can measure recorded behaviors.
- *Technology-based tests* are used to evaluate all types of measurements.

After considering the characteristics of each of these tools individually, their relative strengths and weaknesses are summarized to provide practical comparisons. These comparisons can be helpful when selecting an evaluation methodology within the context of a specific project.

APPROACHES AND TOOLS

A concise synopsis of evaluation approaches and tools is provided in Table 14-1. The strengths and limitations of these tools are outlined in the chapter. Table 14-2 reviews the practical factors that are important to consider when choosing evaluation approaches and tools.

The authors refer readers to the *McMaster Handbook*[4] and to the workbook, *Evaluating Educational Outcomes: A Workbook for*

TABLE 14-1

Evaluation Approaches and Tools

Approach/Procedure	Tool
Survey methods	**Structured survey** (personal interview, telephone interview, written questionnaire, Internet questionnaire) **Unstructured interview** **Semi-structured interview**
Knowledge tests	**OSCE—objective structured clinical examination** [checklist, peer assessment and review, Likert scale (5 point scale), standardized patients] **Written test with restricted answer options** ■ Multiple choice questions (MCQs) ■ True/false ■ Matchings ■ Fill-in-the-blank **Patient management problems** **Essays (and modified essays)** **Oral exam** (see section below)
Observation tools (both direct and recorded behavior, including behavioral analysis)	**Observation of current behavior** ■ Direct observation ■ Structured (eg, checklists, rating scales) observation ■ Semi-structured (eg, oral exams) observation ■ Unstructured observation **Participant observation** **Observation of recorded behavior** ■ Videotape, audiotape, and text analysis **Standardized patients** (see above—OSCE) **Critical incident techniques** **Chart-stimulated recall** (see below)
Archives/documents	**Chart audit** **Chart-stimulated recall** **Secondary databases—administrative, clinical, and other**
Technology-assisted evaluation methods	**Computer simulations** **Computer-aided testing**

Continuing Medical Education Providers[5] for a comprehensive and in-depth examination of evaluation approaches and tools. Key references are provided within these resource materials.

Survey Methods

Surveys are the systematic collection of reports from people. Surveys generally ask people about their beliefs, attitudes, behaviors, feelings, perceptions, motivations, or plans. However, surveys can vary widely in the specificity of content, ranging from unstructured

TABLE 14-2

Factors Affecting the Choice of An Approach/Tool

Approach/ Procedure	Tool	Factors Affecting Choice of Approach/Tool				
		Expense	Validity	Reliability	Acceptability to Users	Feedback opportunity
Survey methods	**Structured interview:**					
	■ Personal interview	+++	+++	+++	+++	+++
	■ Telephone interview	++	++	++	++	+++
	■ Written interview	+	++	++	++	+
	■ Internet questionnaire interview	+	++	++	++	+
	Unstructured interview	++	++	++	++	+++
	Semi-structured interview	++	++	++	++	+++
Knowledge tests	**Objective structured clinical examination**	++	++	+++	++	++
	Written test with restrictive answers:					
	■ Multiple choice questions	+	+	+++	++	+
	■ True/false	+	+	++	+	+
	■ Matching questions	+	+	++	+	+
	■ Fill-in-the-blank	++	+	++	+	+
	Patient management problems/case studies	++	++	++	++	+
	Essays (and modified essay questions)	+++	+	++	+	+
	Oral examinations	+++	++	+	+	++
Observation tools	**Direct observation**	+++	++	++	+	+
	Structured observation	++	++	++	+	++
	Semi-structured observation	++	+	+	+	++
	Unstructured observation	+++	+	+	+	++
	Participant observation	+++	++	+	+	+++
	Videotape, audiotape, and text analysis	++	++	++	++	++
	Standardized patients	+++	+++	+++	+++	+++
	Critical incident technique	++	+++	++	++	+++
Archives/ documents	**Chart audit (review)**	+	++	++	+++	+++
	Chart-stimulated recall	++	+++	++	++	+++
	Administrative, clinical, and other secondary databases	+	+	+	+++	+
Technology-assisted evaluation methods	**Computer simulations**	+++	+++	++	++	+++
	Computer-aided testing	+++	+	++	+	+++

Key: + low; ++ moderate; +++ high.

interviews, to semi-structured interviews, to almost completely structured surveys.

Tools

Structured Survey

Definition, Description, and Uses. Structured surveys have questions and options for answers that are mostly predetermined. The investigator has developed specific hypotheses and identified questions and answers that measure identified variables in specified ways.

Strengths and Limitations. Structured surveys have two major advantages. One advantage is that responses can be compared, aggregated, and analyzed across respondents. Results concerning measures and their relationships can be quantitatively summarized and communicated. Another advantage is that the survey may be administered through procedures that are less expensive than personal interviews performed by a professional familiar with the topics. With the questions-and-answer options specified, administration possibilities include personal interviews by interviewers with limited training, telephone interviews, written questionnaires, and questionnaires completed via the Internet. The strengths and limitations of these methods of administration are addressed separately below.

Structured surveys have two major limitations. One is that the survey developers are assumed to understand correctly the general views of the people being surveyed. The specific questions and answers reflect this understanding. Mistakes in assumptions could result in respondents not correctly interpreting questions and the investigators not correctly interpreting responses. The other limitation is that quantitative data for specified variables may not capture qualitative circumstances occurring for unique cases.

See Table 14-3 for strengths and limitations of structured interviews or questionnaires.

TABLE 14-3

Strengths and Limitations of Structured Interviews or Questionnaires

	Strength	**Limitation**
Structured interviews or questionnaires	■ Measures can be quantitative ■ Responses can be compared and aggregated ■ Less expensive to administer; interviewers need only limited training, telephone interviews, written questionnaires, and Internet questionnaires are option	■ Incorrect assumptions in questions or response options adversely affect results ■ Fixed questions and responses may overlook qualitative aspects of the situation

Source: Compiled from Judd CM, Smith ER, and Kidder LH. *Research Methods in Social Relations.* 6th ed. Fort Worth: Harcourt Brace Jovanovich; 1991.

Methods of Administration.   More personal involvement in administering the survey tends to engage the respondent more fully but also increases the cost of administering the survey. Personal interviews have the most involvement, with the interviewer likely to obtain a high response rate, to maintain interest during long interviews, and to clarify questions for confused respondents. However, the costs for arranging for personal interviews, travel, and the interviewing time result in each interview being expensive to perform.

In contrast, written questionnaires are likely to have lower response rates, engage respondents for only a short time, and have no possibility for clarification. However, written questionnaires are much less costly to administer. Limitations on available resources often restrict investigators to written questionnaires when data are to be collected from a large number of people or to be repeatedly collected from a smaller number of people. Investigators using written questionnaires must understand their limitations and address them in developing specific studies, eg, recognize dependence on respondent's reading ability, determine how to distribute questionnaires and receive responses, increase motivation to respond, and keep length short. In regard to anonymous surveys, answers to personal questions are more likely to be true, eg, if you are asking about practices that people might not admit to if their identity were known.

Telephone interviews occupy a position between personal interviews and questionnaires—they are less personal but not impersonal. Response rates are moderate to high, the interview can be moderately long, and clarifications can be made. The cost is appreciably less than personal interviews but much more than written questionnaires.

Computers and the Internet are increasingly used to increase administration efficiency and reduce operational cost. When a large number of cases are to be processed, response options can be preprogrammed so that responses are directly entered into portable devices carried by personal interviewers, computers used by telephone interviewers, or computers supporting Web pages for written questionnaires completed over the Internet.

Unstructured Interviews

Definition, Description, and Uses.   For unstructured interviews, the questions and answers are completely free. The interviewer begins with only a general topic or issue in mind. The interviewer poses questions in the context of a discussion with the respondent. Depending on the respondent's answers, the interviewer may probe for more clarification or shift the questions to other aspects of the general topic.

Strengths and Limitations. The major advantage of unstructured interviews is that they provide qualitative insight and help generate hypothesis. Investigators may be interested in a topic but have little information about key aspects of a topic and how they interrelate. Through unstructured interviews, the investigator develops an understanding of respondents' views of a topic and the relevance of factors associated with it. Unstructured interviews can also be used to understand the personal significance of a respondent's attitudes.

A major disadvantage of the unstructured interview is that it may be a poor quantitative measurement tool. The flexibility of the interview usually results in responses that are not comparable, making analysis complex. Unstructured interviews also involve appreciable time, energy, and money, limiting the number that are practical to perform. A professional with sufficient training to understand both the underlying purpose of the interview and the situation of the respondent must perform the interview. The complex interaction between the interviewer and respondent generally requires face-to-face interviews. The open-ended nature of the interview typically requires a great deal of time both to perform the interview and to analyze responses.

See Table 14-4 for strengths and limitations of unstructured interviews.

Semi-structured Interviews

Definition, Description, and Uses. For semi-structured interviews, the interviewer knows in advance the specific topics or aspects of an issue that are important to address. The list of topics is specified, but the interviewer decides the manner and order in which questions are asked during each interview. Respondents can answer however they wish, but the interviewer controls the direction of the interview and decides when to pursue unanticipated

T A B L E 14-4

Strengths and Limitations of Unstructured Interviews

	Strength	**Limitation**
Unstructured interviews	■ Provide qualitative insight ■ Can be used to formulate hypothesis ■ Can be used to examine personal attitudes	■ Poor quantitative measurement ■ Analysis is complex ■ Need qualified interviewer ■ Generally require face-to-face interviews ■ Time consuming

Source: Compiled from Judd CM, Smith ER, and Kidder LH. *Research Methods in Social Relations.* 6th ed. Fort Worth: Harcourt Brace Jovanovich; 1991.

TABLE 14-5

Strengths and Limitations of Semi-Structured Interviews

	Strength	**Limitation**
Semi-structured interviews	■ Provide qualitative insight ■ Can be used to confirm general hypothesis about individuals ■ Can be used to generate more specific hypotheses	■ Limited quantitative measurement ■ Analysis is complex ■ Need qualified interviewer ■ Generally require face-to-face interviews ■ Time consuming

Source: Compiled from Judd CM, Smith ER, and Kidder LH. *Research Methods in Social Relations.* 6th ed. Fort Worth: Harcourt Brace Jovanovich; 1991.

responses. Types of semi-structured interviews include "focus groups" for marketing research and clinical interviews for health problems.

Strengths and Limitations.   The major advantage of semi-structured interviews is that they can refine qualitative insights and identify general priorities regarding a topic. The interviewer can ask questions about specific topics to confirm general hypotheses and to generate more detailed hypotheses. When the interviewer needs only to identify a general preference without quantifying it, respondents' unstructured answers may be adequate.

A disadvantage of the semi-structured interview is that it is a limited measurement tool. The open format for responses often makes it difficult to compare or aggregate them across individuals. General patterns or preferences may be evident, but detailed quantitative distinctions and interrelationships are not. Semi-structured interviews involve appreciable resources, limiting the number that is practical to perform. An individual with sufficient training to understand the topics of interest and to follow up on unexpected responses must perform the interview. The complex interaction generally requires face-to-face interviews. The open-ended nature of the interview typically requires appreciable time to perform the interview and to analyze responses.

See Table 14-5 for strengths and limitations of semi-structured interviews.

Relationship Across Levels of Structure

A single project or a program of study may involve unstructured, semi-structured, and structured surveys planned and carried out to support each other. An investigator may use unstructured interviews to develop hypotheses, semi-structured interviews to refine them, and structured surveys to quantify results and relationships across a large, diverse sample of individuals. The development of a structured survey typically involves pilot testing with semi-structured interviews to ask respondents how they interpret the written questions and response options. Unexpected results in a structured survey may lead to further inquiry through unstructured or semi-structured surveys. The level of structure is determined by the investigator's purpose at the time.

Key references

Harrison RV. Simple questionnaire studies. *J Contin Educ Health Prof.* 1997;17:228–238.

Judd CM, Smith ER, Kidder LH. *Research Methods in Social Relations.* 6th ed. Fort Worth, TX: Harcourt Brace Jovanovich; 1991.

Salant P, Dillman DA. *How to Conduct Your Own Survey.* New York, NY: John Wiley & Sons; 1994.

Knowledge Tests

Tests are a methodology for evaluating factual knowledge, interview skills, clinical skills, problem-solving ability, and judgment. Tools and question types used for testing include objective structural clinical examinations (OSCE), multiple-choice questions (MCQ), true/false, matching, fill-in-the-blank, audiotape analysis, patient management problems (PMP)/case studies, essays, modified essay questions (MEQ), and oral examinations.

Tools

Objective Structured Clinical Examinations

Definition, Description, and Uses. Salvatori, Roberts, and Brown[6] define OSCE as "an objective evaluation measure used to assess components of clinical competence." "The OSCE is structured is such a way as to sample student performance in a variety of areas."[6] Examinees rotate through a series of testing stations, in a set time, and are asked to perform specific tasks.

The OSCE format can be used for evaluating a variety of skills including patient history-taking, patient interaction, treatment techniques, clinical procedures, lab test interpretation, and diagnostic analyses. The OSCE can be used to evaluate a wide range of areas and has become a standard in professional programs across Canada.[6] Furthermore, OSCEs can be used to evaluate performance at all levels of professional education (undergraduate, graduate, continuing education, licensure, and certification).

See Table 14-6 for strengths and limitations of objective structured clinical examination.

TABLE 14-6

Strengths and Limitations of Objective Structured Clinical Examination

	Strength	Limitation
Objective structured clinical examination checklist, peer assessment and review, Likert scale (5-point scale), standardized patients	■ High reliability and high validity ■ Potential for testing a wide range of knowledge and clinical skills ■ Flexible (number of stations, duration of stations, etc) ■ Can be used as a formative or summative measure of student performance in a relatively short period of time ■ Establishes pre-set standards of competence ■ Permits immediate and meaningful feedback for students and/or faculty (eg, for purposes of curriculum review) ■ Can reduce evaluation preparation time (through development of a bank of OSCE stations)	■ Difficult to evaluate student's approach to patient with compartmentalized skills ■ Requires internal consistency (ie, sampling enough times to get a reliable estimate of overall competence) for summative evaluation of clinical competence (such as a certification examination) ■ Requires increased staffing, development, and implementation ■ Requires time for evaluation training and criteria/checklist development

Source: Compiled from Ali J, Cohen R, Adam R et al. Teaching effectiveness of the advanced trauma life support program as demonstrated by an objective structured clinical examination for practicing physicians. *World J Surg.* 1996;20:1121–1125; and Salvatori P, Roberts J, Brown B. Objective structured clinical examinations (OSCE). In: Norman G, Shannon S, eds. *Evaluation Methods: A Resource Handbook.* Hamilton, Ont: The Program for Educational Development, McMaster University; 1995.

Key references

Ali J, Cohen R, Adam R, Gana TJ, Pierre I, Bedaysie H, Ali E, West U, Winn J. Teaching effectiveness of the advanced trauma life support program as demonstrated by an objective structured clinical examination for practicing physicians. *World J Surg.* 1996;20:1121–1125.

Salvatori P, Roberts J, Brown B. Objective structured clinical examinations (OSCE). In: Norman G, Shannon S, eds. *Evaluation Methods: A Resource Handbook.* Hamilton, Ont: The Program for Educational Development, McMaster University; 1995.

Multiple-Choice Questions

Definition, Description, and Uses. Robert Ebel,[7] in *Essentials of Educational Outcomes,* indicates that a multiple-choice test item has two parts: (a) the stem, which consists of a direct question or an incomplete statement; and (b) two or more options, consisting of potential answers to the question or completions of statements. Several, all, or none of the possible options may be correct in variations of the MCQ.[8]

The MCQ tool can be used to test understanding and ability, which are also tested by short-answer, true-false, matching, and essay questions.[7] Multiple-choice questions can be used to assess or

TABLE 14-7

Strengths and Limitations of Multiple Choice Questions

	Strength	Limitation
Multiple choice questions	■ Provides objectivity and validity ■ Specifically high content validity (large numbers of items included in the assessment) ■ Establishes high internal consistency reliability ■ Effective means to assess knowledge ■ Low cost ■ Able to sample large content domains efficiently and in relatively short testing times ■ Provides objective scoring in mass testing situations ■ High correlation with performance in practice ■ Is easily, quickly, and accurately scored (using computerized scoring, which has extremely high accuracy)	■ Has lower face and real-world validity ■ Requires extended time to construct in order to avoid arbitrary and ambiguous questions ■ Requires adjustment for positive scores that may be achieved by chance or by guessing ■ Provides cues that are unavailable in practice ■ Have a measurable and likely negative steering effect on student learning (students do study differently when MCQs are used as a major component of evaluation) ■ Focuses on recall of facts and recognition of the "right" answer over higher level thinking

Source: Compiled from Norman G. Multiple choice questions. In: Norman G, Shannon S, eds. *Evaluation Methods: A Resource Handbook.* Hamilton, Ont: The Program for Educational Development, McMaster University; 1995; and Pfeifle WG. *TIPS: Teaching Improvements Project Systems for Health Care Educators.* Lexington, KY: Center for Learning Resources & Office of Educational Development, College of Allied Health Professions, University of Kentucky; 1989.

measure knowledge, understanding, judgment, and general problem-solving ability.[7]

See Table 14-7 for strengths and limitations of multiple-choice questions.

Key references

Assessment Strategies. *A Brief Overview of Assessment Issues and Methods.* Ottawa: Assessment Strategies Inc; 1999.

Ebel RL. *Essentials of Educational Measurement,* 3rd ed. Englewood Cliffs, NJ: Prentice-Hall; 1979.

Norman G. Multiple choice questions. In: Norman G, Shannon S, eds. *Evaluation Methods: A Resource Handbook.* Hamilton, Ont: The Program for Educational Development, McMaster University; 1995.

Pfeifle WG. *TIPS: Teaching Improvements Project Systems for Health Care Educators.* Lexington, KY: Center for Learning Resources & Office of Educational Development, College of Allied Health Professions, University of Kentucky; 1989.

True/False

Definition, Description, and Uses.   In *Essentials of Educational Measurement*, Robert Ebel[7] defines a true/false test item as a statement that an examinee must determine to be either true or false. In addition to being expressed simply and concisely, well-written true/false questions should test an examinee's knowledge of a relevant or significant topic, require understanding and memory, be easily defendable to critics, and be apparent only to examinees with a good command of the required subject.[7] Well-written true/false questions can be used to evaluate an examinee's ability to understand complex ideas and solve problems.[7]

True/false items are not limited to testing for factual knowledge; as with well-written MCQs, they can be used for testing complex and difficult problems.[7]

See Table 14-8 for strengths and limitations of true and false test items.

Key reference

Ebel RL. *Essentials of Educational Measurement*, 3rd ed. Englewood Cliffs, NJ: Prentice-Hall; 1979.

Matching Questions

Definition, Description, and Uses.   Matching test items are comprised of separate lists of statements, terms, names, definitions, or symbols (termed premises and responses) and matching

TABLE 14-8

Strengths and Limitations of True and False

	Strength	Limitation
True and false	■ Provide relevant measure of educational achievement ■ Provide information on basic performance more efficiently than other tests ■ Are efficient (The number of scorable responses per hour of test time tends to be much higher than for MCQ.) ■ Are relatively easy to write in comparison to other test forms ■ Informed guesses are indicative of achievement ■ Does not require correction for guessing (Probability of achieving a high score by guessing is extremely low.) ■ Can identify ambiguous questions (pilot study)	■ Require time and effort to avoid producing items that are ambiguous or trivial ■ Can grossly oversimplify concept of truth ■ Expose examinee to error and falsehoods (This may be educationally harmful.)

Source: Compiled from Ebel RL. *Essentials of Educational Measurement.* 3rd ed. Englewood Cliffs, NJ: Prentice-Hall; 1979.

instructions.[7] A typical matching question should be made up of homogeneous lists of short premises and responses with clear instructions for matching.

Matching questions can be used for rapidly and efficiently testing the factual knowledge of an examinee.[7] As with MCQs, matching questions can be used to test knowledge in anatomy, physiology, and clinical diagnoses.

See Table 14-9 for strengths and limitations of matching questions.

Key reference

Ebel RL. *Essentials of Educational Measurement*, 3rd ed. Englewood Cliffs, NJ: Prentice-Hall; 1979.

Fill-in-the-Blank

Definition, Description, and Uses.   Fill-in-the-blank or short-answer questions test knowledge by requiring examinees to provide a word, number, or phrase to respond to a question or to complete a sentence.[7] Questions must be carefully written so that only one correct answer is possible.

Fill-in-the-blank questions are a rapid and efficient means of testing understanding of factual information.

See Table 14-10 for strengths and limitations of fill-in-the-blank questions.

TABLE 14-9

Strengths and Limitations of Matching Questions

	Strength	Limitation
Matching questions	■ Are efficient and yield many scorable responses per unit of testing time ■ Motivate examinees to integrate their knowledge and consider relations among items in lists	■ Are often limited to specific factual information ■ Are poorly suited for testing understanding and unique ideas

Source: Compiled from Ebel RL. *Essentials of Educational Measurement.* 3rd ed. Englewood Cliffs, NJ: Prentice-Hall; 1979.

TABLE 14-10

Strengths and Limitations of Fill-in-the-Blank Questions

	Strength	Limitation
Fill-in-the-blank questions	■ Are used to test for factual information ■ Are efficient and fairly easy to write	■ Need to be written carefully and conceived with the answer in mind to avoid multiple correct answers ■ Can only be used to test for factual information

Source: Compiled from Ebel RL. *Essentials of Educational Measurement.* 3rd ed. Englewood Cliffs, NJ: Prentice-Hall; 1979.

Key reference

Ebel RL. *Essentials of Educational Measurement*, 3rd ed. Englewood Cliffs, NJ: Prentice-Hall; 1979.

Patient Management Problems/Case Studies

Definition, Description, and Uses.   Patient management problems or case studies are the recreation of complete patient cases in which data related to the case are given at intervals.[9] The case study is a variation of traditional pen-and-paper testing schemes. Case studies are ideal for assessing the ability to think critically and apply knowledge.[5]

Case studies provide a patient-centered approach to CPD and offer an acceptable replacement to the large-group lecture format. The format is associated with a significant effect on knowledge skills and behavior and is usually rated highly satisfactory by participants.[10,11]

See Table 14-11 for strengths and limitations of patient management problems/case studies.

Key references

Assessment Strategies. *A Brief Overview of Assessment Issues and Methods.* Ottawa: Assessment Strategies Inc; 1999.

Davis D, Moore D, Sinclair L, Taylor-Vaisey A, Tipping J. *Evaluating Educational Outcomes: A Workbook for Continuing Medical Education Providers.* Toronto: University of Toronto, Faculty of Medicine, Office of Continuing Education. (Electronic publication; available www.acme-assn.org.)

TABLE 14-11

Strengths and Limitations of Patient Management Problems/Case Studies

	Strength	Limitation
Patient management problems/case studies	■ Moderate validity and reliability ■ Well-suited to assessing critical thinking skills and to evaluating applied knowledge ■ Can provide useful feedback to students	■ Requires a demanding design and complex scoring ■ Mass numbers of cases may be needed to obtain acceptable reliability estimates ■ Has a content validity mid-way between work simulations and MC questions ■ More costly than a MCQ examination

Source: Compiled from Norman GR. Defining competence: a methodological review. In: Neufeld VR, Norman GR, eds. *Assessing Clinical Competence.* New York, NY: Springer; 1985.

McArdle PJ. Innovations in undergraduate medical education and in graduate medical training. *J Contin Educ Health Prof.* 1997;17:214–223.

Norman GR. Defining competence: a methodological review. In: Neufeld VR, Norman GR, eds. *Assessing Clinical Competence.* New York, NY: Springer; 1985.

Premi J. Problem based, self-directed continuing medical education in a group of practicing family physicians. *J Med Educ.* 1988;63:484–486.

Premi J, Shannon S, Hartwick K, Lamb S, Wakefield J, Williams J. Practice-based small-group CME. *Acad Med.* 1994;69(10):800–802.

Essays

Definition, Description, and Uses. An essay test poses a question or problem that requires an extended written response from the examinee.[7] This form allows the evaluator to observe or determine the examinee's ability to synthesize ideas and information, argue points-of-view, integrate relevant information, and develop conclusions with supporting evidence.[12] In the McMaster handbook, Palmer and Rideout state that "the term 'essay' refers to a variety of kinds of written discourse" that vary "according to the degree of freedom enjoyed by the writer in the treatment of the subject" (1995, p. 59).

The essay can be used to assess organizational and communication skills that are not easily tested by other means.[7]

See Table 14-12 for strengths and limitations of essays (and modified essays).

TABLE 14-12

Strengths and Limitations of Essays (and Modified Essays)

	Strength	Limitation
Essays (and modified essays)	▪ Provide opportunity for candidates to indicate knowledge and organizational ideas with effective explanations ▪ Attempt to assess kinds of thinking and communication skills and abilities not generally demanded by other evaluation methods ▪ Are especially suitable for courses that encourage self-directed learning ▪ Are relatively straightforward to devise ▪ Are highly adaptable to different subjects and different levels of sophistication	▪ Low reliability and low validity ▪ Limit severely the total work sampled ▪ Lacks objectivity ▪ Presents difficulties in obtaining consistent judgments of performance ▪ Provides negligible feedback ▪ High cost ▪ Takes considerable time and effort to read and mark

Source: Compiled from Palmer D, Rideout E. Essays. In: Norman G, Shannon S, eds. *Evaluation Methods: A Resource Handbook.* Hamilton, Ont: The Program for Educational Development, McMaster University; 1995; and Pfeifle WG. *TIPS: Teaching Improvements Project Systems for Health Care Educators.* Lexington, KY: Center for Learning Resources & Office of Educational Development, College of Allied Health Professions, University of Kentucky; 1989.

Key references

Ebel RL. *Essentials of Educational Measurement*, 3rd ed. Englewood Cliffs, NJ: Prentice-Hall; 1979.

Palmer D, Rideout E. Essays. In: Norman G, Shannon S, eds. *Evaluation Methods: A Resource Handbook*. Hamilton, Ont: The Program for Educational Development, McMaster University; 1995.

Pfeifle WG. *TIPS: Teaching Improvements Project Systems for Health Care Educators*. Lexington, KY: Center for Learning Resources & Office of Educational Development, College of Allied Health Professions, University of Kentucky; 1989.

Modified Essay Question

Definition, Description, and Uses.   The MEQ is defined by Stratford and Smeda[13] in *McMaster's Evaluation Methods: A Resource Handbook* as an examination tool " . . . intended to examine the respondent's ability to solve and manage (at least on paper) clinical problems, and to assess problem related aspects of basic and clinical sciences" (p. 55). In general, an MEQ is made up of a brief passage or scenario followed by questions that are answered by examinees in an independent and self-directed manner.[5]

The MEQ can be constructed as a series of questions related to a single patient encounter scenario. The tool can be used to assess the examinee's knowledge and ability to interpret clinical, laboratory, and diagnostic data and to determine prudent treatment plans.

See Table 14-13 for strengths and limitations of modified essays.

Key references

Davis D, Moore D, Sinclair L, Taylor-Vaisey A, Tipping J. *Evaluating Educational Outcomes: A Workbook for Continuing Medical Education Providers*. Toronto: University of Toronto, Faculty of Medicine, Office of

TABLE 14-13

Strengths and Limitations of Modified Essays

	Strength	Limitation
Modified essays	■ Tool for both formative and summative components of evaluation ■ Demonstrate reasonable psychometric properties ■ Have development time (including criteria setting) comparable to that of the MCQ ■ Problem-based learning style in that test questions are embedded in a problem format	■ Time consuming to grade (hand marked) ■ Cannot sample as much content as MCQ per unit of examination

Source: Compiled from Stratford P, Smeda J. Modified essay question. In: Norman G, Shannon S, eds. *Evaluation Methods: A Resource Handbook*. Hamilton, Ont: The Program for Educational Development, McMaster University; 1995.

Continuing Education. (Electronic publication; available www.acme-assn.org.)

Ebel RL. *Essentials of Educational Measurement*, 3rd ed. Englewood Cliffs, NJ: Prentice-Hall; 1979.

Stratford P, Smeda J. Modified essay question. In: Norman G, Shannon S, eds. *Evaluation Methods: A Resource Handbook*. Hamilton, Ont: The Program for Educational Development, McMaster University; 1995.

Oral (examinations)

Definition, Description, and Uses. An oral examination is a face-to-face evaluation in which the examinee orally responds to questions posed by the examiner(s).[7] A case study is presented and the examinee is asked to answer questions regarding diagnosis, treatment, and other related issues.[5] Medical rounds can be seen as a form of institutionalized oral examination.[14] The oral examination allows for direct and immediate feedback from the examiners to the examinee. The Structured Office Oral was dropped from the Physician Review Program (a professional competency assessment program that utilizes multiple-choice questions, standardized patients, and chart stimulated recall) in 1995, because "it was insufficiently structured to be reliable and because it did not add significantly to the other tools"[15] (p. 9).

See Table 14-14 for strengths and limitations of oral examinations

T A B L E 14-14

Strengths and Limitations of Oral Examinations

	Strength	**Limitation**
Oral examinations	■ Provide direct personal contact with candidates ■ Provide an opportunity to take into account mitigating circumstances ■ Provide flexibility in moving from strong to weak areas ■ Require the candidate to supply his/her own formulation without cues ■ Provide an opportunity to question the candidate about how he/she arrived at an answer ■ Provide opportunity for simultaneous assessment by two examiners ■ Allow direct feedback between the examiners and the learner ■ Measure skills (eg, personal characteristics) missed by other evaluation tools	■ Low reliability ■ Lack standardization ■ Lack objectivity and reproducibility of results ■ Do not have systematic content analysis ■ Possible abuse of the personal contact, undue influence, or irrelevant factors ■ Lack an adequate cadre of trained examiners ■ High cost ■ Not feasible for large populations because of the logistical problems and costs

Source: Compiled from Pfeifle WG. *TIPS: Teaching Improvements Project Systems for Health Care Educators*. Lexington, KY: Center for Learning Resources & Office of Educational Development, College of Allied Health Professions, University of Kentucky; 1989; and Muzzin LJ. Oral examinations. In: Norman G, Shannon S, eds. *Evaluation Methods: A Resource Handbook*. Hamilton, Ont: The Program for Educational Development, McMaster University; 1995.

Key references

Cunnington JP, Hanna E, Turnbull J, Kaigas TB, Norman GR. Defensible assessment of the competency of the practicing physician. *Acad Med.* 1997;72:9–12.

Davis D, Moore D, Sinclair L, Taylor-Vaisey A, Tipping J. *Evaluating Educational Outcomes: A Workbook for Continuing Medical Education Providers.* Toronto: University of Toronto, Faculty of Medicine, Office of Continuing Education. (Electronic publication; available www.acme-assn.org.)

Ebel RL. *Essentials of Educational Measurement,* 3rd ed. Englewood Cliffs, NJ: Prentice-Hall; 1979.

Muzzin LJ. Oral examinations. In: Norman G, Shannon S, eds. *Evaluation Methods: A Resource Handbook.* Hamilton, Ont: The Program for Educational Development, McMaster University; 1995.

Pfeifle WG. *TIPS: Teaching Improvements Project Systems for Health Care Educators.* Lexington, KY: Center for Learning Resources & Office of Educational Development, College of Allied Health Professions, University of Kentucky; 1989.

Observation Tools

Davis et al[5] define observation in the medical education setting as, "scrutiny of a clinical encounter by a trained individual, generally with a checklist based on appropriate clinical guidelines." Encounters can be video- or audiotaped for postencounter review. Observation can be direct or indirect (by way of a two-way mirror). Real or simulated patients can be used. Tools used in observation include direct observation, structured and semistructured observation (checklists and rating scales), unstructured observation, and participant observation.

Key reference

Davis D, Moore D, Sinclair L, Taylor-Vaisey A, Tipping J. *Evaluating Educational Outcomes: A Workbook for Continuing Medical Education Providers.* Toronto: University of Toronto, Faculty of Medicine, Office of Continuing Education. (Electronic publication; available www.acme-assn.org.)

Tools

Direct Observation

Definition, Description, and Uses. Thomson[16] defines direct observation as the observation of learners ". . . in complete encounters, formally or informally, with real or simulated patients"

TABLE 14-15

Strengths and Limitations of Direct Observation

	Strength	**Limitation**
Direct observation	■ Moderate reliability and high validity ■ High content validity ■ Has better reliability for history-taking, physical examination, and communication skills than for differential diagnosis, laboratory utilization, and treatment ■ Is best suited to the evaluation of procedural skills, technical skills, and interpersonal skills ■ Provides the examiner information about visual and auditory processes	■ High cost ■ May influence performance through learner's awareness of observation and assessment ■ Requires orientation/training of the observers ■ Requires sampling of a number of different situations or evaluations for a reliable estimate of overall skills and/or performance ■ Requires informed consent

Source: Compiled from Thomson MA. Direct observation. In: Norman G, Shannon S, eds. *Evaluation Methods: A Resource Handbook.* Hamilton, Ont: The Program for Educational Development, McMaster University; 1995.

(p. 67). This may involve the evaluation of an examinee or learner in a clinical setting by a preceptor, with a rating assigned at the end of the encounter or a more structured test such as the objective structured clinical examination being given (see *Tests*).[16] The observer may be physically present, may view the encounter by video camera, or may evaluate the completed encounter by videotape.

Direct observation is an apt evaluation method for assessing interpersonal skills and procedural or technical skills. Cognitive processes and problem-solving skills are not as easily assessed with direct observation, and this tool should be coupled with other evaluation tools for complete assessments.[16]

See Table 14-15 for strengths and limitations of direct observation.

Key reference

Thomson MA. Direct observation. In: Norman G, Shannon S, eds. *Evaluation Methods: A Resource Handbook.* Hamilton, Ont: The Program for Educational Development, McMaster University; 1995.

Structured and Semi-structured Observation (Checklists and Rating Scales)

Definition, Description, and Uses   Structured and semi-structured observation are variations of observation tools in which the evaluator or observer gathers information about the performance of an examinee in a clinical setting, with a standardized patient, or at a structured test station with a mannequin or patient simulator, using a checklist or rating scale. The use of a checklist or

TABLE 14-16

Strengths and Limitations of Structured and Semi-structured Observations

	Strength	**Limitation**
Structured (eg, checklists, rating scales) **and semi-structured observation**	■ Is simple and efficient and can be completed in minutes ■ Is comprehensive (can range from clinical judgment to interpersonal skills) ■ May use checklists for reduction of inter-observer variation ■ May use structured rating scales for complex tasks	■ Low validity ■ Has low reliability for global ratings despite apparent face validity and completion ease ■ Has problems with domain discrimination and halo effect

Note: To alleviate many of the limitations of observation tools, increase the sample size of observations and number of independent observers used. Also refer to Table 14-15, which shows the strengths and limitations of direct observation.

Source: Compiled from Streiner S. Clinical ratings-ward evaluation. In: Norman G, Shannon S, eds. *Evaluation Methods: A Resource Handbook.* Hamilton, Ont: The Program for Educational Development, McMaster University; 1995; and Thomson MA. Direct observation. In: Norman G, Shannon S, eds. *Evaluation Methods: A Resource Handbook.* Hamilton, Ont: The Program for Educational Development, McMaster University; 1995.

rating scale reduces inter-evaluator variation and narrows the focus of what is being evaluated in a given encounter.[16]

Structured and semi-structured observation are used in standardized skills assessment in which predetermined techniques and physical maneuvers are performed for evaluators who score the examinee on specific and fixed aspects of the technique.[5]

Case presentations, in which the examinee presents a case and then answers questions about his/her understanding of the case, is another method of evaluation using semi-structured observation.

See Table 14-16 for strengths and limitations of structured and semi-structured observations.

Key references

Bucher L. Evaluating the affective domain. Consider a Likert scale. *J Nursing Staff Devel.* 1991;7:234–238.

Davis D, Moore D, Sinclair L, Taylor-Vaisey A, Tipping J. *Evaluating Educational Outcomes: A Workbook for Continuing Medical Education Providers.* Toronto: University of Toronto, Faculty of Medicine, Office of Continuing Education. (Electronic publication; available www.acme-assn.org.)

Streiner S. Clinical ratings-ward evaluation. In: Norman G, Shannon S, eds. *Evaluation Methods: A Resource Handbook.* Hamilton, Ont: The Program for Educational Development, McMaster University; 1995.

Thomson MA. Direct observation. In: Norman G, Shannon S, eds. *Evaluation Methods: A Resource Handbook.* Hamilton, Ont: The Program for Educational Development, McMaster University; 1995.

T A B L E   14-17

Strengths and Limitations of Unstructured Observation

	Strength	Limitation
Unstructured observation	■ Provides more natural evaluation situation and therefore may be more reflective of true clinical performance ■ Qualitative comments provide useful feedback to learner	■ Low validity and reliability ■ Requires time for written assessment and record maintenance ■ High cost ■ Has problems with objectivity and biases of observer/evaluator ■ Must be evaluated in a number of situations over a period of time for reliability

Source: Compiled from Gronlund NE. *Measurement and Evaluation in Teaching.* 2nd ed. New York, NY: Macmillan; 1971.

van Thiel J, Kraan HF, van der Vleuten CP. Reliability and feasibility of measuring medical interviewing skills: the revised Maastricht history-taking and advice checklist. *Med Educ.* 1991;25:224–229.

Unstructured Observation

Definition, Description, and Uses   Unstructured observation is based on teacher or examiner observations in an uncontrolled environment or situation and involves qualitative comments on the examinee's performance.[17] This may involve the evaluation of an examinee's performance in a clinical setting at the end of a period of time.[16]

See Table 14-17 for strengths and limitations of unstructured observation.

Key references

Borg WR, Gall MD. *Educational Research: An Introduction,* 3rd ed. New York, NY: Longman; 1979.

Gronlund NE. *Measurement and Evaluation in Teaching.* 2nd ed. New York, NY: Macmillan; 1971.

Thomson MA. Direct observation. In: Norman G, Shannon S, eds. *Evaluation Methods: A Resource Handbook.* Hamilton, Ont: The Program for Educational Development, McMaster University; 1995.

Participant Observation

Definition, Description, and Uses.   Participant observation is a method of researching or evaluating a specific group through observation of/interaction with the subjects who make up the group.[18] Over a long period of time, a researcher observes group members, participates in activities, and systematically collects data.[19]

TABLE 14-18

Strengths and Limitations of Participant Observation

	Strength	Limitation
Participant observation	■ Has less likelihood of subject altering their behavior in the presence of observer as time passes ■ Allows differences between described behavior and actual behavior to become apparent ■ Allows contextual understanding of actions and performance ■ Allows complete picture of the health care encounter	■ May be obtrusive to subjects ■ Requires patient consent ■ Lacks standardization ■ Has variations in observer methodology and documentation ■ High cost ■ Time consuming ■ Requires a lot of documentation

Source: Compiled from Crabtree BF, Miller WL, eds. *Doing Qualitative Research: Research Methods for Primary Care, vol. 3.* Newbury Park, Calif: Sage Publications; 1992.

The method of participant observation is appropriate for any research question addressing social or group situations that requires an understanding of processes, events, and relationships.[19]

See Table 14-18 for strengths and limitations of participant observation.

Key references

Crabtree BF, Miller WL, eds. *Doing Qualitative Research: Research Methods for Primary Care, vol. 3.* Newbury Park, Calif: Sage Publications; 1992.

Helman CG. Research in primary care: the qualitative approach. In: Norton PG, Stewart M, Tudiver F, Bass MJ, Dunn EV, eds. *Primary Care Research: Traditional and Innovative Approaches, Research Methods for Primary Care, vol. 1.* Newbury Park, Calif: Sage Publications; 1991.

Videotape, Audiotape, and Text Analysis

Definition, Description, and Uses. Davis et al.[5] define videotape analysis as an "examination of a clinical encounter using a video-camera, or videotaping equipment, permitting a review of the encounter, with the clinician, at a later date." In general, video observations, in conjunction with audiotape and, in some cases, text analysis (the review of transcripts that are prepared from videotape and audiotape data using a system of codes), are used in residency training settings. However, they can also be used to practice and review many basic clinical skills.[5,19]

Videotape, audiotape, and text analysis can be used as powerful teaching tools that provide examinees with an accurate picture of their performance in a given circumstance. They can also be used as evaluation tools for interpersonal, clinical, technical, and patient

TABLE 14-19

Strengths and Limitations of Videotape, Audiotape, and Text Analysis

	Strength	**Limitation**
Videotape, audiotape, and text analysis	■ Moderate validity and reliability ■ Good feedback tool ■ Can produce very accurate data (except in the case of text analysis) ■ Provides a natural setting ■ Provides an opportunity for verification of analysis	■ Requires patient consent ■ High cost (assessor, travel time, equipment, and transcription of tapes) ■ Only evaluate what can be seen or heard on tape

Source: Compiled from Cox J. An instrument for assessment of videotapes of general practitioners' performance. *BMJ.* 1993;306:1043–1046; Davis D, Moore D, Sinclair L, Taylor-Vaisey A, Tipping J. *Evaluating Educational Outcomes: A Workbook for Continuing Medical Education Providers.* Toronto: University of Toronto, Faculty of Medicine, Office of Continuing Education; and Ram P, Grol R, Rethans JJ, Schouten B, van der Vleuten CV, Kester A. Assessment of general practitioners by video observation of communicative and medical performance in daily practice: issues of validity, reliability and feasibility. *Med Educ.* 31999;3:447–454.

interview skills. These types of analyses can be used in conjunction with many other assessment strategies including direct observation, participant observation, OSCE, and standardized patients.

See Table 14-19 for strengths and limitations of videotape, audiotape, and text analysis.

Key references

Cox J. An instrument for assessment of videotapes of general practitioners' performance. *BMJ.* 1993;306:1043–1046.

Crabtree BF, Miller WL, eds. *Doing Qualitative Research: Research Methods for Primary Care, vol. 3.* Newbury Park, Calif: Sage Publications; 1992.

Davis D, Moore D, Sinclair L, Taylor-Vaisey A, Tipping J. *Evaluating Educational Outcomes: A Workbook for Continuing Medical Education Providers.* Toronto: University of Toronto, Faculty of Medicine, Office of Continuing Education. (Electronic publication; available www.acme-assn.org.)

Ram P, Grol R, Rethans JJ, Schouten B, van der Vleuten CV, Kester A. Assessment of general practitioners by video observation of communicative and medical performance in daily practice: issues of validity, reliability and feasibility. *Med Educ.* 31999;3:447–454.

Standardized patients

Definition, Description, and Uses.   Standardized patients are individuals trained to portray specific clinical symptoms and histories in a standard way or actual patients trained to present their illness in a consistent and standard way.[20] The examinee is evaluated for his/her clinical skills and effective evaluation and management of the patient's problems by the examiner, who may directly observe

T A B L E   14-20

Strengths and Limitations of Standardized Patients

	Strength	**Limitation**
Standardized patients	■ Can discriminate wide range of examinee's clinical performances ■ Can be valid and reliable tool ■ Are realistic and accurate in portrayal of cases ■ Can reliably and accurately evaluate clinical skills ■ Are consistent and multiple SPs have little or no effect on reliability	■ High cost to train and employ ■ Time consuming ■ Require training (and even then there are significant differences in accurate portrayal of illnesses) ■ Time consuming because several SPs must be seen for reliable evaluation ■ Are sensitive to breaches of test security

Source: Compiled from Colliver JA, Williams RG. Technical issues: test application. *Acad Med.* 1993;68:454–460; and Vu NV, Barrows HS, Marcy ML, Verhulst SJ, Colliver JA, Travis T. Six years of comprehensive, clinical performance-based assessment using standardized patients at the Southern Illinois University School of Medicine. *Acad Med.* 1992; 67:42–50.

(or observe by camera or two-way mirror). The standardized patient evaluates the interpersonal skills and effectiveness of the examinee.[20] The standardized patient can be used in conjunction with videotape, audiotape, and text analysis to maximize the learning experience and evaluation effectiveness. Standardized patients are also known as simulated patients, pseudo-patients, programmed patients, and surrogate patients.

The standardized patient is a powerful assessment tool that allows examiners to assess ". . . the physician's ability to effectively evaluate and manage the patients' problems, and a non-cognitive one defined as the physicians attitudes, work habits, and interpersonal skill or their effectiveness in physician-patient relationships."[21]

See Table 14-20 for strengths and limitations of standardized patients.

Key references

Barrows HS. An overview of the uses of standardized patients for teaching and evaluating clinical skills. *Acad Med.* 1993;68:443–451.

Colliver JA, Williams RG. Technical issues: test application. *Acad Med.* 1993;68:454–460.

Davis D, Moore D, Sinclair L, Taylor-Vaisey A, Tipping J. *Evaluating Educational Outcomes: A Workbook for Continuing Medical Education Providers.* Toronto: University of Toronto, Faculty of Medicine, Office of Continuing Education. (Electronic publication; available www.acme-assn.org.)

Ram P, van der Vleuten C, Rethans JJ, Grol R, Aretz K. Assessment of practicing family physicians: comparison of observation in a multiple-station examination using standardized patients with observation of consultations in daily practice. *Acad Med*. 1999;74:62–69.

van der Vleuten CP, Swanson DB. Assessment of clinical skills with standardized patients: state of the art. *Teaching Learning in Med*. 1990;2:58–76.

Vu NV, Barrows HS, Marcy ML, Verhulst SJ, Colliver JA, Travis T. Six years of comprehensive, clinical performance-based assessment using standardized patients at the Southern Illinois University School of Medicine. *Acad Med*. 1992;67:42–50.

Vu NV, Marcy ML, Verhulst SJ, Barrows HS. Generalizability of standardized patients' satisfaction ratings of their clinical encounter with fourth-year medical students. *Acad Med*.1990;65(Suppl):S29–S30.

Critical Incidents Technique

Definition, Description, and Uses.   Critical incidents technique, a form of observational rating, is the review of situations or documented events that hold significance for interviewees and are vividly remembered.[22] Concise instructions with clear purpose are given to participants to facilitate recall of crucial details related to an event.[22] The responses from a population are collated and examined for similar themes.

For example, a group of physicians or nurses may be asked to identify events involving interns who had significant effects (positive or negative) on the quality of care delivered to a patient. These anecdotes can then be grouped according to theme and prevalent concerns or comments identified. There is some overlap between this technique and the review of incident logs or incident reports, which fall under the heading of Analysis of Administrative, Clinical and Secondary Databases.

See Table 14-21 for strengths and limitations of critical incidents technique.

Key references

Allery LA, Owen PA, Robling MR: Why general practitioners and consultants change their clinical practice: a critical incident study. *BMJ*. 1997;314:870–874.

Borg WR, Gall MD. *Educational Research: An Introduction*. 3rd ed. New York, NY: Longman; 1979.

Norman GR. Defining competence: a methodological review. In: Neufeld VR, Norman GR, eds. *Assessing Clinical Competence*. New York, NY: Springer; 1985.

TABLE   14-21

Strengths and Limitations of Critical Incidents Technique

	Strength	Limitation
Critical incidents technique	■ Can be used to detect trends that might not be detected with other tools ■ Can identify qualitative concerns that are not easily investigated using quantitative tools ■ Useful method for investigating complex or multi-faceted subjects	■ Lack standardization ■ Problems with validity because bias can be a factor, even in very large groups ■ Anecdotal (dependent on the recall of the participants) ■ Questionable reliability (What sample size is adequate?) ■ Can be too general (respondents must be encouraged to give specific examples of events)

Source: Compiled from Allery LA, Owen PA, Robling MR. Why general practitioners and consultants change their clinical practice: a critical incident study. *BMJ.* 1997;314:870–874; Borg WR, Gall MD. *Educational Research: An Introduction,* 3rd ed. New York, NY: Longman; 1979; and Norman GR. Defining competence: a methodological review. In: Neufeld VR, Norman GR, eds. *Assessing Clinical Competence.* New York, NY: Springer; 1985.

Rosenal L. Exploring the learner's world: critical incident methodology. *J Contin Educ Nursing.* 1995;26:115–118.

Chart-stimulated Recall

The reader is referred to the Archive/Document section for details related to this assessment tool.

Archives/Documents

A document is a written record that can be classified as handwritten or printed, published or unpublished, and confidential or public. Examples of documents include medical charts, prescription slips, diaries, legal records, periodicals, memos, institutional files, tests, etc. Documents can be either primary source (ie, information in the document is described by a person who witnessed an event firsthand) or secondary source (ie, information in the document is described by a person who did not witness the event but learned of it from someone else). An archive is a collection of documents.[17]

Examples of archive/document tools are chart audit (review); chart-stimulated recall; as well as administrative, clinical, and other secondary databases.

Key reference

Borg WR, Gall MD. *Educational Research: An Introduction.* 3rd ed. New York, NY: Longman; 1979.

Tools

Chart Audit (Review)

Definition, Description, and Uses. Tugwell and Dok[23] describe chart audit (CA) as the review and assessment of patient medical records, generally using preset criteria and standards. The CA cycle involves several steps: selecting the subject, criteria, and standards; conducting the audit with data collection; comparing audit findings to standards and criteria; designing and implementing educational programs; and reassessing performance through CA.[24] Explicit or implicit criteria and standards are required against which CA findings can be compared. Preferably, criteria should be developed from scientific evidence. Expert and peer opinion are also used to produce valid standards. The training of chart reviewers in CA activities is required to ensure reliable, consistent, and accurate application of criteria and standards.[24]

Chart audit can be used for assessing needs and evaluating the state of adoption of practice guidelines. In addition, variations in practice and professional competence and performance can be determined. Self-assessment of competence and compliance with standards can also be achieved through self-auditing.[24]

See Table 14-22 for strengths and limitations of chart audit.

Key references

Jennett PA, Affleck L. Chart audit and chart stimulated recall as methods of needs assessment in continuing professional health education. *J Contin Educ Health Prof.* 1998;18:63–171.

Tugwell P, Dok C. Medical record review. In Neufeld VR, Norman GR, eds. *Assessing Clinical Competence.* New York, NY: Springer; 1985.

Chart-stimulated Recall

Definition, Description, and Uses. Jennett and Affleck[24] define chart-stimulated recall (CSR) as a "case-based interviewing technique used to assess the process and nature of clinical decision making" (p. 164). Medical records provide the framework for discussion. A CSR interview around one case generally lasts 15 to 20 minutes. Physicians discuss with trained interviewers the clinical choices they have made in the care of a patient. They use all of the record materials during the interview as a memory jogger. Interviewers review the records for key points prior to the session and use these points, along with predesigned probing questions, as a stimulus and guide for discussion.[25] Questions that explore the diagnostic, investigative, and clinical management choices are used. They are nonbiased (neutral) and nonjudgmental in style. Open-ended questions usually begin the process, and semi-structured questions appear throughout.

TABLE 14-22

Strengths and Limitations of Chart Audit

	Strength	**Limitation**
Chart audit	▪ Less expensive and time consuming than other methods such as interviews and videotaped observation ▪ Relatively easy to perform ▪ Captures data specific to test/medication orders and repeated or continuous visits ▪ Usually accessible ▪ Provides consistent and reliable findings with its standardized approach and use of criteria ▪ Based on relevant daily clinical experience and behavior and therefore is generally acceptable to professionals ▪ Adds face and content validity through the use of actual cases ▪ Allows participation and implementation by professionals ▪ Not usually viewed as invasive or disruptive to practice ▪ Can provide quick feedback and can be used for both formative and summative purposes ▪ Can serve as an active continuing learning technique ▪ Has a generally acceptable inter-rater reliability ▪ Provides personalized and individualized feedback around actual practice and patient charts ▪ Can be used across disciplines and care sites	▪ May be incomplete or inaccurate reflection of the care encounter (can be missing relevant information regarding patient symptoms, communication issues, and care options considered but ruled out) ▪ Does not detail associated reasoning behind choices and negative test results ▪ Can have poor content validity especially due to incomplete recording ▪ Lacks standardization in chart formats, types of filing systems, and in location or retrieval of all parts of the record ▪ Variations in professional recording practices and legibility

Source: Compiled from Jennett PA, Affleck L. Chart audit and chart stimulated recall as methods of needs assessment in continuing professional health education. *J Contin Educ Health Prof.* 1998;18:63–171.

The physician is asked to describe the patient case, outline the approach to the problem, and highlight key points. This information, in addition to other information identified before the interview, is used by the interviewer to guide the remaining time. In order to elicit greater depth to a response, interviewers ask the physicians to outline the diagnostic/management options they considered and ruled out. Physicians are also encouraged to give examples or describe points in more detail. This questioning technique encourages practitioners to reflect upon all the thoughts, feelings, factors, and strategies going through their minds at the time decisions are made. It allows the emergence of professional, social, personal practice, and/or health care system factors.[26]

The CSR tool is frequently used to explore the rationale for and the variation in clinical decision-making. In addition, the method

TABLE 14-23

Strengths and Limitations of Chart Stimulated Recall

	Strength	Limitation
Chart stimulated recall	■ Reliable and valid ■ Good inter-rater reliability with trained interviewers and assessors	■ More costly and time consuming than chart audit alone ■ Too expensive if large numbers of physicians need to be assessed ■ Depends upon self-report and memory of interviewees (subjective) ■ May be obtrusive to interviewees ■ Requires three to six cases for accurate assessment of competence ■ Requires adequate interviewer training

Source: Compiled from Jennett PA, Affleck L. Chart audit and chart stimulated recall as methods of needs assessment in continuing professional health education. *J Contin Educ Health Prof.* 1998;18:63–171.

has been employed to assess needs, clinical competence, and performance in recertification and enhancement programs. It can identify patient, practice, and/or health care system determinants of clinical decisions. It can also reveal the strengths and weaknesses in physicians' knowledge, skills, and attitudes. The power of the CSR technique is in understanding aspects and determinants of competence and performance, as well as in assessing them. It helps capture the complexity of the health care context and culture and, thus, makes explicit those elements neglected by more traditional assessment methods. CSR therefore can be an important adjunct to current assessment methods.[26]

See Table 14-23 for strengths and limitations of chart stimulated recall.

Key references

Jennett PA, Affleck L. Chart audit and chart stimulated recall as methods of needs assessment in continuing professional health education. *J Contin Educ Health Prof.* 1998;18:63–171.

Jennett PA. Chart stimulated recall: a technique to assess clinical competence and performance. *Educ Gen Prac.* 1995;6:30–34.

Jennett PA, Scott SM, Atkinson MA, Crutcher RA, Hogan DB, Elford RW, MacCannel KL, Baumber JS. Patient charts and physician office management decisions: chart audit and chart stimulated recall. *J Contin Educ Health Prof.* 1995;15:31–39.

TABLE 14-24

Strengths and Limitations of Administrative, Clinical, and Secondary Databases

	Strength	Limitation
Administrative, clinical, and secondary databases	■ Can be used to assess performance-related problems that will not be detected using other means (eg, overprescription of antibiotics and other drugs) ■ Low cost because the database has already been developed	■ A crude representation of performance ■ Can be of varying reliability and validity because the investigator using the information did not develop the database ■ Limited in that the person using the database must use the same terms and definitions as the database creator

Source: Compiled from Borg WR, Gall MD. *Educational Research: An Introduction.* 3rd ed. New York, NY: Longman; 1979; and Davis D, Moore D, Sinclair L, Taylor-Vaisey A, Tipping J. *Evaluating Educational Outcomes: A Workbook for Continuing Medical Education Providers.* Toronto: University of Toronto, Faculty of Medicine, Office of Continuing Education. (Electronic publication; available www.acme-assn.org.)

Administrative, Clinical, and Other Secondary Databases

Definition, Description, and Uses. A secondary database is a collection of information and documents in which the writer describing the event was not present but obtained the information from someone else.[17] In the context of the health care environment, a secondary database may contain information about the number of times that specific physicians ordered certain diagnostic tests in a month. Data can be collected continuously and automatically, and analyses of trends can be performed on a regular basis.

Secondary databases may be analyzed for a number of different indicators of a health care professional's performance. Relevant data includes patient length of stay (from hospital records), lab data (eg, physician ordering habits), radiology data (eg, diagnostic ability and preventive care), drug utilization review (eg, antibiotic prescribing behavior), and insurance claim data.

See Table 14-24 for strengths and limitations of administrative, clinical, and secondary databases.

Key references

Borg WR, Gall MD. *Educational Research: An Introduction.* 3rd ed. New York, NY: Longman; 1979.

Davis D, Moore D, Sinclair L, Taylor-Vaisey A, Tipping J. *Evaluating Educational Outcomes: A Workbook for Continuing Medical Education Providers.* Toronto: University of Toronto, Faculty of Medicine, Office of Continuing Education. (Electronic publication; available www.acme-assn.org.)

Technology-Assisted Evaluation Methods

Technology is the application of scientific advances to practical problems. The tools we use with our hands, the way that our systems are organized, and the way that we use records and communication systems are all dependent on technology. Both organizational technology and specific technologies are applied to the fields of health care, medical education, and CPD.[27] Specific examples of technological aids are computer simulations, CD-ROMs, Web-based learn-wares, multimedia tools, telementoring, and telelearning.

The technological methods and tools examined in this section are computer simulations and computer-aided testing or electronic tracking/monitoring systems.

Key reference

McWhinney IR. Primary care research in the next twenty years. In: Norton PG, Stewart M, Tudiver F, Bass MJ, Dunn EV, eds. *Primary Care Research: Traditional and Innovative Approaches, Research Methods for Primary Care, vol. 1*. Newbury Park, Calif: Sage Publications; 1991.

Tools

Computer Simulations

Definition, Description, and Uses. Computer simulations are evaluation/teaching tools that simulate a patient/medical encounter and that deliver medical information relevant to the simulation through the display terminal of a computer or medical monitor.[28] In some cases, the simulator may include pieces of medical equipment (ie, anesthesia machine and monitor, laparoscopic simulators, cardiac patient simulators) or whole body mannequins that are controlled by a computer program. Virtual-reality simulations, haptic devices (forced feedback), and scoring models are presently in place for surgical and medical training and will be an evaluation trend that will be explored in the future.[29]

Computer simulations can be used to portray both procedural problems (ie, surgery, anesthesia) and medical management problems.[30]

See Table 14-25 for strengths and limitations of computer simulations and electronic standardized patients.

Key references

Chopra V, Gesink BJ, De Jong J, Bovill JG, Spierdijk J, Brand R. Does training on an anaesthesia simulator lead to improvement in performance? *Br J Anaesth*. 1994;73:293–297.

Friedman CP. The marvelous medical education machine or how medical education can be unstuck in time. *Acad Med*. 2000;75(Suppl):S137–S142.

TABLE 14-25

Strengths and Limitations of Computer Simulations and Electronic Standardized Patients

	Strength	**Limitation**
Computer simulations and electronic standardized patients	■ Eliminate observer variability ■ Can provide immediate feedback to the learner in learning and evaluation situations ■ Can respond to interventions and develop medical conditions in realistic manner ■ Can automatically collect data and score the examinee as the simulation/test proceeds (eliminate the need for postexam scoring) ■ Fit curriculum needs and schedules as they are available at any time ■ Eliminate risk to patients ■ Allow time compression (several years of a patient's life can pass in a few minutes) ■ Allow reproducibility of problems until learners have mastered the scenario (Also, for evaluation purposes, the same problem can be reproduced for different students.) ■ Can be programmed to simulate any condition or complication ■ Do not require patient consent and do not become embarrassed or stressed as is possible with standardized patients ■ Can be used to assess medical management skills as well as speed, precision, and technique in performing procedural tasks ■ Can integrate testing tools like MCQs for rapidly evaluating problem-solving skills ■ Improve performance and facilitate knowledge retention ■ Flexibility in three dimensions: content, location, and time ■ Low costs, once up-front costs are invested ■ Standardization ■ Collaborative opportunities	■ Expensive to develop ■ High cost of equipment ■ High cost to maintain ■ Cannot be used to assess interpersonal skills or interview techniques (unless the simulated encounter is videotaped and then reviewed by an evaluator) ■ Problems with interoperability ■ Lower validity, reliability, and efficiency than MCQs ■ Technical, economical, organizational, and behavioral barriers that must be overcome for the technology to be accepted ■ Limited with respect to bandwidth and connectivity ■ Require user training and technical support ■ Optimal design ■ Readiness of the medical and health communities ■ Integration into present and future systems

Source: Compiled from Chopra V, Gesink BJ, De Jong J, Bovill JG, Spierdijk J, Brand R. Does training on an anaesthesia simulator lead to improvement in performance? *Br J Anaesth.* 1994;73:293–297; Friedman CP. The marvelous medical education machine or how medical education can be unstuck in time. *Acad Med.* 2000;75(Suppl):S137–S142; Norcini JJ, Meskauskas JA, Langdon LO, Webster GD. An evaluation of a computer simulation in the assessment of physician competence. *Eval Health Prof.,* 1986;9:286–304; Norman GR, Painvin C. Computer simulations. In: Neufeld VR, Norman GR, eds. *Assessing Clinical Competence.* New York, NY: Springer; 1985; and Tanriverdi H, Iacono CS. Diffusion of telemedicine: a knowledge barrier perspective. *Telemed J.* 1999;5:223–244.

Issenberg SB, McGaghie WC, Hart IR, Mayer JW, Felner JM, Petrusa ER, Waugh RA, Brown DD, Safford RR, Gessner IH, Gordon DL, Ewy GA. Simulation technology for health care professional skills training and assessment. *JAMA.* 1999;282:861–866.

Langsley DG. Medical competence and performance assessment. A new era. *JAMA*. 1991;266:977–980.

Norcini JJ, Meskauskas JA, Langdon LO, Webster GD. An evaluation of a computer simulation in the assessment of physician competence. *Eval Health Prof.* 1986;9:286–304.

Norman GR, Painvin C. Computer simulations. In: Neufeld VR, Norman GR, eds. *Assessing Clinical Competence*. New York, NY: Springer; 1985.

Tanriverdi H, Iacono CS. Diffusion of telemedicine: a knowledge barrier perspective. *Telemed J.* 1999;5:223–244.

Computer-Aided Testing

Definition, Description, and Uses. Computer-aided testing is an evaluation/teaching tool that simulates a patient/medical encounter and that delivers medical information relevant to the simulation through the display terminal of a computer.[28] Schuwirth et al.[31] summarize guidelines for designing computerized case-based test materials.

Electronic forms of assessment are currently being designed and employed for both formative and summative types of evaluation activities. Software packages, such as WebCT, are being developed and offer a wide variety of testing options. Electronic tracking/ monitoring systems and self-audited programs are positioned to be evaluation approaches of the future.

See Table 14-26 for strengths and limitations of computer-aided testing.

Key references

Issenberg SB, McGaghie WC, Hart IR, Mayer JW, Felner JM, Petrusa ER, Waugh RA, Brown DD, Safford RR, Gessner IH, Gordon DL, Ewy GA. Simulation technology for health care professional skills training and assessment. *JAMA*. 1999;282:861–866.

Langsley DG. Medical competence and performance assessment. A new era. *JAMA*. 1991;266:977–980.

Norcini JJ, Meskauskas JA, Langdon LO, Webster GD. An evaluation of a computer simulation in the assessment of physician competence. *Eval Health Prof.* 1986;9:286–304.

Norman GR, Painvin C. Computer simulations. In: Neufeld VR, Norman GR, eds. *Assessing Clinical Competence*. New York, NY: Springer; 1985.

Schuwirth LWT, Van der Vleuten CPM, De Kock CA, Peperkamp AGW, Donkers HHLM. Computerized case-based testing: a modern method to assess clinical decision making. *Med Teacher.* 1996;18:294–299.

Tanriverdi H, Iacono CS. Diffusion of telemedicine: a knowledge barrier perspective. *Telemed J.* 1999;5:223–244.

T A B L E   14-26

Strengths and Limitations of Computer-Aided Testing

	Strength	Limitation
Computer-aided testing	■ Eliminate observer variability ■ Can provide immediate feedback to the learner in learning and evaluation situations ■ Can respond to interventions and develop medical conditions in realistic manner ■ Can automatically collect data and score the examinee as the simulation/test proceeds (eliminate the need for postexam scoring) ■ Fit curriculum needs and schedules as they are available at any time ■ Allow reproducibility of problems until learners have mastered the scenario (Also, for evaluation purposes, the same problem can be reproduced for different students.) ■ Can be programmed to simulate any condition or complication ■ Can integrate testing tools like MCQs for rapidly evaluating problem-solving skills ■ Allow sequential questions to be independent of responses (ie, with multipart written exam questions, an incorrect answer may be indicated by the information in a subsequent question; the examinee can then go back and correct answers) by not allowing the user to go back to the previous screen ■ Minimize test security threats because every student can receive a random selection of questions from the test item data bank	■ Expensive to develop ■ High cost of equipment ■ High cost to maintain ■ Problems with interoperability ■ Lower validity, reliability, and efficiency than MCQs ■ Technical, economical, organizational, and behavioral barriers that must be overcome for the technology to be accepted ■ Limited with respect to bandwidth and connectivity ■ Require user training and technical support ■ Have high initial cost for software and hardware ■ Can be more fatiguing to take an examination on a computer screen as opposed to a conventional written exam ■ Difficult and time consuming to mark if open-ended questions are used

Source: Compiled from Issenberg SB, McGaghie WC, Hart IR, et al. Simulation technology for health care professional skills training and assessment. *JAMA.* 1999;282:861–866; Norman GR, Painvin C. Computer simulations. In: Neufeld VR, Norman GR, eds. *Assessing Clinical Competence.* New York, NY: Springer; 1985; Schuwirth LWT, Van der Vleuten CPM, De Kock CA et al. Computerized case-based testing: a modern method to assess clinical decision making. *Med Teacher.* 1996;18:294–299; and Tanriverdi H, Iacono CS. Diffusion of telemedicine: a knowledge barrier perspective. *Telemed J.* 1999;5:223–244.

PRACTICAL ISSUES IN SELECTING EVALUATION METHODOLOGIES

How Do You Go About Selecting Specific Evaluation Methods?

The previous section detailed a variety of evaluation methods (or "tools") to choose from. The selection process involves assessing your context and defining your objectives. Then, you need to determine what objectives can be met with the evaluation methods that you have the resources to use.

Objectives

A first step is to clarify what you are trying to accomplish. Review your situation in its overall context and ask the following questions to clarify your objectives:

- Who is the audience for the evaluation report?
- What are the most important questions that they would like answered?
- How will they use the information?
- How much of and what types of information do they need for their purpose?

Second, clarify specifically what you want to measure.

- Is it attitudes, knowledge, skills, competency, behavior, and/or cost?
- From whose perspective should the measurement be made (self-evaluation, peer, independent source)?

Third, assess your resources.

- What data sources are available (eg, individuals, clinical records)?
- What other resources are available (eg, funding, skilled personnel)?

Fourth, considering your possibilities and tradeoffs, as well as the feasibility and practical constraints, make your choice of an evaluation approach or tool.

Possibilities and Tradeoffs

Keeping in mind what you want to measure and your available resources, review the summary of evaluation methods in Table 14-2. Which methods are appropriate for your purpose and your resources? In many circumstances, more than one method may be satisfactory. For example, if you need only an indicator that some type of change is occurring, you may be able to choose among several of the methods.

Feasibility and Practical Constraints

After determining the method that is likely to be conceptually appropriate for your situation, outline all of the key aspects of the evaluation methodology to confirm that the evaluation project is practically feasible in your circumstances. Consider what is feasible and what is practical given your study design, study population, timeline, and resources. Practical constraints often limit how much can be done in one evaluation project.

The discussion in this chapter has focused on measurement methods, but their reliability and validity depend on the circumstances in which they are used in a specific project. Here are some of the additional methodological issues to consider:

- What is the study design? If it involves a controlled trial, how are groups identified?
- What is the study population? How are they sampled?
- Are the measures appropriate for this population? Will much modification and pretesting be required?
- Are the detailed procedures for collecting the data feasible?
- Are individuals with strong biases involved in administering the evaluation or providing the data?

When faced with an evaluation project where the practical constraints are difficult, reconsider the evaluation methods listed in Table 14-2. What is the most important constraint in your situation (eg, time, money)? What is the second most important constraint? Which methods clearly meet the most important constraint and do a reasonable job of meeting the second constraint? For example, if the most important constraint is money and reliable methods of measuring behavioral change are too expensive, the objective of the evaluation may be limited to showing types of change that precede behavioral change, eg, change in attitudes or change in knowledge. If those changes are demonstrated, they may justify requesting additional funding for a subsequent evaluation project to measure change directly. To paraphrase an example from manufacturing, a common problem is being asked to perform an evaluation project well, quickly, and cheaply. Meeting any two of the requirements is usually reasonable, but meeting all three simultaneously is often difficult.

Key references

Biddle S. Outcome measures in CME: steps along a continuum. *Alliance for CME Almanac*. 1998;20:3.

Casebeer L, Raichle L, Kristofco R, Carillo A. Cost benefit analysis: review of an evaluation methodology for measuring return on investment in continuing education. *J Contin Educ Health Prof*. 1997;17:225–227.

Torgerson D, Raftery J. Economics notes: measuring outcomes in economic evaluations. *BMJ*. 1999;318:1413.

Wilkes M, Bligh J. Evaluating educational interventions. *BMJ*. 1999;318: 1269–1272.

CHALLENGES AND THE FUTURE

Although current evaluation methods are relatively stable, the circumstances affecting their selection are not. Several factors are increasing the importance of evaluation and shifting the potential interest in, and costs of, specific methods. Some forces likely to affect the increased use of evaluation and the selection of methods are discussed in the following paragraphs.

Cost Reduction

Increasing cost constraints on health care are forcing the reexamination of the value of many activities, including CME/CPD activities. Financial pressures will increasingly force CME/CPD activities to include evaluation components that demonstrate that their outcomes justify their costs. For example, does an educational program on appropriate antibiotic use result in physicians using the most cost-effective antibiotics? Evaluations associated with cost reduction will primarily focus on methods that measure actual behavior.

Quality of Care

The public and the purchasers of health care are increasingly concerned that health care be demonstrated to be of acceptable quality (eg, HEDIS®, the Health Plan Employer Data and Information Set). The establishment of standards with rewards and sanctions is resulting in organizational efforts to assure care quality. These organizational efforts often include educational components, linking health services research and CME/CPD evaluation. Evaluations associated with quality-of-care improvement tend to focus on methods that measure actual behavior.

Improved Clinical and Administrative Databases

Pressures to manage care more efficiently have health care providers and third-party payers developing substantially enhanced clinical and administrative databases. The infrastructure and cost to develop and maintain these databases are being paid as part of routine practice expenditures. Evaluation activities need only pay additional marginal costs to abstract and analyze newly available information. Much of these data will be available on an ongoing basis to evaluate improvement across time. These databases will significantly increase the evaluation of care actually provided.

Board Recertification

Medical specialty boards have made an important commitment to require that specialists periodically demonstrate their competence in meeting current standards of practice. The development of recertification programs involves a fresh look at the content to be included (eg, physician–patient communication skills), as well as at the extent to which recertification should reflect knowledge, competence, and actual performance. The specialty boards are investing substantial resources into developing specific applications of evaluation methods that can be performed cost-effectively. Most of the methods in this chapter are being tried. Recertification will most likely be based on the use of several methods to evaluate different aspects of overall requirements.

Practitioner Performance Indicators

Both the United States and Canada are pursuing explicit assessment methods specific to performance indicators. This method of evaluation is deemed to be particularly strong from the perspective of validity, because it links performance and competence within an actual clinical setting.[28,32]

Communication Linkages and Technology-enabled Evaluations

The development of the Internet, teleconferencing, and other technology will enhance the use of evaluation methods that depend on communication. Teleconferencing can reduce the cost of communications-based evaluation approaches, such as focus groups that involve geographically separated individuals. Surveys, knowledge tests, and other written materials can be distributed and collected more economically, because most of the potential respondents have Internet access and are comfortable using it.

Self-Assessment

With the growing complexity of the knowledge base associated with health care, some emphasis is being placed on helping physicians perform more formal self-assessments of their practices, performance, and learning needs. These efforts are resulting in the application of several evaluation methods, including self-audit and peer evaluation. The development of these evaluation applications will be particularly important for physicians who do not work in large organizational settings. They need applications of methodologies that are more suited to individual and small-group practice.

Team Care and Communities of Practice

Communities of practice are emerging in organizations that are knowledge-based. Communities of practice, according to Wenger and Snyder,[33] are "groups of people informally bound together by shared expertise and passion for a joint enterprise." (p.139). Group members "share their experiences and knowledge in free-flowing, creative ways that foster new approaches to problems"[33] (p. 140). Communities of practice add value to organizations. However, the effects of their activities are complex, and the value of these communities is difficult to assess. Nontraditional evaluation methods, such as systematically gathering anecdotal evidence by listening to community of practice members' stories, can "clarify the complex relationships among activities, knowledge, and performance"[33] (p. 145).

Environmental changes can alter many activities related to evaluation. As a CME coordinator, you need to be aware of such changes in your environment when selecting and designing evaluation approaches and tools. Are forces in your environment increasing the importance of evaluation or making new data available that can be used for evaluation? Are any of the above forces evident? Are unique forces or events occurring? Periodically, you will need to reconsider the methods, tools, and techniques of evaluation detailed in this chapter and to reassess their feasibility in meeting your updated objectives with the resources available at that time.

CONCLUSION

This chapter has reviewed some of the major principles and practices that influence the effective and efficient use of evaluation methods, tools, and techniques for assessing the impact of CME/CPD programs. Along with an appreciation of the available approaches and tools relevant to continuing professional education, the effective and efficient use of evaluation tools requires an understanding of evaluation terms, knowledge of what is being evaluated, and knowledge of what questions to ask. Survey tools, knowledge tests, observations, archives/document review, and technology-based tests are five major categories of evaluation approaches and tools that can be used to collect and monitor data about the impact of educational interventions. A synopsis of evaluation approaches and tools, and an assessment of the five categories of tools based on their expense, validity, reliability, acceptability, and feedback opportunity, has been provided for practical comparisons. The CME coordinator can use this information to assess the strengths and limitations of each evaluation approach or tool when selecting or designing measurement instruments for a CME/CPD program.

REFERENCES—CHAPTER 14

1. Scriven M. *Evaluation Thesaurus.* 4th ed. Newbury Park, Calif: Sage Publications; 1991.

2. Phillips JJ. *Handbook of Training Evaluation and Measurement Methods.* Houston, TX: Gulf Publishing; 1997.

3. Spencer JA, Jordan RG. Learner centered approaches in medical education. *BMJ.* 1999;318:1280–1283.

4. Norman G, Shannon S, eds. *Evaluation Methods: A Resource Handbook.* Hamilton, Ont: The Program for Educational Development, McMaster University; 1995.

5. Davis D, Moore D, Sinclair L, Taylor-Vaisey A, Tipping J. *Evaluating Educational Outcomes: A Workbook for Continuing Medical Education Providers.* Toronto: University of Toronto, Faculty of Medicine, Office of Continuing Education. (Electronic publication; available www.acme-assn.org.)

6. Salvatori P, Roberts J, Brown B. Objective structured clinical examinations (OSCE). In: Norman G, Shannon S, eds. *Evaluation Methods: A Resource Handbook.* Hamilton, Ont: The Program for Educational Development, McMaster University; 1995.

7. Ebel RL. *Essentials of Educational Measurement,* 3rd ed. Englewood Cliffs, NJ: Prentice-Hall; 1979.

8. Norman G. Multiple choice questions. In: Norman G, Shannon S, eds. *Evaluation Methods: A Resource Handbook.* Hamilton, Ont: The Program for Educational Development, McMaster University; 1995.

9. McArdle PJ. Innovations in undergraduate medical education and in graduate medical training. *J Contin Educ Health Prof.* 1997;17:214–223.

10. Premi J. Problem based, self-directed continuing medical education in a group of practicing family physicians. *J Med Educ.* 1988;63:484–486.

11. Premi J, Shannon S, Hartwick K, Lamb S, Wakefield J, Williams J. Practice-based small-group CME. *Acad Med.* 1994;69:800–802.

12. Palmer D, Rideout E. Essays. In: Norman G, Shannon S, eds. *Evaluation Methods: A Resource Handbook.* Hamilton, Ont: The Program for Educational Development, McMaster University; 1995.

13. Stratford P, Smeda J. Modified essay question. In: Norman G, Shannon S, eds. *Evaluation Methods: A Resource Handbook.* Hamilton, Ont: The Program for Educational Development, McMaster University; 1995.

14. Muzzin LJ. Oral examinations. In: Norman G, Shannon S, eds. *Evaluation Methods: A Resource Handbook.* Hamilton, Ont: The Program for Educational Development, McMaster University; 1995.

15. Cunnington JP, Hanna E, Turnbull J, Kaigas TB, Norman GR. Defensible assessment of the competency of the practicing physician. *Acad Med.* 1997;72:9–12.

16. Thomson MA. Direct observation. In: Norman G, Shannon S, eds. *Evaluation Methods: A Resource Handbook.* Hamilton, Ont: The Program for Educational Development, McMaster University; 1995.

17. Borg WR, Gall MD. *Educational Research: An Introduction.* 3rd ed. New York, NY: Longman; 1979.

18. Helman CG. Research in primary care: the qualitative approach. In: Norton PG, Stewart M, Tudiver F, Bass MJ, Dunn EV, eds. *Primary Care Research: Traditional and Innovative Approaches, Research Methods for Primary Care, vol. 1.* Newbury Park, Calif: Sage Publications; 1991.

19. Crabtree BF, Miller WL, eds. *Doing Qualitative Research: Research Methods for Primary Care, vol. 3.* Newbury Park, Calif: Sage Publications; 1992.

20. Barrows HS. An overview of the uses of standardized patients for teaching and evaluating clinical skills. *Acad Med.* 1993;68:443–451.

21. Vu NV, Marcy ML, Verhulst SJ, Barrows HS. Generalizability of standardized patients' satisfaction ratings of their clinical encounter with fourth-year medical students. *Acad Med.* 1990;65:S29–S30.

22. Rosenal L. Exploring the learner's world: critical incident methodology. *J Contin Educ Nursing.* 1995;26:115–118.

23. Tugwell P, Dok C. Medical record review. In Neufeld VR, Norman GR, eds. *Assessing Clinical Competence.* New York, NY: Springer; 1985.

24. Jennett PA, Affleck L. Chart audit and chart stimulated recall as methods of needs assessment in continuing professional health education. *J Contin Educ Health Prof.* 1998;18:63–171.

25. Jennett PA, Scott SM, Atkinson MA, Crutcher RA, Hogan DB, Elford RW, MacCannel KL, Baumber JS. Patient charts and physician office management decisions: chart audit and chart stimulated recall. *J Contin Educ Health Prof.* 1995;15:31–39.

26. Jennett PA. Chart stimulated recall: a technique to assess clinical competence and performance. *Educ Gen Prac.* 1995;6:30–34.

27. McWhinney IR. Primary care research in the next twenty years. In: Norton PG, Stewart M, Tudiver F, Bass MJ, Dunn EV, eds. *Primary Care Research: Traditional and Innovative Approaches, Research Methods for Primary Care, vol. 1.* Newbury Park, Calif: Sage Publications; 1991.

28. Langsley DG. Medical competence and performance assessment. A new era. *JAMA.* 1991;266:977–980.

29. Friedman CP. The marvelous medical education machine or how medical education can be unstuck in time. *Acad Med.* 2000;75:S137–S142.

30. Issenberg SB, McGaghie WC, Hart IR, Mayer JW, Felner JM, Petrusa ER, Waugh RA, Brown DD, Safford RR, Gessner IH, Gordon DL, Ewy GA. Simulation technology for health care professional skills training and assessment. *JAMA.* 1999;282:861–866.

31. Schuwirth LWT, Van der Vleuten CPM, De Kock CA, Peperkamp AGW, Donkers HHLM. Computerized case-based testing: a modern

method to assess clinical decision making. *Med Teacher*. 1996;18:294–299.

32. Hall W, Violato C, Lewkonia R, Lockyer J, Filder H, Toews J, Jennett P, Donoff M, Moores D. Assessment of physician performance in Alberta: the physician achievement review. *Can Med Assoc J*. 1999;161:52–57.

33. Wenger ET, Snyder WM. Communities of practice: the organizational frontier. *Harvard Business News*. Jan–Feb, 2000.

chapter 15

Advancing the Body of Knowledge: Evidence and Study Design for Quality Improvement*

Paul E. Mazmanian, PhD

Since accepting this position in continuing medical education, I have been under constant pressure to demonstrate that my programs make a difference in the ways that physicians practice and in the health of their patients. Pre- and post-tests, course evaluations, and a few grants have enabled me to show that there is usually some educational benefit for physicians and there are some health care improvements for patients, but not always. But there is a mixed message here. On one hand, department heads appear happy with the way things are; on the other hand, they complain about my suggestions for how important it is to assess needs, structure programs, and teach with interaction. When they ask me why, I try to explain that these things make a difference in quality, but they want more evidence to support my stand. My evaluations are not serving me, because when I finish, I only know whether the program appears to have succeeded or not, at pretty basic levels. I don't know why or how they've succeeded; and I only rarely know if they have a broader impact.

INTRODUCTION

There is increasing recognition of a half-life to medical school and graduate training and a growing sense that the attitudes and skills ordinarily associated with lifelong, self-directed learning will enable physicians to improve the health of the public. Physicians are expected to influence health by staying abreast of the most valid and reliable scientific advances for clinical care. However, less than half of a physician's daily practice appears based in solid scientific

---

*I am grateful to my colleague, Anton Kuzel, MD, for his review and comments on early drafts of this chapter.

evidence.[1] Instead, it involves continually searching to match globally incomplete scientific knowledge of disease and treatment with incomplete local knowledge about individual patients.[2]

Despite growing pressure to guarantee patient safety—with limited data to assure performance—systems providing health care and programs offering education are compelled to demonstrate effectiveness and continuous improvement.[3,4] Evaluation is central to the effort. As physicians are encouraged to use the best scientific evidence for patient care and to test clinical innovations within the health care systems where they work, thoughtful evaluators reason that such locally executed studies not only lead to improvements in the day-to-day provision of health services,[2] they also add to what is known about physician learning and change.[5] An opposing school of thought contends that those studies add very little to what is known about physicians or health care, because the study designs fall outside the traditional belief system that upholds the education and training of most professionals in the biological, physical, and social sciences.[1,6] Once providers and evaluators of continuing medical education (CME) and continuing professional development (CPD) become skilled with an armamentarium of diverse study designs, they may find themselves more comfortable and effective in their leadership roles, planning solutions to daily clinical problems and promoting sound health policy.

For this chapter, evaluative research includes assessments of educational programs and health services involving physician learning, behavior, and change. The philosophical foundations of evaluative research are discussed, linking them to perspectives on causal relations. The essential features of evaluation in two popular approaches to quality improvement—evidence-based medicine (EBM) and total quality management (TQM)—are appraised for their potential contributions to global understandings of day-to-day practice and policy development. In addition, newer competencies are suggested for those who evaluate CME, CPD, or conduct health services research that involves physicians in learning or behavioral change.

EVALUATIVE RESEARCH IN HEALTH CARE: WHAT IS IT? WHAT CAN IT DO?

An arguably disjointed and markedly mercantile approach to continuing education is organized nearly parallel to an increasingly coordinated and thoughtfully legitimized system of health services research. Both systems share concerns regarding the quality of health care and both see evidence, research, and evaluation as means to improvement. Research in CME and CPD addresses the physician per se. It speaks to adult development, learning, competency assessment, and programs designed to effect change in performance and patient outcomes.[7] In contrast, health services research intends to improve the quality of health care, reduce its cost, improve patient safety, decrease medical errors, and broaden access to essential services. Research in CME and CPD helps physicians, administrators, and planners tell about educational programs that serve as instruments of change and about physicians who participate as learners. Health services research helps patients, clinicians, policy makers, educators, and health care system leaders to make informed decisions aimed at improving the quality of the health services they provide.[8] The goals of all these—CPD, CME, and health services research—comprise the content of evaluative research in health care. Because it discovers and tests knowledge, evaluative research can be a powerful tool in promulgating and measuring change. To be effective proponents of evaluative research in health care, CME and CPD leaders must recognize the limits of evaluation as well as the promise it brings to improvement.

THE CONTEXT OF DISCOVERY

Each evaluative research project presents an opportunity for learning about inquiry itself, and probing the origins of inquiry often leads to the discovery of relationships involving science and philosophy. For many, it never has been clear where thinking and philosophy give way to science. For example, both John Dewey,[9] philosopher (1859–1952), and Albert Einstein,[10] physicist (1879–1955), variously expressed a struggle to answer the question, "What is thought?" Niels Bohr (1885–1962),[11] a nuclear physicist who maintained a lifelong interest in biology and psychology, speculated about the implications of quantum mechanics for living systems and the applicability of quantum mechanical concepts to the explanation of biological systems and behavior.

Does science include the private, speculative, largely nonverbal activity carried on with its own motivations, free of self-consciously examined methods?[12] Plato (427–347 BC) offered that there could be no real definition of things perceived by the senses. *Or is science solely the clarified, codified, refined concepts that are passed through a process of peer review and public scrutiny?* Plato's pupil, Aristotle (384–322 BC), worked at studies to organize things into classes and subclasses, to enumerate their qualities, and to recognize the distinction between essential and nonessential qualities.[13,14] The private aspect does not need to remain silent or unattended, nor should it be discredited as inaccessible to rational study. It should be searched out and defended in order that the context of discovery and the justification of reasons why scientists embrace their guiding ideas may be better understood.[12]

Why are understandings of scientific thought important to evaluation? *Each evaluative research project presents an opportunity to contribute to the body of knowledge regarding physicians, learning, and change and each is complicated by influences that range from abstract philosophical issues regarding what is knowable, to methodological and technical questions that are subject to the practicalities of each project itself.* The director in the opening vignette of the present chapter and those who evaluate continuing education and CPD must become facile with diverse research designs in order to explain when and how select methods can enable the identification of need and the solution of problems found variously in education and health care.

WHAT IS THE MEANING OF EVALUATIVE RESEARCH?

History shows that a body of scientific knowledge that ceases to develop ceases to be science at all, in part, because science is not a static body of knowledge but rather an active process of knowledge making.[14] To add to what is known about physicians in practice, those who provide or evaluate CPD must articulate sound explanations and realistic expectations for the utility of their work. *Responsibility to the public requires knowledge and philosophical grounding to site rational limits and realistic expectations for education and health services.*

During the twentieth century, a philosophical system of positivist beliefs alternately informed and even dominated medical and social sciences research. Summarized, the positivist school holds that there is a single reality governed by natural laws independent of any observer's interest. John Stuart Mill[6] (1806–1873) was a major proponent of positivism in behavioral science. He believed that positive explanation derives from objective examination of social phenomena. In contrast to positivist philosophy, a school of constructivist beliefs[15,16] is gaining recent attention. Constructivism asserts multiple realities, socially formed and ungoverned by natural laws. The positivist and constructivist schools are steeped in traditions of inquiry that seek truths and principles of being, knowledge, and conduct. The inquiry involves fundamental questions that perplexed Western thinkers such as Kepler (1571–1630), Descartes (1596–1650), and Newton (1642–1727), and the questions are those that challenge the scientific and philosophical foundations of investigation today:

1. What is there that can be known?
2. What is the relationship of the knower to the known or the knowable?
3. What are the ways of finding out knowledge?

The first question is ontological, concerned with issues of existence or being. The second question is epistemological, dealing with the origin, nature, and limits of human knowledge. The third question is methodological, addressing methods, systems, and rules for the conduct of inquiry. There are many tenets or convictions one might invoke to answer these fundamental questions, but, at this writing, none appears subject to proof.[17] Instead, the set of answers one gives reveals a basic belief system rooted in inference, probability, or faith. And for those who must evaluate progress in education or health services, the choices of questions to study and methods to apply may conflict not only with prior training but also with personal philosophical beliefs. How each of the two major schools, the positivist and the constructivist, deals with these questions is explored in Table 15–1.

Positivist beliefs hold that quantitative methods of inquiry can be used to verify truth, explaining naturally occurring relationships by collecting empirical evidence organized around possible explanations.

TABLE 15-1

The Contrasting Positivist and Constructivist Belief Systems

Positivist Belief	Constructivist Belief
Ontology: *A realist ontology* asserts that there exists a single reality that is independent of any observer's interest in it and that operates according to immutable natural laws, many of which take cause–effect form. Truth is defined as that set of statements that is isomorphic to reality.	*A relativist ontology* asserts that there exist multiple, socially constructed realities ungoverned by any natural laws, causal or otherwise. "Truth" is defined as the best informed (amount and quality of information) and most sophisticated (power with which the information is understood and used) construction on which there is consensus (although there may be several constructions extant that simultaneously meet that criterion).
Epistemology: *A dualist objectivist epistemology* asserts that it is possible (indeed, mandatory) for an observer to exteriorize the phenomenon studied, remaining detached and distant from it (a state often called "subject–object dualism"), and excluding any value considerations from influencing it.	*A monistic, subjectivist epistemology* asserts that an inquirer and the inquired-into are interlocked in such a way that the findings of an investigation are the *literal creation* of the inquiry process.
Methodology: *An interventionist methodology* strips context of its contaminating (confounding) influences (variables) so that the inquiry can converge on truth and explain nature as it really is and really works, leading to the capability to predict and to control.	*A hermeneutic methodology* involves a continuing dialectic of iteration, analysis, critique, reiteration, reanalysis, and so on, leading to the emergence of a joint (among all the inquirers and respondents) construction of a case.

Source: Adapted from Guba EG, Lincoln YS. *Fourth Generation Evaluation.* Newbury Park, Calif: Sage Publications, 1989; 84.

The constructivist school holds that rigorous inquiry into the nature of the real world can be used to identify and develop mutually held meanings that, in turn, describe and explain naturally occurring phenomena. Although many studies of continuing education and CPD are founded on positivist beliefs that rely on quantification to verify explanations of behavior,[18–20] many others involve constructivist thinking to learn how or why selected social phenomena occur.[21–23] The positivist and constructivist schools occupy central roles in evaluation of CPD, continuing education, and health services and both may contribute to theory.[5,24–27] The positivist paradigm presents compelling evidence for the success of its chiefly recognized scientific tool—the randomized controlled trial. However, the constructivist paradigm is gaining in use and understanding, in part, because it succeeds at filling in knowledge gaps left by randomized controlled trials or in outlining complex questions that may be subjected to further study by accepted means of the positivist school.[28]

CAUSE, EFFECT, AND CONTEMPORARY APPROACHES TO QUALITY IMPROVEMENT

What is the value of continuing education? Of continuing professional development? Or of health care? These questions are asked freely and frequently by those who expect improved services or certain returns on their investments. *In answering these questions, practitioners and evaluators endeavor to control variables to isolate the causal effects of the programs or services they provide. Yet, if one accepts: a) the conventional wisdom that art and science comprise the practice of medicine, and b) the evidence that most current medical practice is not based on solid science, then c) chasing after cause and effect in health care presents a formidable challenge.* Part of the challenge appears to involve the background, training, and expectations of most professionals in the health sciences and in education. For them, prospective experimentation is synonymous with research, the possibility of learning causal relationships through probability theory, and statistical analyses leading to inferences from observations. For others, explanation and meaning can be taken from several differing study designs.

Since research in continuing education and health services is tied closely to the problems of day-to-day practice, it also can contribute to understandings of human action. Theory is the medium that enables a contribution; yet, theory may be valued differently, depending upon one's personal system of beliefs. To the positivist, a theory is a set of interrelated constructs, definitions, and propositions that present a systematic view of phenomena by specifying relations among variables, with the purpose of explaining and predicting the phenomena.[29] Hypotheses are conjectural statements of relations between two or more variables, either asserted provisionally to guide investigation or accepted as highly probable in the light of established facts.[29] Investigators ordinarily use quantitative research designs to test hypotheses, with the quality of the theory being judged by its explanatory or predictive power. The evidence for cause and effect is self-explanatory, found in the proof that exactly corresponds with the theoretical assertion.

From the constructivist perspective, a theory is a mental plan.[26] It is not reality but a perception or organization of reality, perhaps closely resembling reality, but not reality per se. It remains a representation of reality, malleable and modifiable. Constructivists hold that systems and organisms cannot be separated from their environments because their meaning and existence depend upon interaction with other systems and organizations. The doctrine of constructivism offers that systems and organisms evolve and change in such ways as to make the distinction between cause and effect meaningless.[5]

How are these theoretical precepts of research put into practice? What do they mean to those with responsibility for planning and evaluation in continuing education, CPD, and health services research?

Two major strategies presently define the essentials of health quality improvement. One strategy is evidence-based medicine (EBM),[1] which holds that critical appraisals of scientific evidence may be transformed directly into clinical action. The other is total quality management (TQM),[30] including the plan-do-study-act (PDSA) learning cycle ordinarily associated with the quality improvement programs of manufacturing and selected service industries. Both strategies emphasize factual information and the use of reason and reflection to learn from experience. Positivism provides the basis for prospective interventional studies that are vital to EBM; proponents of TQM suggest that correlational studies also report causal relations they are defined by pragmatic, compelling, and implicitly shared constructivist realities.

Evidence-based Medicine

Proponents of EBM[1] describe it as a process of lifelong, self-directed learning in which caring for patients creates the need for clinically important, valid, and reliable information about diagnosis, prognosis, therapy, and other clinical and health care issues. Physicians practicing EBM:

1. Convert their information needs into answerable questions.
2. Track down, with maximum efficiency, the best evidence with which to answer the questions (whether from the clinical

examination, the diagnostic laboratory, research evidence, or other sources).

3. Critically appraise the evidence for its validity (closeness to the truth) and usefulness (clinical applicability).
4. Apply the results of the appraisal in clinical practice.
5. Evaluate performance.

EBM may be seen as the most recent representation of positivist thinking to drive the medical profession. It also may be seen as a method of continuing education or CPD, driven by the ideals of continuous inquiry and provision of the best scientifically based care.

With EBM, randomized controlled trials (RCTs) or systematic reviews of RCTs receive the highest priority in the physician's search to verify the recency, accuracy, and applicability of an effectiveness claim. The design of RCTs involves random assignment of subjects matched on selected background characteristics such as age, gender, and occupation into treatment and control groups. Baseline measures are acquired for dependent variables associated with the subjects in both groups. An intervention is introduced. Its effect is measured upon the dependent variable in the subjects of each group. Statistical tests of correlation determine whether the association of the intervention and its effect on the dependent variable are significant. The principles of EBM allow that evidence resources include textbooks as well as generalized or specialized bibliographic databases in print or electronic form. Other information sources may not provide evidence to support claims of effectiveness.

Although the decision to embark upon the practice of EBM may appear to be individual in nature, it also involves an assessment of clinical practice systems, including organizational and other barriers and a determination of whether they can be overcome; possible collaboration of key colleagues; and the likelihood that the educational, administrative, and economic resources required for success are available. EBM holds that quality-improving strategies are more likely to succeed if they are based on credible syntheses of evidence developed by respected bodies and if influential local colleagues already are implementing them.[1] It is expected that success is more likely to occur when physicians receive consistent information from several sources and when quality-improving strategies are directed toward a targeted group of clinicians who does not require collaboration with clinicians or administrators that function outside the ordinary organizational boundaries. Finally, changes are more likely to be implemented if they do not conflict with local economic or administrative incentives and patient expectations or community expectations.[1] In this sense, the practice of EBM presents a compelling case for understanding systems, which is the focus of TQM.

FIGURE 15-1

Deming Wheel (PDSA cycle)

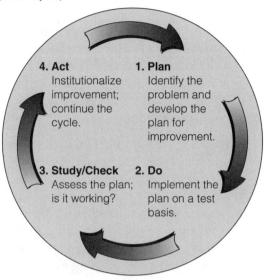

Total Quality Management

TQM uses evidence and research to assure that products and services reach an intended level of quality. TQM features a set of management principles that converges with commitment to quality improvement to become a driving force throughout all functions of an organization. In a recent report, the Institute of Medicine[3] took lessons to improve safety from other high-risk enterprises. Five principles were identified as crucial to the design of safe health care, whether in a small group practice, a hospital, or a large health system. The principles assert that an effective system should: (1) provide leadership, (2) respect human limits in the design process, (3) promote effective team functioning, (4) anticipate the unexpected, and (5) create a learning environment. Such a strategy for improvement of health practices and outcomes depends on thoughtful development of information about the effectiveness of the system itself.

Edward Deming is credited with development of the PDSA cycle for quality improvement (Figure 15-1). The rationale for PDSA cycles comes largely from systems theory that suggests that systems perform according to their designs; therefore, refinement of outcomes is a function of refinement of design. The four stages of PDSA are

1. *Plan*: In this stage, a process or situation is studied, problems are identified, and plans are made to solve them.
2. *Do*: The plan is implemented on a test basis, improvement is measured, and the results documented.

3. *Study:* The plan is assessed to see if it is achieving the goals established in stage 1 and to see if any new problems have developed.

4. *Act:* In the final stage, the plan is implemented, and quality improvement is made part of the normal operation. The process then returns to stage 1 to start the cycle over again, to identify new quality problems and develop plans to solve them— the continuous improvement of a committed quality management program.[30]

To evaluate the PDSA cycle as an approach to improving health care, most physicians must depart from reliance on the results of randomized controlled trials to define and explain outcomes. Proponents of TQM assert that those who find small-scale PDSA cycles insufficiently rigorous need only contemplate the lack of discipline that produces widespread variation in practices to understand the improvement the PDSA system provides.[2] They suggest the PDSA cycle is far more rigorous an approach than most physicians have used historically to justify changes they make in their practices; and the outcomes from the PDSA cycle, though perhaps only locally reproducible, are as valid as those of any RCT. To the extent the PDSA cycle engages physicians in learning to effect change in performance and patient outcomes, it may be seen as CME or CPD. To the extent that practitioners of PDSA design studies intended to improve the quality of care, it may be declared TQM. *Where the functions of quality improvement and learning overlap, the differences in health services research and evaluation of continuing education and CPD seem nominal.*

Many experts[2,31–34] are beginning to assert that improvement in practice derives more from reflection on thoughtful experience and new options and less from erratic trial and error or from randomized controlled experimentation. Reflecting upon one's actions appears central to improvement. It may occur during the delivery of care (reflection in action) or afterward (reflection on action). In his review of the PDSA cycle in quality improvement, Berwick[2] concludes:

> Guiding medical cultures—whether in large, formal organizations or in office practices—to accept and value small-scale tests of change as part of the daily routine and as essential steps in the continuous search for improvement is a daunting task. The alternatives, however, can be worse: to accept an inadequate status quo or to take blind, wholesale stabs at change in complex, non-linear systems where consequences can be dire and hard to predict. Physicians play a crucial role and have a great stake in the choice of the approach that is taken: status quo, "shot in the dark" changes, or the real-time signs of the PDSA cycle.

Since minor clinical actions can have major consequences, remote in space and time, prospective interventional studies often take too long for the immediate needs of day-to-day quality improvement.[2] As an option, proponents of TQM advocate for a series of small-scale tests that build knowledge sequentially to yield useful information in a timely fashion. They believe cohort studies, case controlled studies, and survey research completed over time can be equally conclusive in local settings.

CAUSALITY IN QUANTITATIVE AND QUALITATIVE STUDY DESIGN

The ideal of a health care or educational system influenced by EBM or TQM demands acceptance of causal explanations and clarification of the causal role played by health care practitioners or educators. To endorse this notion of causality, one must accept that the same cause always produces the same effect. In the health care systems of EBM and TQM, one must hold a philosophical belief that there are effects associated with the actions of health care providers, learning can effect behavioral change in physicians, and interventions applied by educators can effect change in physician behavior and patient outcomes.

In practical applications of ideal systems, administrators, educators, and others interested in measures of the PDSA cycle use several criteria to decide whether associations of variables are causal. The three most commonly recognized and influential criteria are: strength of association, dose-response, and biological plausibility.[35] When the relative risk or relative odds are high, the argument for cause gains support. In the association between cigarette smoking and lung cancer, risk ratios as high as 30 to 1 have been found. The statement that a heavy cigarette smoker is 30 times more likely to contract lung cancer than a nonsmoker is difficult to ignore. Conversely, the case for causation is weakened when the magnitude of risk is assessed at lower ratios.[35]

Any time a risk factor comes in doses or gradients of exposure, it is reasonable to expect that the risk of disease should increase with higher levels of exposure. Again, cigarette smoking and lung cancer provide an excellent example. The more cigarettes people smoke, the more death rates from cancer go up, implying causality.[35] Similarly, those who plan and study educational interventions find it reasonable to expect learning and change to occur as a result of carefully sequenced exposures delivered over time and designed to cause behavioral change. For example, Chassin and McCue,[36] using didactic sessions, printed material, and feedback, altered pelvimetry rates in an obstetrical setting.

In health services, the associations of variables should make biological sense. They should be consistent with information available from the related worlds of physiology, pharmacology, and anatomy. An argument that strengthens the case for estrogens as a cause for endometrial cancer is the demonstration of concordance between the duration of exposure and development of disease. What is known about neoplasia suggests that cancers are not triggered immediately on exposure to a carcinogen but develop after a latent period. One would expect that women exposed to estrogens would contract the neoplasm only some years after initial exposure. *Similarly, in studies of learning and behavior, the associations of variables should be consistent with knowledge in physiology, psychology, sociology, and ethics.* What is known about the adoption of a new procedure is that it must be compatible with existing practice and bear relative advantage over current practices. It should be observable and perceived as simple, whenever possible allowing learners a chance to attempt the procedure and to make mistakes during a trial period.[37,38] Each of these features has a direct bearing on the evaluation of CPD and CME and on the ability of the director to account for change associated with behavioral interventions.

Measuring Causation: Quantitative Study Design

RCTs, cohort studies, case-control studies, and surveys are considered examples of quantitative research. The reliability of the RCT is especially strong in pharmaceutical studies that search for the safety and efficacy of one medicine or another. Its ability to isolate the effect of an intervention on human physiology has been widely debated but generally accepted as a staple of the RCT study design. To answer the question, What works and does not work in CME?, reviews of RCTs in continuing medical education[18,19,37,39] have enabled CME practitioners and researchers to advance toward instructional designs that often include educational interventions combined with increased opportunities for human interaction. However, there are many other types of quantitative studies, the value of which must be recognized by planners and evaluators.

The cohort study is similar to the experimental study or clinical trial. Although there are several different types of cohort studies, the general concept of a cohort is reasonably straightforward.[35,40] A sample of the population is selected and information is obtained to determine which persons are exposed to a particular characteristic; similar life events, such as an educational session; or possible etiologic agents. The sample of individuals is followed for a period of time to observe who develops or dies from the disease of interest or how they experience other events or stages of personal, professional, or social development. Effects such as incidence and mortality rates or performance changes are then calculated for each exposure group and compared to determine if a statistical association exists. As one measure of their success, many medical schools follow their graduating students to determine whether they match with residency programs of their choice. Later, they check with residency program directors to assess the performance of their graduated medical students and to judge the success of their own undergraduate training programs.

In contrast to cohort studies in which individuals are selected into a study according to their exposure status, in case-control studies, the selection is based on disease status.[35] Individuals with a specific disease or condition (the cases) are compared with individuals without the disease or condition (the controls). Past exposures to potential risk factors are determined for each group and compared. Case-control studies are retrospective. They document and analyze previous occurrences in order to confirm or refute suspicion or to determine at what level of exposure effects might be found. Retrospective studies may be made by examining records or reports or by interviewing those involved and affected. For advocates of TQM, it is cohort and case-control studies sustained by theoretical probability and standard statistical analyses that help clinicians and other decision-makers to arrive at conclusions regarding behaviors measured and to be measured for improvement. Case-control studies offer educators an opportunity to assess needs, design learning interventions, and track their possible effects upon physicians and patients. In one recent study,[41] medical students were followed through residency into practice. The study revealed the physicians' prescribing habits for treating anxiety in older adults differed according to the training curriculum of their undergraduate medical school.

Survey research also depends upon statistics and probability.[42] It is like a census, differing primarily in that a survey typically examines a sample from a population while a census generally implies an enumeration of the entire population. Survey research is especially useful in learning the opinions or attitudes of large groups of persons with interests in health care. Just as it may be used to determine patient satisfaction, it may also be used to test hypotheses regarding the rate that physicians adopt clinical innovations or to verify physicians' differing motivations to change. Survey research may collect data that is prospective or retrospective or that reflects real events or attitudes and motivation. Surveys include written questionnaires, telephone interviews, or face-to-face interviews. Survey research is used often in continuing education and CPD to assess learning needs or to determine the effects of selected educational activities.

Qualitative Study Design

As a field, health services research frequently involves physicians and other health care providers as investigators, participants, and reviewers. Yet, some of the most important questions in health services concern the organization and culture of those who provide the care. For example, many investigators believe it is important to learn why physicians who are trained to respect the highest quality scientific research so often do not apply the best scientific evidence in day-to-day clinical practice. The methods appropriate to study such phenomena are different from the methods familiar to most health professionals. They may be traced to the social sciences. Often, they are called qualitative research methods. Causal presumption is unnecessary to qualitative research, because all entities are seen in a state of mutual simultaneous shaping, so that it is impossible to distinguish causes from effects.[5] As a result, there is no qualitative analogy to the gold standard of quantitative studies, the randomized controlled trial.[24] Quantitative and qualitative approaches to research differ in assumptions, methods, and outlook. A common feature of qualitative methods is that they do not primarily seek to provide quantified answers to research questions. Instead, the goal of qualitative research is to develop concepts that enable understanding of social phenomena in natural settings. Emphasis is afforded to the meanings, experiences, and views of the participating subjects.

Certain research questions are especially suited to qualitative study designs. For example, there is little doubt that quantitative methods, including randomized controlled trials, have contributed to advances in the treatment of diabetes mellitus. However, for a primary care physician who already learned that intensive insulin therapy works to reduce long-term complications, the more immediate question may be knowing whether a patient will comply with the treatment. In health services research, there are qualitative studies to examine and explain why patients do not comply with treatment regimens. In CPD, there are qualitative studies to explain why physicians do or do not change in practice.

A simplified comparison of qualitative and quantitative research[24] is featured in Table 15-2. It suggests that qualitative methods address one or a few cases and that quantitative research involves populations. Qualitative research includes observation and interview compared to measurement and survey methods of quantitative studies.

Qualitative research uses interpretation for analysis; quantitative research applies statistics. The reasoning of quantitative research is deductive; both inductive and deductive reasoning may apply in qualitative studies. Typical qualitative research questions aim to learn what is happening or what phenomena might mean; quantitative research asks what causes a selected effect or which treatment is more effective. The qualitative researcher is encouraged not to separate the stages of design, data collection, and analysis but to go backward and forward between raw data and the process of

T A B L E 15-2

Characteristics of Qualitative vs Quantitative Research

Characteristic	Qualitative Research	Quantitative Research
Domain	One or a few cases	Population
Typical methods	Observation	Measurement
	Interview	Survey
Means of analysis	Interpretation	Statistics
Logic of analysis	Induction and deduction	Deduction
Typical questions	What's going on?	What causes_____?
	What does this mean?	Which treatment is more effective?

Source: Adapted from A J Kuzel et al. Desirable features of qualitative research. *Fam Pract Res J.* 1994;14:369–378.

conceptualization, thereby making sense of the data throughout the period of data collection. Strategies frequently used to accomplish the work include in-depth interviews, face-to-face conversations with the purpose of elaborating issues or topics in detail; focus groups, group interviews explicitly including and using group interaction to generate data; and participant observation, the act of noticing during which the researcher occupies a role or part in the setting in addition to observing.

In CPD and health services, research must be tethered to practice. Studies in these fields often are driven not by the theoretical stance of the investigator but by a specific practical problem that is turned into a research question. Regardless of whether the data accrue from qualitative or quantitative approaches to data collection, the study design must match what is being studied, rather than the disciplinary or methodological leanings of the researcher. Qualitative research can be preliminary to quantitative studies, providing descriptions and understanding of situations or behaviors. Also, it can be used to supplement quantitative studies through triangulation, a strategy wherein three or more methods are used and the results compared for convergence of meaning and validation. Finally, qualitative research can complement quantitative studies by exploring complex phenomena or areas not amenable to quantitative research.[26–28]

WHAT LEADERS NEED TO KNOW ABOUT ORGANIZATIONS PROVIDING HEALTH CARE

To succeed, the director who opened this chapter, unable to explain the importance of needs assessment and instructional design, must recognize the organizational systems that enable improvement in health care. Health care services need to be organized and financed in systems that make sense to patients and clinicians and that encourage the coordination of care and collaborative work.[4] Whatever their form, health care organizations need to meet challenges that cut across different health conditions; types of care, such as preventive, acute, and chronic; and health care settings. The challenges include:[4]

- Redesigning processes of care;
- Making effective use of information technologies;
- Managing clinical knowledge and skills;
- Developing effective teams;
- Coordinating care across patient conditions, services, and settings over time; and
- Incorporating performance and outcome measurements for improvement and accountability.

It is not contradictory to say that learning causes action and that action causes learning, and it is likely that both learning and action will be required to meet these challenges. It is possible that continual learning will enable health care organizations to survive through sensing and adapting to changes in the organizational environment.

Peter Senge,[43-44] a well-recognized advocate of organizational learning, asserts that organizations and the people comprising them were designed for learning, coming fully equipped with an insatiable drive to explore and experiment. He describes three core capabilities that determine the ability of organizations to learn:[44] *aspiration*, the extent to which people are oriented toward creating what they truly care about; *reflective conversation*, the ways people talk with one another about conflict and complex issues, setting the tone for collective learning; and *understanding complexity*, recognizing how the world becomes more interconnected and dynamic as compared to presently conditioned ways of thinking. Senge suggests these capabilities involve particular skills and internalized knowledge that can be built over time and that without genuine aspiration, there is no real reason for learning, especially if the learning is difficult. Without reflectiveness and the capacity for conversation, there is limited opportunity to connect people to projects and plans for change, and without conversation, there may be many visions but no shared vision. Finally, without a collective capability for conversation, promising strategic insights will end up creating polarization, as people try to impose their ideas on one another. And without the capability to understand complexity, there is no insight into the deeper causes of problems: quick-fix solutions dominate, and even powerful visions become connected to dangerously oversimplified views of reality.[44]

Those who provide clinical care operate at the heart of the value-creation process in health care organizations. Those who plan, implement, and evaluate learning and behavioral change may foster a culture of learning by nurturing the core capabilities that form the foundation for organizations that learn.

WHAT CAN THE DIRECTOR DO TO ASSURE BROADER IMPACT?

Although CME planners and CPD professionals ordinarily engage in reflective conversation, seeking and culling the ideas of others and providing service to enable learning and change, the inherently social, political, and ethical practice of planning involves participants in deliberation and judgment. Program planners make judgments based on personal, organizational, and social interests.[45] They must be sensitive to the issues surrounding an educational activity. They are not free agents able to choose any course of action they want, nor, are their actions wholly determined by the social and institutional structures in which they work. Planners negotiate the interests of other people acting within their organizations; if they don't, their programs fail.[45] The interests embedded in their organizational systems constrain what is possible and desirable so that only a certain range of actions is conceivable. The norms of what is possible and desirable are rooted in the systems within which planners act. Consequently, by recognizing the interests that guide planning practice, planners can understand why programs end up with certain purposes, content, audiences, and formats. In turn, planners are prepared to participate in the design of evaluative activities intended to explain strengths and weaknesses of program planning and changes possibly resulting from program implementation.

The number of leaders in continuing education and CPD with formal degrees, including coursework or theses specific to education or evaluation, is very small compared to the number who enter with experience or terminal degrees in the health professions. As the opening vignette to this chapter suggests, the longstanding expectation of CME planners is that they deliver service. The success of the planner is measured by consumers and colleagues, and often the measure includes how well the logistics of a meeting were carried out. Responsibility for the effect of a course or conference on learning, physician behavior, or patient outcomes is resisted, overlooked, or simply denied by many, including the planners themselves. Yet, the influence of the planner's actions on outcomes and the opportunity to influence instructional design are undeniable.[45] For example, the planner can conduct follow-up tests of knowledge; surveys of physicians, patients, and medical staff; or reviews of patient records to help prove the value of educational activities

FIGURE 15-2

Performance Data Linking CME/CPD and Health Services Research

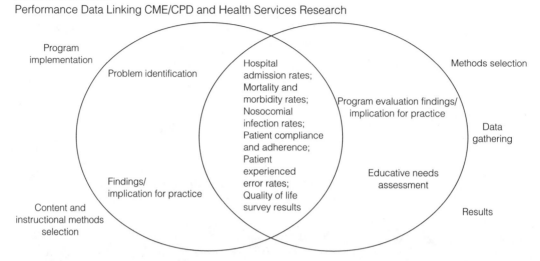

Continuing Medical Education/Performance Data
Continuing Professional Development

Health Services Research

intended to promote learning, cause change in clinical behavior, or influence patient outcomes.[46]

The performance data to link clinical care and health outcomes focuses continuing education, CPD, and health services research on quality improvement. As physicians practice within the organizational boundaries of health care systems, hospital admission rates, mortality and morbidity rates, nosocomial infection rates, patient compliance and adherence, patient-experienced error rates, and quality of life survey results are examples of performance data that may disclose opportunities for clinical improvement,[47] intermittently revealing learning needs and educational outcomes for the practicing physicians. And because CME is forcefully driven by success with the markets it serves, performance data for its physicians and health systems clients can be added to the mix of physician participation and satisfaction rates ordinarily collected by planners (Figure 15-2). Together, these data may be used to carefully specify and inform the budgetary, financial, and market performance goals of the CME, CPD, or health services research programs themselves.[47]

It may be necessary to redirect some of the energy spent collecting participation and satisfaction data in CME toward an increasingly rigorous effort to evaluate CPD and health services. Because so many in CME, CPD, and health services research share interests in performance data, the transition from current evaluative behavior ought not to be strained. To enable the transition, leaders must:

■ recognize the philosophical biases central to inquiry, knowledge interpretation, and methods;

- recognize their role and influence in setting priorities for planning and evaluation decisions;

- articulate sound explanations and realistic expectations for the use of evaluative research to improve learning and health care;

- select the evaluative study design that best fits the practical problem;

- command enough knowledge of clinical performance indicators to recognize their value in:

  —measuring the results of educational activities intended to improve clinical care in the health system, and

  —assessing the effects of educational and clinical improvements with regard to CME and health system financial, budgetary, and market performance, and

- participate in collaborative efforts that enable personal and organizational learning; and

- submit reports of personal and organizational learning to peer evaluation and public scrutiny.

If ever it was unique to them, it is no longer that CME planners are singly qualified to advise which educational activities work best to solve selected problems in health care. Leaders must continue to conduct critical appraisals of the literature to determine the educational interventions that work best in selected contexts. Randomized controlled trials must be completed to measure the effects of CME, and evidence-based guidelines must be identified to inform not only health care but also educational practice. Hypotheses tested under controlled conditions can add to theoretical understandings of physician learning, behavior, and planned change. Those with special responsibility in evaluation must acquire facility with cohort, case-controlled, and survey research to participate in decisions regarding the quality of care and the influence of educational interventions in health care systems. Qualitative studies involving focus groups, in-depth interviews, and participant observation can enable richer theoretical understandings, not only of learning and change but also of the CPD of physicians. The ultimate value of all these applied skills is determined by their usefulness in addressing the concerns of patients, practitioners, and policy makers in systems of care.

THE LONG VIEW

For the director whose vignette opened this chapter, the data on how physicians learn and change are recent and sparse, offering a restricted benchmark for the future. Long-term perspective[48] may free his thinking and that of those who demand to know why determinations of learning needs are important to education, patient safety, and the health of the public. Involving interested stakeholders in generating goals to describe the health care and educational services to be provided and to identify the thresholds of error to be tolerated ought to enable formulation of a shared vision for success. To enable achievement of the vision, all those with an interest may agree to function on a day-to-day basis in service to the vision. For example, if the vision includes elimination of all medication errors 100 years from now, progress may be measured and followed using the quantitative and qualitative study designs presently available to evaluative researchers.

Improvement in health care and the education services required to accomplish the 100-year goal will depend, in part, upon the collective will of all those who agree to cooperate or to compete in order to realize the vision. Responsibility of planners in CME and CPD may include learning the complexities, identifying the aspirations, and leading the reflexive conversation toward achievement of the vision, including development of the educational infrastructure to assure its attainment. It may also include negotiation of the interests of stakeholders toward achievement of the vision and development of an evaluative research design. In such a project, there can be no loss for failed studies, only evidence to guide improvement and to serve as markers for empiricists of the future. As the project moves toward total elimination of medication errors by 2103, planners must assure the availability of a long line of useful data that explain for future generations the emotions and intellectual contributions that define present-day successes and failures. At present, the highest quality evidence applied in contemporary evaluation of CME and CPD and of health services research involving physicians' learning and behavior includes social and psychological studies of change in the clinical behavior of physicians and associated patient outcomes. Continually revisiting the problems of patient safety, quality improvement, and education, while looking across disciplines that include not only psychology and sociology but also ethics, biology, biomedical imaging, and heritability, may lead to improved policy, increased productivity, additional knowledge of human behavior, and progress in teaching and learning that is intended to eliminate error and improve health care.

REFERENCES—CHAPTER 15

1. Sackett DL, Richardson WS, Rosenberg W, Haynes RB. *Evidence Based Medicine: How to Practice and Teach EBM.* New York, NY: Churchill Livingstone; 1997.

2. Berwick DM. Developing and testing changes in delivery of care. *Ann Intern Med.* 1998;128:651–656.

3. Institute of Medicine. *To Err Is Human: Building a Safer Health System.* Kohn LT, Corrigan JM, Donaldson MS, eds. Washington, DC: National Academy Press; 2000.

4. Institute of Medicine. *Crossing the Quality Chasm: A New Health System for the 21st Century.* Corrigan JM, Donaldson MS, Kohn LI, Maguire SK, Pike KC, eds. Washington, DC: National Academy Press; 2001.

5. Lincoln YS, Guba EG. *Naturalistic Inquiry.* Newbury Park, Calif: Sage Publications; 1985.

6. Mill JS. *A System of Logic.* London: Longmans Green; 1906 (original work published 1843).

7. Houle CO. *Continuing Learning in the Professions.* San Francisco, Calif: Jossey-Bass Publishers; 1980.

8. www.ahcpr.gov/about/stratpln.htm#mission

9. Dewey J. *How We Think.* Amherst, NY: Prometheus Books; 1991.

10. Einstein A. *Ideas and Opinions.* New York, NY: Modern Library; 1994 (originally published in 1954 by Crown Publishers).

11. Bohr N. *Atomic Theory and the Description of Nature.* Cambridge, Mass: The University Press; 1961.

12. Holton G. *Thematic Origins of Scientific Thought.* Cambridge, Mass: Harvard University Press; 1973.

13. Wolf A. *A History of Science, Technology, and Philosophy in the 16th and 17th Centuries.* London: George Allen & Unwin Ltd; 1935.

14. Singer C. *A Short History of Scientific Ideas to 1900.* London: Oxford University Press; 1959.

15. Geertz C. *The Interpretation of Cultures: Selected Essays.* New York, NY: Basic Books; 1973.

16. Geertz C. *Local Knowledge: Further Essays in Interpretative Anthropology.* New York, NY: Basic Books; 1983.

17. Guba EG, Lincoln YS. *Fourth Generation Evaluation.* Newbury Park, Calif: Sage Publications; 1989.

18. Davis DA, Thomson MA, Oxman AD and Haynes B. Changing physician performance. *JAMA.* 1995;274:700–705.

19. Davis DA, Thompson O'Brien MA, Freemantle N, Wolf FM, Mazmanian P, Taylor-Vaisey A. Impact of formal continuing medical education: do conferences, workshops, rounds, and other traditional continuing education activities change physician behavior or health care outcomes? *JAMA.* 1999;282:867–874.

20. Grol R. Improving the quality of medical care: building bridges among professional pride, payer profit, and patient satisfaction. *JAMA.* 2001;286:2578–2585.

21. Fox RD, Mazmanian PE, Putnam RW. *Changing and Learning in the Lives of Physicians.* New York, NY: Praeger Publishers; 1989.

22. Campbell CM, Parboosingh J, Gondocz T, Babitskaya G, Pham B. Study of the factors influencing the stimulus to learning recorded by physicians keeping a learning portfolio. *J Contin Educ Health Prof.* 1999;19:16–24.

23. Knox AB, Underbaake G, McBride PE, Mejicano GC. Organization development strategies for continuing medical education. *J Contin Educ Health Prof.* 2001;21:15–23.

24. Kuzel AJ, Engel JD, Addison, RB, Bogdewic ST. Desirable features of qualitative research. *Fam Pract Res J.* 1994;14:369–378.

25. Pope C and Mays N. Reaching the parts other methods cannot reach: an introduction to qualitative methods in health and health services research. *BMJ.* 1995;311:42–45.

26. Morse JM. Considering theory derived from qualitative research. In: Morse JM, ed. *Completing a Qualitative Project.* Thousand Oaks, Calif: Sage Publications; 1997.

27. Kuzel AJ. Some pragmatic thoughts about evaluating qualitative health research. In: Morse JM, Swanson JM, and Kuzel AJ, eds. *The Nature of Qualitative Evidence.* Thousand Oaks, Calif: Sage Publications; 2001.

28. Swanson JM. The nature of outcomes. In: Morse JM, Swanson JM, and Kuzel AJ, eds. *The Nature of Qualitative Evidence.* Thousand Oaks, Calif: Sage Publications; 2001.

29. Kerlinger FN. *Foundations of Behavioral Research.* New York, NY: Holt, Rinehart and Winston, Inc; 1973.

30. Russell RS, Taylor BW III. *Operations Management: Focusing on Quality and Competitiveness.* Upper Saddle River, NJ: Prentice-Hall; 1998.

31. Brigley S, Young Y, Littlejohn P, McEwen J. Continuing education for medical professionals: a reflective model. *Postgrad Med J.* 1997;73:23–26.

32. Brookfield SD. Critically reflective practice. *J Contin Educ Health Prof.* 1998;18:197–205.

33. Frankford DM, Patterson MS, Konrad TR. Transforming practice organizations to foster lifelong learning and commitment to medical professionalism. *Acad Med.* 2000;75:708–717.

34. Mott VW. The development of professional expertise in the workplace. In: Mott VW, Daley BJ, eds. *Charting a Course for Continuing Professional Education: Reframing Professional Practice.* San Francisco, Calif: Jossey-Bass Publishers; 2000.

35. Gehlbach SH. *Interpreting the Literature: A Clinician's Guide.* New York, NY: Macmillan; 1982.

36. Chassin MR, McCue SM. A randomized trial of medical quality assurance. *JAMA.* 1986;256:1012–1016.

37. Davis DA, Taylor-Vaisey A. Translating guidelines into practice. A systemic review of theoretic concepts, practical experience and research evidence in the adoption of clinical practice guidelines. *Can Med Assoc J.* 1997;157:408–416.

38. Rogers EM. *Diffusion of Innovations.* 4th ed. New York, NY: The Free Press; 1995.

39. Davis DA, Thomson MA, Oxman AD, Haynes RB. Evidence for the effectiveness of CME: a review of 50 randomized controlled trials. *JAMA.* 1992;268:1111–1117.

40. Harris SA. Epidemiology: Theory, study design, and planning for education. *J Contin Educ Health Prof.* 2000;20:133–145.

41. Monette J, Tamblyn RM, McCleod PJ, Gayton DC. Characteristics of physicians who frequently prescribe long-acting benzodiazepines for the elderly. *Eval Health Prof.* 1997;20L2:115–130.

42. Babbie ER. *Survey Research Methods.* Belmont, Calif: Wadsworth; 1973.

43. Senge PM. The leader's new work: building learning organizations. In: Steers RM, Porter LW, Bigley GA, eds. *Motivation and Leadership at Work.* New York, NY: McGraw-Hill; 1996.

44. Senge PM. The Academy as Learning Community: Contradiction in Terms or Realizable Future? In: Lucas AF and Associates, *Leading Academic Change.* San Francisco, Calif: Jossey-Bass Publishers; 2000.

45. Cervero RM, Wilson AL. *Planning Responsibly for Adult Education.* San Francisco, Calif: Jossey-Bass Publishers; 1994.

46. Mazmanian PE, Davis DA. Continuing medical education and the physician as learner: a guide to the evidence. *JAMA.* 2002;288:1057–1060.

47. Baldridge National Quality Program 2001. Health Care Criteria for Performance Excellence. www.quality.nist.gov 2001.

48. Brand S. *The Clock of the Long Now.* New York, NY: Basic Books; 1999.

chapter 16

Integrating Theory and Practice: Toward Practical Scholarship and Scholarly Practice

Robert Fox, EdD; Dave Davis, MD; Barbara E. Barnes, MD

INTRODUCTION

The context of research and the context of practice present two distinct and unique sets of problems for the interaction of theory and practice. To some extent, it is a matter of perspective and purpose; the researcher is engaged in a search for clearer and more accurate explanations of phenomena. The principle tasks of the researcher are to construct and evaluate the plausibility of these explanations in terms of their rationality and the extent to which there is or could be empirical evidence of relationships described in the explanation. This formal explanation of a set of relationships that can be verified in reality is theory.[1] For the scientist/researcher, the construction, development, and deflection of a theory are the principle challenges behind all research.

For example, a scholar may understand that there are differences in the level of motivation of learners who are participating in a continuing medical education (CME) program. The scholar's overall purpose is to understand this difference so clearly and accurately that she can explain it correctly and consistently. The more differences (variation) that can be explained, the more accurate and dependable is the explanation (theory). Evaluation of accuracy and dependability is based on attempts to either control reality (through experiments or quasi-experiments) to fit the explanation or to examine the parts of an ongoing reality in a way that excludes distractions from the explanation (eg, using statistical controls). Some qualitative approaches collect all of reality, use what is useful to construct an explanation of differences, and discard the rest. In the end, the product is the theory, developed from empirical evidence, modified or left alone because of evidence, having endured a test of reality.

The practitioner works immersed in the reality, interacting and attempting to change it in a meaningful way. The principle task of the practitioner is to address a set of problems that fall within the scope of his responsibilities. This involves a process that includes gathering information about a particular problem or set of problems, applying that information in the form of decisions about what to do about the problems, managing the actions and resources that follow from the decisions, and monitoring and correcting as the process unfolds. The principle challenges for the practitioner of continuing professional development (CPD) are developing a clear view of reality and translating what is seen in that view into decisions and actions that allow for success in developing and evaluating interventions. The view almost always includes some informal explanation of the problem or problems of CPD practice and a logical process connecting informal explanations to decisions and actions intended to solve the practice problem.

For example, for the practitioner, the problem of motivation may be seen as a problem of attendance; some physicians come to the program and some do not. Moreover, some learn and some do not. It is up to the CPD practitioner to collect information about the problem, perhaps from reflection on past experiences and from observations made related to planning an educational program. This may mean collecting information related to the kinds of learners that are sought—their states of mind, their experiences with the issue, the contents and formats of preprogram materials (eg, brochures, self-assessments, needs assessments, opinion leaders, quality assurance activities), and the overall design of the effort. Like scholars, they try to explain the problem of low motivation, and they do it systematically. However, rather than organizing their information and evidence from reality around the explanation, they organize everything around the problem and happily discard anything that does not add to the clarity of their vision of the problem. Explanations tend to be constructed extemporaneously, as "straw men" to be discarded and replaced as they fail to add to the solution or fit the information from reality.

Theory and data are representations of the real world for both the scholar and the practitioner. However, they serve different masters. For the scholar, a theory is a formal explanation of a set of phenomena that is constructed out of concepts and leads to one or more hypotheses that can be tested against data (information). For the practitioner, a theory is a best guess as to what causes a problem or constitutes a solution to a problem. It guides practices as long as it stands the test of application and holds up as a useful explanation. Although there are differences in the meaning of theory, both use ideas and both evaluate them against reality. The gap between the scholar and the practitioner is one of purpose and degree more than of fundamental process. The problem is how do we reduce the gap without damaging the value of each perspective, thereby undermining either research, or practice, or both.

THREE AREAS OF DEVELOPMENT

One way to examine more closely the problem of integrating theory and practice is to look at several issues for both scholars and practitioners. The focus of this discussion is on how research and theory may lead to changes in three areas: the tools of practice, the processes CPD practitioners use, and the way the elements that support CPD are designed and organized.

DEVELOPING THE TOOLS OF CPD

Like all professional activities, CPD uses artifacts to accomplish its purposes. Because the primary problems faced in the practice of CPD have to do with gathering and understanding information to be used to develop and evaluate programs and services related to facilitating learning and change, research-like tools are important artifacts associated with this purpose.

The literature of adult learning and CPD is not organized in a way that makes it possible to create a catalogue of tools for the CPD professional. Often tools are developed for one task (ie, a survey) and discarded after the task. No record of its use, its value, or its purpose are left behind or communicated to anyone else. Because of the extemporaneous nature of the processes associated with many CPD strategies, everything associated with it tends to be developed as a throwaway. This is in contrast to the enduring, sometimes intractable nature of undergraduate and graduate curricula, where everything is permanent until substantial evidence or political force moves it out, in favor of replacement. Overcoming this problem requires CPD professionals, scholars, and practitioners alike to begin to use theory as a superstructure for the tools of the enterprise and as a system for labeling, grouping, and applying tools to practice problems. Of course, this means tools and theories must interact in a way that each affects the other.

This book is another kind of tool. It is organized into three fundamental parts based on a very simple idea about how the practice of CPD is organized. It presumes that every practitioner can view their efforts as oriented toward solving three fundamental problems: How do I decide what to do next year? How do I decide how to do it? And, how do I decide if I was successful? There are many ways that the book could have been constructed, but this one was selected to facilitate the transformation of research and theory into practices and to enable the authors to organize knowledge and theory around practices. The principle is one of attending to the ultimate value of the knowledge base; research and theory are present to generate explanations and predictions that form the basis of action. If the ultimate purpose is to have an effect on the actions of those who are engaged in the CPD enterprise, knowledge should be organized around those actions and around the problems those actions are intended to resolve.

Tools that need to be in the practitioner's toolbox, those that relate to deciding what to do, can be gleaned from the first section of this text. Emphasis in each chapter is on the elements and processes that may be used to decide what to do. It also highlights how different perspectives point one in different directions. The information and the interpretation of information are different if one is working from the perspective of population health, the institutions of health care, the performance of physicians in practice, and the needs of learners. Each perspective implies different kinds of tools. From the perspective of population health, the CPD professional needs to be able to gain reports, use statistics and population health techniques, and even develop screens to assist in interpreting the data available. She also needs to be able to replicate or approximate the tools of population health research on different levels, from macro to micro. Likewise, in terms of the needs of organizations and health care systems, tools to help audit charts or track costs or outcomes need to be developed. Tools for assessing performance and for identifying learner need can range from chart-stimulated recall interviews to computerized prescription systems. These tools look to the actual behavior that may lead to the performance and on to the hospital's cost of care and the incidence and prevalence of disease in a province or state.

One very explicit example of a tool that has been developed systematically from a body of theory and research is the change readiness inventory (CRI).[2] This instrument examines different elements of change and learning theory in order to provide a profile of a physician's self-perceived readiness to change. Converting the theory into a tool for CPD practitioners involved comparing surveys to interviews and case studies of change and engaging in extensive reflective utilization and experimentation related to the use of the tool in CPD. Oriented toward providing useful information based on both evidence and theory, the tool was not designed primarily as a valid scientific device in the traditional sense. Rather, its purpose was to give a voice to physicians regarding their perceptions of the issues involved in changing their practices. It was valuable because it was better than giving them no voice and it responded to the requirements of practicing CPD rather than only that of science.

Another example of a tool useful to practitioners is the "commitment to change" survey.[3] It was used to reinforce educational strategies for change and to estimate the relative effect of a change strategy on behavior and performance. Like the CRI, the commitment to change inventory is a set of questions in survey format, developed out of a body of research and theory and designed to fit the problems of practice, namely, How does one learn about the potential outcomes of CPD? and How does one encourage change in practice? It is now widely used for both purposes because it has transformed a body of theory into a tool that fits the needs of CPD.

Among the areas for future development are the need to design useful everyday instruments, such as surveys, interview guides, checklists, computer software and educational formats, methods, and techniques, from some of the major theories that are cited in the literature. Prochaska[4] and Rogers[5] offer different perspectives, eg, on stages of change. Both theories could be translated into schemes, techniques, or information-collection strategies that may better inform CPD professionals about status, progress, and outcomes associated with change strategies. For example, both areas of theory include attempts to explain how change is a result of several strategies for learning rather than a single event. The need to monitor the progress and direction of change across these strategies is readily apparent, but the adaptation of the literature on stages of change or on stages of learning, as articulated by Putnam,[6] initially, and later by Fox,[7] and Slotnick,[8] into useful instruments or other tools of practice has not been forthcoming.

Chapter 14 in this text describes a rich inventory of methods and techniques for data collection and analysis. A system for developing and integrating typologies and theoretical models with these techniques would facilitate a more sound and useful way for practitioners to match their information needs to methods for explaining results. This need to develop the intellectual hardware of CPD should dominate the landscape of change in CPD.

THE REDESIGN OF PROCESSES FOR CPD

There is also a powerful need to redefine the role of the CPD practitioner in a way that reflects the present fund of knowledge in the field and the directions development of new knowledge will take over the next decade. The process for program planning and evaluation used in most CPD efforts over the past 40-plus years was initially articulated by Tyler[9] as a simple, linear model for planning curricula and instruction in public schools. It was a powerful force, primarily because it was a simple, digestible guide that had the advantage of organizing actions around decisions. It also focused on planning for classes, groups of 20 or more, to maximize effectiveness in this context. Like most clear, simple, and useful perspectives, it spread quickly from public schools to vocational programs, community colleges, universities, training programs, and CME.

The model prescribes that one should:

- assess competence,
- design objectives,
- design instruction, and
- evaluate effectiveness.

The model also discusses principles of teaching that have endured over time, including attention to continuity sequence and integration as principles of organization. It was especially useful for teaching directed toward adding new knowledge and for moving a group of learners from novice to expert. It was not designed or intended to be used as a way to deal with the complexities of unlearning, replacing skills or habits, translating knowledge into professional behavior, or reforming performance. Because adults, in general, and professionals, in particular, are engaged in the application of knowledge to performance, which affects outcomes in terms of the well-being of their clients and client systems, behavioral change is not a matter of pouring new behavior into half-full vessels. Usually, something must go to make space for new behaviors. In addition, many things in old behavior, social and practice contexts, professional culture, and the behavior of clients may need to change to allow this new, changed behavior to endure. This means that processes used to design and implement CPD must focus more on the collection and interpretation of information about the learner and the context of practice than on the psychology of learning. This also means that new models of managing the change and learning processes must be used to accommodate what we have learned about change and learning in practice.

CME has a long tradition of using educational models to foster changes is physicians' behaviors. These approaches have often focused on the individual practitioner operating a "cottage industry" style of practice. The physician was viewed as an independent professional with wide discretion as to what he or she did and how it was done. Providers of CME offered educational programs "on a buffet line" for consumption by independent physicians in individual or small-group practices. However, research showed little effect of singular programs on individual practices.[10] Multiple interventions seemed to be necessary to foster change in performance.

One way to foster planned and purposeful change in any setting is through process consultation. This approach to planned change is based on initial work by Schein[11] and more recent work by Cockman et al.[12] and Block.[13] Schein[11] offered process consultation as a model for managing change. It has been widely used and adapted to fit the problems of organizational change and professional performance change. An extensive discussion of this perspective was offered in Chapter 6.

Process consultation as applied to CPD takes the perspective that change in performance and outcomes is a complex phenomenon that occurs in stages.[13] The model emphasizes change strategies built from a series of steps, including:

- gaining entry into a client organization, which includes being allowed to assist the learners with clinical or other professional problems in the context of practice with its needs for changes;

- contracting a relationship with the client system that focuses on coming to an agreement as to who will do what, when, where, why, and how;

- collecting data about the organization's problems, which requires being able to describe the problems in terms of antecedents, consequences, elements, and processes;

- analyzing data so as to understand the problems;

- designing interventions by selecting and revising educational and other strategies for changing competence and performance;

- implementing interventions in a way that ensures that the strategies are translated into the actions that represent the context of application;

- evaluating outcomes by describing and explaining the differences that result from the effort;

- disengaging or renegotiating the contract to formalize revision of the plan or collecting new data to improve the way one describes the situation and the problem.

The process focuses on the need for understanding and explanation as the basis for decisions about what to do, how to do it, and how to determine the effects of the strategy in terms of outcomes. In this process, the CPD professional works with client systems (learners, patients, managed care systems, collegial systems, third parties, or institutions of care). The notion that underlies this perspective is that although all change strategies do not necessarily lead to change, change is always the issue. It is also assumed that change in practice requires multiple actors and multiple strategies. Finally, it assumes that the outcomes and the processes are information-driven. In process consultation, a CPD professional

FIGURE 16-1

Process Consultation as Applied to CPD

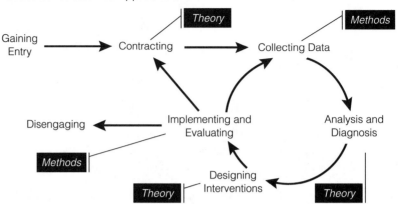

Source: Adapted from Cockman P, Reynolds P Evans B. *Clients-Centered Consulting; Getting Your Expertise Used When You're Not in Charge.* New York, NY McGraw Hill; 1996:17.

is a change consultant who acts as a "smart" lens, taking in and analyzing information in a collaborative fashion that enables the client systems (from the learner to the other stakeholders) to make good decisions that facilitate CPD and practice improvement.

The perspective assumes that information is essential to problem solving, that information can be collected and analyzed in a fair way, and that collaborative strategies for collecting and applying information increase motivation and commitment. This enhances the chances for success. It also assumes that attempts to change performance need to be collaborative acts, engaged in with the consent of clients and accomplished in a way that enhances the competencies of the client to manage the processes of change and learning in the future.

Figure 16-1 describes this process, as portrayed by Cockman[12] but with modifications to demonstrate the place of theory in the process of facilitating change and learning in medical practices and medical systems.

As is evident, the CPD professional acting in this way must apply theory and knowledge of educational and research methodology at several key points:

- In contracting, one must understand the whole process, including the process consultation cycle, the factors that may impinge upon behavior, the principles of learning and change, and the range of methods and techniques that may be applied.

- In collecting data, one must understand the strengths and weaknesses of different strategies, methods, and techniques for collecting data related to performance and competence in clinical and other professional practices.

■ In analysis and diagnosis, one must be able to relate the results to the problem and the potential explanations of the problem in clinical performance. It is also important to see how the results resemble other similar efforts to change behavior and the body of evidence related to behavior change.

■ In designing interventions, one must be able to use evidence-based criteria to select the methods and techniques that will have an impact on the issues of performance that are indicated by the analysis and diagnosis. This stage recognizes competencies in the CPD professional, not only in educational change strategies but also in such strategies as reminders and feedback systems, as described in Chapter 10.

■ In implementing and evaluating interventions, one must possess competencies in a range of evaluation methods and techniques (see Chapter 14) as well as a conceptual model that relates outcomes to antecedent conditions (see Chapter 13).

Process consultation is one of several process models that may guide the work of CPD in the future. Other process models include models of facilitated self-directed learning (see Chapters 7 and 8), program planning,[14,15] innovation diffusion,[5] and planned change.[16] Each deserves attention for its implications for managing the roles and responsibilities of the CPD professional.

THE REDESIGN OF SYSTEMS FOR CPD

In order to better integrate theory and practice, it is necessary to reform the systems that support, sponsor, and offer strategies and programs designed to help physicians learn and change. Currently, CPD systems are organized around political and economic models rather than models that are generated from the CPD literature. The organization of CPD today emphasizes the lateral differentiation of systems, each making specialized efforts to change clinical outcomes and medical performance. There are quality-assurance systems that lean on the physician's behavior by comparing and contrasting performance and outcomes with peers or with guidelines, usually without sophistication in their explanations of how the outcome or performance came to be. There are also policy approaches that lean on behavior by making rules and regulations, usually accompanied by threats and coercion in the form of consequences for failure to comply. Sometimes these systems use feedback or reminders as accompaniments to the coercion. Finally, there are information-dissemination systems, like traditional CME programs in hospitals, specialty societies, and medical schools, that operate under the assumption that if the practitioners get the information and it makes sense, they will change.

Studies of the effectiveness of CME have pointed out the weaknesses of simple information diffusion, single strategies for change, and strategies that are designed without the benefit of knowledge about need or explanations of why the performance is as it is.[10] CPD will need to be organized around the complexities of our understanding of performance change and learning in practice if it is to allow for the application of knowledge to the problems of physician performance.

There are three kinds of systems that can benefit from changes that encourage the application of theory to practice: delivery systems, knowledge systems, and quality-control systems. Each system uses research and new knowledge differently, but each can play a role in knowledge generation and application.

Delivery Systems

Delivery systems are those organizations and their system of organizational processes that make CPD programs. These processes include planning, designing, financing, marketing, implementing, and evaluating systematic efforts to alter inappropriate performance or assure appropriate performance by the application of knowledge to medical practice. Delivery systems include medical schools, hospitals, specialty and other professional associations, communication or other medical education companies, major clinics, governments, and managed care organizations. Delivery systems may also be units within pharmaceutical or equipment companies, Internet companies, publishers, and advocacy groups. However, not all of these groups have a high stake in the development and implementation of a system for delivering continuing education. Not all believe that their organization should play a role in the generation and integration of knowledge and theory. Some may not believe that knowledge and theory should form the basis of practice. However, some (such as medical schools, professional associations, and academic hospitals) have a higher stake in the development of the art and science of CPD than others, who may be content to view CPD programs as products within a marketplace or tools to achieve other goals.

There are two roles that delivery systems can play in building and integrating theory into practice; they can thoughtfully experiment with the transformation of knowledge into new processes and tools for CPD and they can practice CPD in a systematic manner that includes the documentation of the "art of CPD." Thoughtful experimentation refers to the development of processes and skills that enable adaptation of the evidence and theoretical foundations into actions that lead to better strategies for CPD. For example, understanding that motivation is a "function of the drive to reduce a sense of anxiety arising from the perception that one's performance is not as it should be"[2] cannot really affect practice until someone "experiments" with this in a CPD system. In this case, an organization with a mission related to application of theory to practice must discover opportunities to apply this idea to its work, select an opportunity, record the conditions of application, and decide on how to determine if the "experimental application" of this idea to CPD is appropriate. It may mean developing a way of estimating the gap between where one's performance is and where it ought to be, developing a tool for estimating consequences of different levels, and altering presentations in the CPD program so that some enhanced self-estimation of this discrepancy occurs.

Presently, there are lots of little and big experiments with ideas and applications under way, but there are few opportunities to share these methods or their results. Part of this problem is simply a failure to recognize that "reflective practice" of this kind can lead to learning across delivery systems, but part of it also may be that there is little effort to document these exercises in the art of applying theory to practice.

Documenting the actions, conditions, and outcomes of attempts to transform theory into practice is as important to learning and developing CPD as experimental application. Without documentation, both errors and successes go undetected and learning from them is impossible. This dilemma is made more problematic by a culture of health care that has developed a tendency to disseminate its successes rather than its failures and to reward right answers and, via a variety of expressions, its intolerance for wrong answers. This kind of context makes it difficult to refine practices. Errors are not explained and corrections are not recorded, assuring that the errors and the failed attempts to correct them will be repeated. Medicine would not have become as adept as it is at putting science to work in practice if it had not also become good at documenting the problems and the attempts at solutions of all who intervene. CPD can learn from this.

Documentation of successes is also necessary to understanding how to integrate theory and research with CPD practice. The emerging emphasis on "best practices" has helped with this problem, as books, articles, and conferences related to CPD have picked up on the value of sharing successes. What may be needed that is not present in many of these discussions is more direct reference and discrete attention to the description of the ideas and explanations that form the basis of these presentations. Except in cases where mimicking the practices of others is enough for success, lack of structured incorporation of theory into discussions of best practices inhibits the success of scholars or practitioners to improve the theory or delivery of CPD. The problem with mimicking the practices of others is that the problems and contexts of practice are often different in meaningful ways from one point of application to the other. The incorporation of theory into practice by thoughtful experimentation and careful documentation by CPD delivery systems is an essential element in developing a body of practice that is founded on knowledge because it allows for practices based on ideas and reasons.

THE REDESIGN OF KNOWLEDGE SYSTEMS

If knowledge is to be applied to practice, there must be a system for generating and disseminating new knowledge. There must be research units, new and revised knowledge and theory emanating from research units, and a body of literature that reflects the place of new knowledge in the overall body of knowledge. The development of knowledge systems has begun in CPD with a scattering of research units within medical schools and a few university departments of adult education. But these units are dependent upon the leadership of the departments that house them and the competence of the researchers within them. The research function has not been embedded in the enterprise. It is still peripheral in many ways, subject to the first budget cut or to a change in the preference or requirements of institutional leadership. Add to the sporadic efforts to establish research units a growing interest in research as a secondary responsibility on the part of many CPD practitioners in a variety of settings. These may be the disorganized beginnings of an international "college of continuing professional development" that may someday see itself as the responsible party in the knowledge generation enterprise in CPD. Before this can happen, cohesion among systems must develop around the value of this enterprise to the world of CPD for physicians. This means that the world of delivery systems, described above, must begin to see the work of the research enterprise as valuable to the practice of CPD. In turn, this research must be generated from the problems of CPD practice and must always return to it in the final analysis with contributions to the solutions of problems of practice. Without this relevance, the community of researchers will continue to languish in hopes of a better foundation of support and a larger audience of interested consumers of new knowledge.

The CPD literature for physicians must also reflect a concern for the problems of practice. Researchers must look to the world of practice for needs and priorities related to new knowledge. They must begin to see that the principle role of theory in CPD, as in any other area of practice in education, is to explain the problems of practice. Therefore, research questions and research priorities that reflect the problems of practices and include in their goals the

F I G U R E 16-2

The Place of Theory and Practice in Research

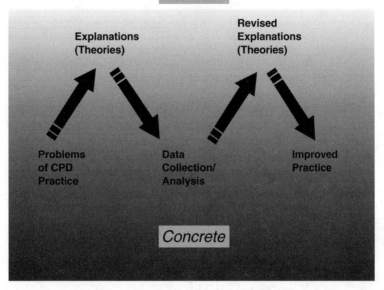

development and discussion of principles and practices that may solve similar problems is essential. This approach of placing problems, like brackets, at the front and at the end of research embeds the generation of new knowledge with the practice. If one embeds research so that every study starts with a problem, finds the best existing explanation of the problem, studies the value of this explanation, revises the explanation, and sets actions from it to solve problems, the study will be embedded in practice and the practice will be connected to theory. In this process, scholarship is evident in both the research and the transformation of knowledge to integrate it with application (Figure 16-2).

The figure represents the dialectical interaction among the five stages of the research process. Fundamentally, the research enterprise in an applied field, such as CPD is always a function of the resolution of conflict between that which is imagined and that which is real. Research that fosters scholarly application begins with problems and ends with problems but proceeds with interaction between ideas and events, concepts and data, and explanations and practices. It is this dialectic resolution of conflicting ways of viewing the world that makes the research and the practice continue to develop.

CPD for physicians should begin to structure ways to ensure that practice and theory are part of a formal plan for the CPD of the knowledge professionals working within the CPD enterprise. This means developing ways of cataloging both practice problems and bodies of knowledge. It also means that the knowledge base in journals, research presentations, keynotes, or workshops for CPD professionals should be held to the standards that the offering:

■ must reflect the problems of practice in the beginning and the end, and

■ must reflect sound theories and ideas related to the problem in the beginning and the end.

This simple addition to the ethos of theory to practice would advance application of knowledge to practice to a large measure and in an important way.

The current knowledge base of CPD for physicians should also be reorganized. In other fields, it is the work of texts to organize knowledge and present it in a way that is relevant to practice. This text takes one step toward the integration of theory and practice. It has attempted to do this by steadfastly holding to an organization that requires that all literature be attached to three primary problems faced in practice:

■ How do I decide what to do?

■ How do I decide how to do it?

■ How do I decide the extent to which I have succeeded?

In this way, the relevance of the literature, the variety of theories related to CPD, and the philosophical underpinnings are tested and evaluated and given new meanings within this mandate.

The *Journal of Continuing Education in the Health Professions* has also attempted to organize literature of the field by offering new knowledge within a framework. There are usually articles in each issue that review and reflect on theory, describe new knowledge generated from studies, and critically review existing knowledge. It also offers literature summaries and new scholarly tools that are commented on for their worth. It has resisted reduction to a "practice-only" perspective and has held to the requirement that there must be evidence in the manuscript of the dialectic interconnection between theory and practice.

THE REFORMATION OF QUALITY ASSURANCE SYSTEMS IN CPD

The last area of reformation that is needed is of systems for developing and assuring quality CPD processes and programs. The quality-assurance systems in different countries are those entities that decide about the credit physicians receive for their efforts to learn and change and the qualities that must be in place for these credits to be a dependable currency of CPD. The problem is that many of these systems have developed in a political model rather than a professional development model. Politics is commonly referred to as the sum total of methods that come into play when determining who gets what. Regulation is a coercive act designed to enforce who gets what. Those accreditation systems that focus more on politics, policing, and the compliance of delivery systems often do not use the knowledge base or advance knowledge in any serious way. However, systems like those of the Royal College of Physicians and Surgeons of Canada and the Royal Australasian College of Physicians base the awarding of credit on processes that reflect the knowledge base. These systems lean on research related to reflective practice and change and learning as well as information on needs and outcomes from the clinical world of medical practice. This embeds knowledge in practice and fosters the development of scholarship among practitioners of CPD. It also allows these systems to play a part in the growth and development of the CPD enterprise.

Accreditation systems can also serve a developmental purpose if they can act to codify and educate CPD practitioners regarding the processes of education, learning, and performance change. Codification of processes and outcomes is the initial stage of theory building. After codification comes concept formation and the development of propositions that explain relationships. These explanations, generated from practice experience, enable the writing of new or revised formal theory that explains and predicts the relationships among actions and outcomes in practice. In turn, the principles derived from these explanations can inform practice and bring about a greater connection of scholarship to application.

NEXT STEPS FOR THE INTEGRATION OF THEORY AND PRACTICE: THE SCHOLARLY PRACTITIONER

In order to form interactive effects from the bonding of theory and practice, certain steps are worthwhile. These are not the only steps that the reader may identify or necessarily the best steps. However, these steps seem to be reasonable and potentially valuable for building a more scholarly practitioner and a more pertinent research enterprise in CPD.

The Professional Associations for CPD Professionals

Professional associations whose mission includes the development of personnel who work with CPD must begin to incorporate the development and promotion of scholarly practice into their educational programs for CPD practitioners. This means that the practice of CPD must be appreciated for its ties to a body of evidence, literature, and theory that allow for the generalization of right actions across settings, practitioners, and problems. This is not to argue that theory should dominate. On the contrary, practice should dominate but not to the exclusion or disregard for the research and theory that apply to practice. The danger of a world full of best practices but missing the evidence and ideas that inform and connect practices is self-evident. Without common knowledge, every experience is new and every success and failure is unique. There is nothing to be learned in this world and nothing to guide the interpretation of the problems of practice. Without explanations that may be generalized or used as a framework and applied to CPD practice, practice becomes a series of discrete problem-solving exercises informed by experience without any potential for growth and development. The community of practice becomes a collection of individuals who are disconnected from each other because their work has no common ground. Not a community at all.

Theory and research complement experience to form a common ground made not only from sharing best practices but also from learning and sharing explanations for why things succeed and why they fail. The propositions and concepts that make up formal explanations are the linchpins among the actions of a community of practice. Just as those who fail to study history are destined to repeat it, those who fail to generate, apply, and evaluate theory are destined to make the same mistakes again and again. The formal educational efforts at annual meetings and special workshops in CPD for physicians should incorporate evidence and theory with practice principles to display the scholarship of practice in CPD.

The Formation of Development Teams

Another step that may lead to greater integration of theory and practice is the formation of development teams in a variety of settings for the explicit purpose of transforming theory into practice and practice into theory. These teams may represent small groups of investigators and practitioners who come together to:

- generate, from the documentation of practice and its outcomes, a set of ideas, concepts, and propositions that merit investigation;
- transform the concepts from theory into principles for practice with an emphasis on the question, What does this all mean for me when I try to facilitate change in the medical practices of my clients?
- reform existing theories to reflect evidence from practice and the experiences of CPD practitioners; and

■ set goals, objectives, and priorities for research, practice, and the reformation of knowledge based on the perspectives of investigators and practitioners.

Development teams make the integration and invention of theory and of new practices possible by accepting, from the start, that these two worlds are connected and interdependent and that this fact is a strength and a foundation for enhancing the quality of both theory and practice.

MOVING TO A NEW WORLD OF CPD AS COMMUNITIES OF PRACTICE

Nowlen[17] describes the development of a professional performance as the product of a double helix of personal history and professional culture. If one considers *culture* as defined in the *Merriam-Webster's Collegiate Dictionary*, it includes:[18]

> (a) the integrated pattern of human knowledge, belief, and behavior that depends upon man's capacity for learning and transmitting knowledge to succeeding generations; (b) the customary beliefs, social forms, and material traits of a racial, religious, or social group; (c) the set of shared attitudes, values, goals, and practices that characterizes a company or corporation.

This view of culture as the outcome of a process of development and acquisition of meaning is at the heart of a community of practice in CPD. If CPD for physicians is to take on the mantle of a professional activity, it must build and share its culture among the community of practitioners who engage in efforts to foster the CPD of physicians. This means an active transformative enterprise that involves the development and assignment of meaning to knowledge about practice and theory. For example, Schon's model of learning from experience can have different meanings according to the attitudes, values, and practices of the recipient of the knowledge. In medical practice, a clinician assigns meaning to the Schon model by using it to explain how the art of practice interacts with the science. This assignment of meaning changes the uses of the model and, in fact, alters the relative weight of different concepts within it. For example, the notion that professionals frame problems according to the solutions they have at their disposal helps a medical practitioner understand why some problems are harder to work on than others. For the CPD practitioner, the same statement means that teaching new frameworks for problems depends on teaching new solutions. This is a very different meaning for the same theoretical proposition, indicating that in at least two ways the knowledge is altered as it is applied within two different cultures—the culture of medicine and the culture of CPD.

The development of CPD for physicians as a community of practice requires the recognition and continuing development of the values, attitudes, beliefs, goals, and behaviors that emerge from the domains of research and the domains of application. Boyer[19] refers to scholarship as being made of four domains: the scholarship of discovery, of teaching, of integration, and of application. It is the last that is most relevant to the application of theory to practice because it suggests that knowledge and theory do not translate directly into practice anymore than one language can be translated word for word into another. Knowledge must be interpreted and modified to account for the meanings that the words have in context rather than their literal equivalent. All knowledge is subject to "meaning making" as it is transformed into knowledge that is useful in culture. In CPD, there is a culture of practice that makes meaning from the artifacts, language, values, attitudes, and behaviors associated with the practice of developing and delivering CPD for physicians. Knowledge in the culture of practice is not used in the same way as knowledge in culture of research. It must be remade to fit the context.

A community of scholarly application is the answer to the riddle of translation and transformation. Rather than the simple transmission of information that characterizes the current situation, this requires a deeper and more profound collaboration. It also requires the dissolution of any hierarchy that puts either research or practice at the top, authoritatively directing the activities of others. It means creating a scholarship of application that focuses not only on the generation of new knowledge and the utilization of new knowledge but the active and interactive transformation of both the knowledge of practice and the knowledge of theory. It is appropriate for an applied field like CPD to ask that practice and theory be equal partners in the generation and application of sound, empirically grounded principles of practice and professional behavior. This text has sought to foster the development of a scholarship of application and the emergence of the scholarly practitioner by holding theory accountable to practice and holding practice accountable to theory. Its success will be measured by the changes it fosters.

It also calls for the transformation of the norms, values, and competencies that define the professional performance of those who seek to assist physicians with their CPD. It means a transformation of the role of knowledge professional in CPD from a profession that makes meetings to a profession that studies, understands, and intervenes in a way that facilitates the CPD of physicians. In this new role, the scholarly practitioner is an active problem-solver and change agent, working with physicians to transform practices as need and opportunity provide.

REFERENCES—CHAPTER 16

1. Kerlinger FN. *Foundations of Behavioral Research*. 2nd ed. New York, NY: Holt, Rinehart and Winston; 1973.

2. Fox RD, Miner C. Motivation and the facilitation of change, learning, and participation in educational programs for health professionals. *J Contin Educ Health Prof*. 1999;19:132–141.

3. Mazmanian PE, Ratcliff SR, Johnson RE, Davis DA, Kantrowitz MP. Information about barriers to planned change: a randomized controlled clinical trial involving continuing medical education lectures and commitment to change. *Acad Med*. 1998;73:882–886.

4. Prochaska JO, DiClemente CC, Norcross JC. In search of how people change. Applications to addictive behaviors. *American Psychologist*. 1992;47:1102–1114.

5. Rogers EM. *Diffusion of Innovations*. 4th ed. New York, NY: Free Press; 1995.

6. Putnam RW, Campbell MD. Competence in Fox RD, Mazmanian PE, Putnam RW. *Changing and Learning in the Lives of Physicians*. New York, NY: Praeger Publishers; 1989.

7. Fox RD, Bennett NL: Learning and change: implications for continuing medical. *BMJ*. 1998;316:466–468

8. Slotnick HB. How doctors learn: physicians' self-directed learning episodes. *Acad Med*. 1999;74:1106–1117.

9. Tyler RW. *Basic Principles of Curriculum and Instruction*. Chicago, Ill: University of Chicago Press; 1949.

10. Davis DA, Thompson O'Brien MA, Freemantle N, Wolf FM, Mazmanian P, Taylor-Vaisey A. Impact of formal continuing medical education: do conferences, workshops, rounds, and other traditional continuing education activities change physician behavior or health care outcomes? *JAMA*. 1999;282:867–874.

11. Schein EH. *Process Consultation: Lessons for Managers and Consultants*. New York, NY: Addison-Wesley Publishing Company; 1987.

12. Cockman P, Reynolds P, Evans B. *Client-Centered Consulting; Getting Your Expertise Used When You're Not in Charge*. New York, NY: McGraw Hill; 1996.

13. Block P. *Flawless Consulting: A Guide to Getting Your Expertise Used*. 2nd ed. San Francisco, Calif: Jossey-Bass Publishers; 1999.

14. Caffarella RS. *Program Planning for Adults: A Comprehensive Guide for Adult Educators, Trainers, and Staff Developers*. San Francisco, Calif: Jossey-Bass Publishers; 1994.

15. Cervero R. *Effective Continuing Education for Professionals*. San Francisco, Calif: Jossey-Bass Publishers; 1988.

16. Bennis WG, Benne KD, Chin R. *The Planning of Change*. 4th ed. New York, NY: Holt, Rinehart and Winston; 1985.

17.   Nowlen PM. *A New Approach to Continuing Education for Business and the Professions: The Performance Model.* New York, NY: American Council on Education and Macmillan Publishing Company; 1988.

18.   *Merriam-Webster's Collegiate Dictionary.* 10th ed. Springfield, Mass: Merriam-Webster, Incorporated; 1999:282.

19.   Boyer EL. *Scholarship Reconsidered: Priorities of the Professoriate.* Princeton, NJ: Carnegie Foundation for the Advancement of Teaching; 1990.

Resources—Books and Articles

The following list of books and articles, generated by the authors, are considered essential for reflection on the state of the art of continuing health professional education. Some of the entries have been annotated.

BOOKS AND CHAPTERS

Abernathy C. *Surgical Intuition: What It Is and How to Get It*. Philadelphia, Pa: Hanley & Belfus (Mosby); 1995.

Aristotle. *Nichomachean Ethics* [translated by M. Ostwald]. New York, NY: Macmillan Publishing; 1962.

> *Comment:* Re Book VI—Choice is the starting point of action. It is the source of human action but not the end. The starting point of choice is desire and reasoning directed toward some end. There can be no choice without intelligence and thought or without some moral characteristic. Human action requires thought and character.

Balestracci D, Barlow JL. *Quality Improvement: Practical Applications for Medical Group Practice*. Englewood, Colo: Center for Research in Ambulatory Care Administration; 1996.

Bandura A. *Self Efficacy: The Exercise of Control*. New York, NY: W.H. Freeman; 1997.

Bastable SB. *Nurse as Educator: Principles of Teaching and Learning*. Sudbury, Mass: Jones and Bartlett Publishers; 1997.

Boud D, Keogh R, Walker D. *Reflection: Turning Experience into Learning*. London: Kogan Page; 1985.

Boyle PJ. *Getting Doctors to Listen: Ethics and Outcomes Data in Context*. Washington, DC: Georgetown University Press; 1998.

Chaiklin S, Lave J. *Understanding Practice: Perspectives on Activity and Context*. New York, NY: Cambridge University Press; 1993.

Davis DA, Fox RD. *The Physician as Learner: Linking Research to Practice*. Chicago, Ill: American Medical Association; 1994.

DiBella AJ, Nevis EC. *How Organizations Learn: An Integrated Strategy for Building Learning Capability*. San Francisco, Calif: Jossey-Bass Publishers; 1998.

Fox RD, Mazmanian PE, Putnam RW. *Changing and Learning in the Lives of Physicians*. New York, NY: Praeger Publications; 1989.

> *Abstract:* This volume makes at least four unique contributions to the literature of adult education in general and continuing medical education in particular. 1) It provides a wide array of descriptions of techniques and resources that continuing learners have found to be helpful. 2) It models a qualitative approach to social science research that offers a more productive way of discovering the important variables in the processes and dynamics of lifelong learning than the traditional quantitative and correlational approaches and, at the same time, lays a rich foundation of potential hypotheses for subsequent empirical research. 3) It offers the beginning of a theoretical framework for conceptualizing the phenomena of continuing education and serves as a guide for practical experimentation and further development of theory. 4) It presents continuing education as a highly human, personal, and creative enterprise in contrast to the more institutionalized, prescriptive, and mechanistic undertaking often depicted.

Green JS, Grosswald SJ, Suter E, Walthall DB. *Continuing Education for the Health Professions*. San Francisco, Calif: Jossey-Bass Publishers; 1984.

Green LW, Kreuter MW. *Health Promotion Planning: An Educational and Environmental Approach*. 2nd ed. Mountain View, Calif: Mayfield Publishing Company; 1991.

Haines A, Donald A. *Getting Research Findings into Practice*. London: BMJ Books; 1998.

Jahn RG, Dunne BJ. Consciousness, particles, and waves. In: *Margins of Reality: The Role of Consciousness in the Physical World*. New York, NY: Harcourt, Brace and Company; 1999;208–219.

> *Comment:* Generalizing the concept of observation to encompass all information-processing capacities of consciousness—cognition, emotion, behavior, and any other form of experience—the same pragmatic interpretations may be obtained. Just as there may be a probability of observation waves, there may be a probability of experience waves.

Kane RL. *Understanding Health Care Outcomes Research*. Germantown, Md: Aspen; 1997.

King PM, Kitchener KS. *Developing Reflective Judgement*. San Francisco, Calif: Jossey-Bass Publishers; 1994.

Lave J, Wenger E. *Situated Learning: Legitimate Peripheral Participation*. New York, NY: Cambridge University Press; 1991.

Posner MI, DiGirolamo GJ. Executive attention: conflict, target detection, and cognitive control. In: *The Attentive Brain*. Cambridge, Mass: MIT Press; 1998.

> *Comment:* Cognitive models suggest executive attention is required when tasks involve planning, error detection, novelty, difficult processing, or conflict. In processing one target event at a time, neuroimaging studies have found activation in frontal midline areas; yet, a longstanding and controversial issue remains. Is attention a causal force that influences other activities such as perception or is attention a by-product of other

processes such as stimulus priming or competitive neural interactions? The issue of whether attention is a cause or an effect is closely related to the question of whether attentional systems exist separate from other sensory and motor systems in the brain.

Prochaska JO. Revolution in health promotion. In: *Health Psychology Through the Lifespan: Practice and Research Opportunities.* Washington, DC: American Psychological Association; 1996.

Robinson DG, Robinson JC. *Performance Consulting: Moving Beyond Training.* San Francisco, Calif: Berrett-Koehler; 1996.

Rogers EM. *Diffusion of Innovations.* 4th ed. New York, NY: The Free Press; 1995.

Rosof AB, Felch WC. *Continuing Medical Education: A Primer.* 2nd ed. Westport, Conn: Praeger Publications; 1992.

Schön DA. *Educating the Reflective Practitioner: Toward a New Design for Teaching and Learning in the Professions.* San Francisco, Calif: Jossey-Bass Publishers; 1990.

Vaill PB. *Learning as a Way of Being.* San Francisco, Calif: Jossey-Bass Publishers; 1996.

Yinger JM. *Toward a Field Theory of Behavior: Personality and Social Structure.* New York, NY: McGraw-Hill; 1965.

> *Comment:* The introductory chapters present a good overview of "behavioral science and analytic science," "levels of analysis," and multidisciplinary approaches to practical problems.

ARTICLES

Note: Abstracts included when available.

Allery LA, Owen PA, Robling MR. Why general practitioners and consultants change their clinical practice: a critical incident study. *BMJ.* 1997;314:870–874.

> *Abstract:* OBJECTIVE: To describe the complete range of factors which physicians recognize as changing their clinical practice and provide a measure of how often education is involved in change. DESIGN: Interviews using the critical incident technique. SETTING: Primary and secondary care. SUBJECTS: Random sample of 50 general practitioners and 50 consultants. MAIN OUTCOME MEASURES: Categories of reasons for change in clinical practice. RESULTS: Doctors described 361 changes in clinical practice, with an average of 3.0 reasons per change. The three most frequently mentioned reasons were organizational factors, education, and contact with professionals, together accounting for 47.9% of the total number of reasons for change. Education accounted for one sixth (16.9%) of the reasons for change and was involved in one third (37.1%) of the changes. Education was seldom mentioned as a reason for change in referral practice but was more often mentioned in management and prescribing changes. Consultants were influenced by medical journals and scientific conferences, while general practitioners were more influenced by medical newspapers and postgraduate meetings.

CONCLUSIONS: Education is involved in about a third of changes in clinical practice. The wide range of other factors affecting changes in practice need to be taken into account in providing and evaluating education. The role of education in the numerous changes in clinical practice that currently have no educational component should also be considered.

Allison JJ, Kiefe CI, Cook EF, Gerrity MS, Orav EJ, Centor R. The association of physician attitudes about uncertainty and risk taking with resource use in a Medicare HMO. *Med Decis Making.* 1998;18:320–329.

Abstract: PURPOSE: To explore the association between the attitudes of primary care physicians toward uncertainty and risk taking, as measured by a validated survey, with resource use in a Medicare HMO. DESIGN: All primary-care internists (n = 20) in a large, multi-specialty clinic were surveyed to measure their attitudes about uncertainty and risk taking using three previously developed scales. Results were linked with administrative data for 792 consecutive patients in a recently created Medicare HMO. The patients' index visits occurred between April 1, 1995, and November 30, 1995. ANALYSIS: Charges stemming from several claim types (primary care and subspecialty physician, laboratory, radiology, and ambulatory procedures) in the 30 days following the index visit were summed. The physician scales were dichotomized at the median to seek unadjusted associations with charges. Generalized estimation equations were used to account for the correlation of charges resulting from patients' being nested within physicians and adjusted for physician characteristics (age, sex, years in practice) and patient characteristics (age, sex, comorbidity). MAIN RESULTS: The physician response rate was 90%. Most physicians (90%) were male. The mean age of the patients was 74 years, and 69% were female. The mean cost (+/−SD) per patient was \$621.61 +/− 1,737.31. From the unadjusted analysis, high "anxiety due to uncertainty" was associated with higher patient charges (\$197.85 vs \$158.21, p = 0.01). From the multivariable analysis, each standard deviation increase in "anxiety due to uncertainty" (3.5 points) corresponded to a 17% increase in mean charges (p < 0.01) and each similar increase in "reluctance to disclose uncertainty to patients" (1.92 points) corresponded to a 12% increase (p = 0.03). However, increasing "reluctance to disclose mistakes to physicians" and increasing physician risk-taking propensity were associated with decreased total charges [−10% per standard deviation (1.34 points), p = 0.02, and −8% per standard deviation (3.26 points), p = 0.02, respectively]. CONCLUSION: Physician attitudes toward uncertainty were significantly associated with patient charges. Further investigation may improve prediction of patient-care charges, offer insight into the medical decision-making process, and perhaps clarify the relationship between cost, uncertainty, and quality of care.

Bero LA, Grilli R, Grimshaw JM, Harvey E, Oxman AD, Thomson MA. Closing the gap between research and practice: an overview of systematic reviews of interventions to promote the implementation of research findings. The Cochrane Effective Practice and Organization of Care Review Group. *BMJ.* 1998;317:465–468.

Brigley S, Young Y, Littlejohns P, McEwen J. Continuing education for medical professionals: a reflective model. *Postgrad Med J.* 1997;73:23–26.

Abstract: The Royal Colleges and their Faculties have moved continuing professional development up the agenda of doctors in the UK. The low educational value and failure to change professional practice of much continuing medical education has led to criticism of its emphasis on formal, didactic teaching and academic knowledge. The ubiquitous scientific or technical bias in medical education makes questionable assumptions about the nature of professional knowledge, how professionals learn, and the linkage of theory and practice in professional work. Given its narrow conception of professional knowledge, it is hardly surprising that the effectiveness of continuing medical education has proven difficult to evaluate. These points of criticism suggest that a more systematic and coherent approach to continuing education is required. The adoption of the concept of continuing professional development, which draws on learning by reflective practice, marks an important step in this direction. Continuing professional development emphasizes self-directed learning, professional self-awareness, learning developed in context, multidisciplinary and multilevel collaboration, the learning needs of individuals and their organizations, and an inquiry-based concept of professionalism. It also involves a widening of accountability to patients, the community, managers and policymakers, and a form of evaluation that is internal, participatory, and collaborative rather than external and scientific in character. COMMENT: This article highlights the essential differences between traditional CME and CPD or workplace learning.

Brookfield SD. Critically reflective practice. *J Contin Educ Health Prof.* 1998;18:197–205.

Abstract: The concept of critical reflection is frequently invoked as a distinguishing feature of good practice in continuing health education. But what exactly is critical reflection? How is it recognized? What are its benefits? How can it be incorporated into professional practice? This article explains the constituent elements of critical reflection and provides an example of how a critically reflective approach can be taken toward continuous, formative evaluation. Four lenses through which educators can view their practice critically are outlined and the critical incident questionnaire is described. The critically reflective habit is proposed as a survival necessity for continuing health educators.

Butler C, Rollnick S, Stott N. The practitioner, the patient and resistance to change: recent ideas on compliance. *CMAJ.* 1996;154:1357–1362.

Abstract: Despite the explosion of research into the effect of medical advice on patient behavior, only about 50% of patients comply with long-term drug regimens. And when it comes to changes in lifestyle, the percentage of patients who comply with medical advice often falls to single figures. Review articles on compliance have traditionally concentrated on factors that make it easier for patients to adhere to medical advice. However, recent articles urge clinicians to be more understanding of the wider implications of compliance in their patients' lives. This article focuses on how clinicians' consulting methods can affect patients' behavior. Specifically, the authors consider the patient-centered clinical method as well as insights from and consulting techniques pioneered in the addictions field that can help to bring ambivalent patients closer to decisions about change. Instead of seeing resistance to change as rooted entirely in the patient, the authors view it as stemming partly from the way clinicians talk to patients. An advice-giving approach is usually inadequate to motivate people to embark on major lifestyle changes. Instead, the authors propose a negotiation-based framework that harnesses patients' intrinsic motivation to make their own decisions. This approach also promotes clinicians' acceptance of patients' decisions, even if these decisions run counter to current medical wisdom.

Campbell CM, Parboosingh JT, Gondocz ST, et al. Study of physicians' use of a software program to create a portfolio of their self-directed learning. *Acad Med.* 1996;71:S49–S51.

Carpenter CE, Johnson NE, Rosenfeld JF. The impact of clinical guidelines on practice patterns: doing more versus doing less. *American Journal of Medical Quality.* 1998;13:98–103.

Abstract: This study examined the determinants of compliance with clinical guidelines for glucocyte colony-stimulating factor (GCSF), a biotechnology product designed to reduce postchemotherapy infections. The pattern of compliance did change over time. After the guidelines were disseminated, appropriate use of GCSF increased. However, inappropriate use also increased. Patients who were younger and had an attending physician who was an oncologist or hematologist were more likely to receive GCSF whether they met the guideline criteria or not. Our findings suggest that older patients may be treated less aggressively than others and that physicians who are the most knowledgeable about guidelines may feel the most qualified to override the guidelines when they believe they do not apply. Our findings also demonstrate that it is easier to encourage physicians to do more for patients rather than less.

Christensen CM, Armstrong EG. Disruptive technologies: a credible threat to leading programs in continuing medical education? *J Contin Educ Health Prof.* 1998;18:69–80.

Abstract: Recent research into the history of some of the most prominent and successful firms in the for-profit sector has shown that industry leadership is extraordinarily fragile. Over and over, in industries as diverse as microelectronics, steel, motorcycles, and software, leading firms whose management practices at one point were widely admired and imitated have stumbled badly and even failed. The factor that consistently has triggered these failures has not been complacent, arrogant, or bureaucratic management. It has been the emergence in their markets of disruptive technology-simple, convenient-to-use innovations that initially are used only by unsophisticated customers at the low end of markets. Ironically, two of the fundamental paradigms of good management—the importance of listening closely to customers and the necessity of bringing to market a regular flow of improved products that can be sold at higher profit margins—are the reasons why well-managed companies have consistently failed when confronted by disruptive technologies in their markets. This paper asserts that in a very analogous way, disruptive innovations in continuing education for managers and for health care professionals pose a significant threat to the impact and profitability of the continuing education programs of the leading schools of medicine and business. Through their focus on the leading edges of technology, therapy, and practice, many of these programs have lost sight of a very different set of educational needs among the fastest growing health care institutions in our environment. The paper suggests that unless leading providers of continuing medical education at medical schools aggressively begin offering courses that are customized to the needs of specific health care providers, in formats and venues that are conveniently accessible, they will increasingly be displaced by new providers of these services.

Chueh H, Barnett GO. "Just-in-time" clinical information. *Acad Med*. 1997;72:512–517.

Abstract: The just-in-time (JIT) model originated in the manufacturing industry as a way to manage parts inventories process so that specific components could be made available at the appropriate times (that is, "just in time"). This JIT model can be applied to the management of clinical information inventories, so that clinicians can have more immediate access to the most current and relevant information at the time they most need it—when making clinical care decisions. The authors discuss traditional modes of managing clinical information, and then describe how a new JIT model may be developed and implemented. They describe three modes of clinician-information interactions that a JIT model might employ, the scope of information that may be made available in a JIT model (global information or local, case-specific information), and the challenges posed by the implementation of such an information-access model. Finally, they discuss how JIT information access may change how physicians practice medicine, various ways JIT information may be delivered, and concerns about the trust-worthiness of electronically published and accessed information resources.

Cohen SJ, Halvorson HW, Gosselink CA. Changing physician behavior to improve disease prevention. *Prev Med*. 1994;23:284–291.

Abstract: Physicians often fail to provide nationally recommended preventive services for their patients. Addressing this, we have reviewed selected literature on changing physician behavior using the organizational construct of the readiness for change transtheoretical model. This model suggests that behavior evolves through stages from precontemplation, to contemplation, to preparation, to initiation, and to maintenance of change. Traditional continuing medical education may affect knowledge and beliefs, but rarely results in behavior change. However, motivational strategies such as practice feedback reports and influential peers can foster stage change. Successful interventions aimed at physicians preparing for change frequently use an office-system approach that targets not only physicians, but office staff and patients as well. Illustrating how the readiness to change model can guide the design and implementation of interventions, we describe strategies being used in a statewide randomized controlled trial to improve cancer prevention counseling and early detection by primary care physicians. The multistage interventions of Partners for Prevention include support from a medical liability carrier, a motivational videotape, a task-delineated office manual, chart flowsheets, patient activation forms, practice feedback reports, a designated prevention coordinator within each practice and regular telephone calls and office visits by project staff.

Confessore SJ. Building a learning organization: communities of practice, self-directed learning, and continuing medical education. *J Contin Educ Health Prof.* 1997;17:5–11.

Abstract: Learning organizations may provide a mechanism by which physicians can meet the challenges currently occurring in the medical profession, such as the emergence of HMOs, increased concern over medical costs, and the need to maintain continuing competence in increasingly complex environments. Learning organizations are generative; they are responsive and have been used effectively during times of rapid change and in chaotic, highly competitive environments. This paper describes the learning organization and discusses how self-directed learning and communities of practice provide the beginnings for the establishment of a learning organization in the medical profession. Continuing medical education (CME) is seen as the mechanism to transfer new knowledge across all members of the community of practice and become a key component in building learning organizations.

Davis DA, Thomson MA, Oxman AD, Haynes RB. Evidence for the effectiveness of CME. A review of 50 randomized controlled trials. *JAMA.* 1992;268:1111–1117.

Abstract: OBJECTIVE: To assess the impact of diverse continuing medical education (CME) interventions on physician performance and health care outcomes. DATA SOURCES: Using continuing medical education and related phrases, we performed regular searches of the indexed literature (MEDLINE, Social Science Index, the National Technical Information Service, and Educational Research Information Clearinghouse) from 1975 through 1991. In addition, for these years, we used manual searches, key informats, and requests to authors to locate other indexed articles and the nonindexed literature of adult and continuing professional education. STUDY SELECTION: From the resulting database we selected studies that meet the following criteria: randomized controlled trials; educational programs; activities, or other interventions; studies that included 50% or more physicians; follow-up assessments of at least 75% of study subjects; and objective assessment of either physician performance or health care outcomes. DATA EXTRACTION: Studies were reviewed for data related to physician specialty and setting. Continuing medical education interventions were classified by their mode(s) of activity as being predisposing, enabling, or facilitating. Using the statistical tests supplied by the original investigators, physician performance outcomes and patients outcomes were classified as positive, negative, or inconclusive. DATA SYNTHESIS: We located 777 CME studies, of which 50 met all criteria. Thirty-two of these analyzed physician performance; seven evaluated patient outcomes; 11 examined both measures. The majority of 43 studies of physician performance showed positive results in some important measures of resource utilization, counseling strategies, and preventive medicine. Of the 18 studies of health care outcomes, eight demonstrated positive changes in patients' health care outcomes. CONCLUSION: Broadly defined CME interventions using practice-enabling or reinforcing strategies consistently improve physician performance and, in some instances, health care outcomes.

Davis DA, Thomson MA, Oxman AD, Haynes RB. Changing physician performance: a systematic review of the effect of continuing medical education strategies. *JAMA*. 1995;274:700–705.

Abstract: OBJECTIVE: To review the literature relating to the effectiveness of education strategies designed to change physician performance and health care outcomes. DATA SOURCES: We searched MEDLINE, ERIC, NTIS, the Research and Development Resource Base in Continuing Medical Education, and other relevant data sources from 1975 to 1994, using "continuing medical education (CME)" and related terms as keywords. We manually searched journals and the bibliographies of other review articles and called on the opinions of recognized experts. STUDY SELECTION: We reviewed studies that met the following criteria: randomized controlled trials of education strategies or interventions that objectively assessed physician performance and/or health care outcomes. These intervention strategies included (alone and in combination) educational materials, formal CME activities, outreach visits such as academic detailing, opinion leaders, patient-mediated strategies, audit with feedback, and reminders. Studies were selected only if more than 50% of the subjects were either practicing physicians or medical residents. DATA EXTRACTION: We extracted the specialty of the physicians targeted by the interventions and the clinical domain and setting of the trial. We also determined the details of the educational intervention, the extent to which needs or barriers to change had been ascertained prior to the intervention, and the main outcome measure(s). DATA SYNTHESIS: We found 99 trials, containing 160 interventions, which met our criteria. Almost two thirds of the interventions (101 of 160) displayed an improvement in at least one major outcome measure: 70% demonstrated a change in physician performance, and 48% of interventions aimed at health care outcomes produced a positive change. Effective change strategies included reminders, patient-mediated interventions, outreach visits, opinion leaders, and multifaceted activities. Audit with feedback and educational materials were less effective, and formal CME conferences or activities, without enabling or practice-reinforcing strategies, had relatively little impact. CONCLUSION: Widely used CME delivery methods such as conferences have little direct impact on improving professional practice. More effective methods such as systematic practice-based interventions and outreach visits are seldom used by CME providers.

Davis DA, Taylor-Vaisey AL. Translating guidelines into practice: a systematic review of theoretic concepts, practical experience and research evidence in the adoption of clinical practice guidelines. *Can Med Assoc J.* 1997;157:408–416.

Abstract: OBJECTIVE: To recommend effective strategies for implementing clinical practice guidelines (CPGs). DATA SOURCES: The Research and Development Resource Base in Continuing Medical Education (RDRB/CME), maintained by the University of Toronto, was searched, as was MEDLINE, using the MeSH term "practice guidelines" and relevant text words. STUDY SELECTION: Studies of CPG implementation strategies and reviews of such studies were selected. Randomized controlled trials and trials that objectively measured physicians' performance or health care outcomes were emphasized. DATA EXTRACTION: Articles were reviewed to determine the effect of various factors on the adoption of guidelines. DATA SYNTHESIS: The articles showed that CPG dissemination or implementation processes have mixed results. Variables that affect the adoption of guidelines include qualities of the guidelines, characteristics of the health care professionals, characteristics of the practice setting, incentives, regulation and patient factors. Specific strategies fell into two categories: primary strategies involving mailing or publication of the actual guidelines and secondary interventional strategies to reinforce the guidelines. The interventions were shown to be weak (didactic, traditional CME and mailings), moderately effective (audit and feedback, especially concurrent, targeted to specific providers and delivered by peers or opinion leaders) and relatively strong (reminder systems, academic detailing and multiple interventions). CONCLUSIONS: The evidence shows serious deficiencies in the adoption of CPGs in practice. Future implementation strategies must overcome this failure through an understanding of the forces and variables influencing practice and through the use of methods that are practice- and community-based rather than didactic.

Davydov VV. The influence of L. S. Vygotsky on education theory, research, and practice. *Educational Researcher.* 1995;24:12–21.

Abstract: Discusses L. S. Vygotsky's theories and explores why these theories can affect the improvement and reform of contemporary education and research, both in Russia and in the United States. The author also examines the main theses behind Vygotsky's cultural historical theory of the psychological development of personality and how these theses are being used in Russian educational reform.

Donen N. No to mandatory continuing medical education, yes to mandatory practice auditing and professional educational development. *CMAJ.* 1998;158:1044–1046.

Abstract: The issue of mandatory continuing medical education (CME) is controversial. Traditional measures mandate only attendance, not learning, and have no measurable performance end points. There is no evidence that current approaches to CME, mandatory or voluntary, produce sustainable changes in physician practices or application of current knowledge. Ongoing educational development is an important value in a professional, and there is an ethical obligation to keep up-to-date. Mandating self-audit of the effect of individual learning on physician's practices and evaluation by the licensing authority are effective ways of ensuring the public are protected. The author recommends the use of a personal portfolio to document sources of learning, the effect of learning and the auditing of their applications on practice patterns and patient outcomes. A series of principles are proposed to govern its application.

Fischer KW, Granott N. Beyond one-dimensional change: parallel, concurrent, socially distributed processes in learning and development. *Human Development.* 1995;38:302–314.

Abstract: The study of microdevelopment offers a potentially powerful way to relate learning and development in which similar changes occur but in differing time frames. Microdevelopment analyzes short-term changes as developmental functions. Individuals and groups function at widely different developmental levels and grow in diverse nonlinear dynamic shapes.

Fox RD. Implications of the model of change and learning for undergraduate medical education. *J Contin Educ Health Prof.* 1996;16:144–151.

Abstract: This essay responds to the need for closer intellectual ties between continuing medical education (CME) and the undergraduate experience. Medical educators in each of these two phases of lifelong learning are often unfamiliar with the implications of research in each phase for the other. In order to redress this, this essay describes one of the major explanations for change and learning in clinical practice and draws implications of this model for the education of undergraduate medical students. The model includes the role of forces for change, image of change, assessment of needs for learning, and the use of learning resources in a self-directed curriculum. Specific implications for each of the phases of the change process are offered. General implications of the model and a set of new assumptions for the development of formal curriculum in undergraduate medicine are also described.

Fox RD, Bennett NL. Learning and change: implications for continuing medical education. *BMJ.* 1998;316:466–468.

Garrison RD. Self-directed learning: toward a comprehensive model. *Adult Education Quarterly.* 1998;48:18–33.

Gerrity MS, DeVellis RF, Earp JA. Physicians' reactions to uncertainty in patient care. A new measure and new insights. *Med Care.* 1990;28:724–736.

Abstract: Although variations in physicians' practice patterns and use of resources are well documented, the reasons for these variations are less well understood. The uncertainty inherent in patient care may be one explanation. Existing measures of intolerance to uncertainty, developed in contexts outside of patient care, fail to explain these variations. To address this limitation, the Physicians' Reactions to Uncertainty scale was developed. A questionnaire containing an initial pool of 61 items was mailed to a random sample of 700 physicians in North Carolina and Oregon, stratified by specialty. The items covered nine areas of physicians' reactions to uncertainty derived from interviews with physicians and a definition of the concept affective reactions to uncertainty in patient care. Factor analysis of the 428 responses received yielded two primary factors that accounted for 58% of the common variance among the 61 items. Items with unambiguous loadings on these factors defined two reliable and readily interpretable subscales: Stress from Uncertainty (Cronbach's alpha = 0.90, 13 items) and Reluctance to Disclose Uncertainty to Others (alpha = 0.75, 9 items). By virtue of its clarity and good psychometric properties, this new measure promises insights into the role that uncertainty plays in physicians' resource utilization and practice patterns.

Goldin-Meadow S. Transitions in concept acquisition: using the hand to read the mind. *Psychological Review.* 1993;100:279–297.

Abstract: A model of the sources and consequences of mismatches between gestures and speech is presented that argues that the transitional knowledge state is the source of the mismatch and that such mismatches signal that a child is in a transitional state of concept acquisition and is ready to learn.

Goulet F, Gagnon RJ, Desrosiers G, Jacques A, Sindon A. Participation in CME activities. *Can Fam Physician.* 1998;44:541–548.

Abstract: OBJECTIVE: To compare the continuing medical education (CME) activities of family physicians in the province of Quebec with more than 25 years in practice with those with less than 25 years in practice. DESIGN: Mailed questionnaire survey. SETTING: Family practices in the province of Quebec. PARTICIPANTS: All physicians (n = 722) with more than 25 years in practice (expressed as older) and a matched sample of 721 physicians with less than 25 years in practice (expressed as younger). MAIN OUTCOME MEASURES: Types of CME activities and time spent on them, participant characteristics. RESULTS: Older physicians spent more time in individual CME activities than younger ones (21 hours vs 18 hours monthly). Younger physicians, however, spent more time in group CME activities than older ones did (100 hours vs 80 hours yearly). Excluding physicians who devoted no time to CME activities, only two activities differentiated between the two groups: older physicians spent more time than their younger colleagues reading and listening to audiocassettes. CONCLUSIONS: Older physicians maintained their clinical competence by participating in different CME activities from younger physicians. They participated in as many CME activities as their younger colleagues.

Green LW, Erikson MP, Schor EL. Preventive practices by physicians: Behavioral determinants and potential interventions. *Am J Prev Med.* 1990;4 (suppl 4):101–107.

Abstract: What makes physicians behave as they do with respect to prevention and health promotion? Although their education and training have not emphasized either, they show growing interest in enhancing their preventive practices. This paper will attempt to assess these conditions and trends and arrive at some principles of behavioral change that will help physicians become more effective in counseling their patients to change lifestyles and specific health practice.

Grilli R, Lomas J. Evaluating the message: the relationship between compliance rate and the subject of a practice guideline. *Med Care.* 1994;32:202–213.

Abstract: To explore the relationship between providers' compliance and some key aspects of the clinical messages in practice guidelines, studies published in the English language medical literature between 1980 and 1991 were retrieved through MEDLINE and through relevant review articles in the field. All published studies providing compliance rates with practice guidelines and endorsed by official organizations were eligible for the study. The clinical content and the reported compliance rate were gathered for each recommendation in the 23 studies selected. The medical and surgical procedures addressed by 143 recommendations were identified according to specialty area, type of procedure (diagnostic, surgical, etc.) and were independently classified by the authors as being high or low on characteristics thought to influence diffusion: complexity, trialability and observability. The mean compliance rate with the 143 clinical recommendations was 54.5% (95% CI: 50.2%–58.9%), with those in the specialty areas of cardiology and oncology showing the highest compliance (mean 63.6% and 62.2%, respectively). Recommendations concerning procedures with high complexity had lower compliance rates than those low on complexity (41.9% vs 55.9%; P = 0.05), and those judged to be high on trialability had higher compliance rates than those low on trialability (55.6% vs 36.8%; P = 0.03). Overall, all the characteristics of the clinical recommendations considered in the practice guidelines could account for no more than 47% of the observed variability in compliance rates. The target area of practice and the complexity and trialability of the recommended procedure appear to be useful, if partial, predictors of the level of compliance with a practice guideline.

Hancock VE. Information literacy for lifelong learning. *ERIC Digest.* ERIC Clearinghouse on Information Resources, Syracuse, NY. 1993. www.ed.gov/databases/ERIC_Digests/ed358870.html

Abstract: Information literacy requires that the learner recognize the need for information, be able to identify and locate it, gain access to it, and then evaluate the quality of the information received before organizing it and using it effectively. In an information literate environment students engage in active and self-directed activities. Information literacy thrives in a resource-based learning environment in which students and teachers make decisions about appropriate sources of information and how to access them. Information literacy benefits students by counteracting the information dependency created by traditional schooling and sets the teacher free to become the facilitator of interaction at the small-group or individual level. Information literate students are more effective consumers of information resources, and become better-prepared citizens, who know how to use information to their best advantage in work and everyday life. The workplace of the future will also demand information literate workers. An early commitment to learning as a process will enable the worker of the future to function effectively. COMMENT: This text describes the competencies required for information literacy and their importance to professionals in the future. It makes me think of the question: what will be learning for professional of the future?

Hoskins G, Neville RG, Smith B, Clark RA. Does participation in distance learning and audit improve the care of patients with acute asthma attacks? The General Practitioners in Asthma Group. *Health Bull (Edinb)*. 1997;55:150–155.

Abstract: OBJECTIVE: To test whether general practitioners who completed an audit cycle encompassing a data recording exercise, distance learning program and personalized feedback changed their management of patients with acute asthma attacks. DESIGN, SETTING AND SUBJECTS: Practice and patient details from two national correspondence surveys of the management of acute asthma attacks in the United Kingdom in 1991–92 and 1992–93 were compared. Main outcome measures were use of nebulised bronchodilators, systemic steroids during an asthma attack, and increased use of prophylactic therapy after attacks. RESULTS: Ninety-one general practitioners completed an audit cycle and reported data on 782 patients with asthma attacks in 1991–92 and 669 in 1992–93. There were no significant changes in practice resources during this time. Management changed in line with recommended guidelines and audit feedback suggestions leading to more use of nebulised bronchodilators [272 (35%) before, 268 (40%) after, Odds Ratio (OR) 0.80, 95% Confidence Intervals (CI) 0.64–0.99], systemic steroids [563 (72%) before, 506 (76%) after, OR 0.83, CI 0.65–1.06], and 'step-up' in preventative therapy [402 (51%) before, 382 (57%) after, OR 0.79, CI 0.64–0.98]. CONCLUSION: General Practitioners who completed an audit cycle showed changes in the management of acute asthma attacks in line with guidelines which may have been caused by participation in distance learning and clinical audit. However, general practitioners motivated to change clinical management may be similarly motivated to take part in audit. Audit may be the catalyst for change rather than the cause of change.

Jennett PA, Affleck L. Chart audit and chart stimulated recall as methods of needs assessment in continuing professional health education. *J Contin Educ Health Prof*. 1998;18:163–171.

Abstract: This article describes the chart audit (CA) and chart stimulated recall (CSR) needs appraisal methods, outlines their strengths and limitations, and provides examples of their applications in the continuing education (CE) environment. Both CA and CSR can be valuable tools for continuing educators and learners in the following activities: the assessment of needs prior to education, the identification of educational needs specific to a particular condition, the reassessment of needs post-education, the study of needs arising from factors influencing management choices, needs assessment associated with professional competence and performance, and the assessment of educational needs specific to practice guidelines. Providing personalized and individualized feedback around actual practice and patients' charts are attractive features shared by both procedures. CA has been used across disciplines and care sites and is viewed as less costly and less intrusive than most needs assessment tools. Its true value lies in the choice of appropriate explicit and implicit criteria and the definition of valid standards, along with the availability of trained abstracters. When compared to CA, CSR potentially increases the content validity and types of information accessible. As well, it explores the reasoning around diagnostic, investigative, and management decisions. Further, CSR permits patient, environmental, system, and other factors that can influence clinical decisions to emerge. Opportunities for professional educators and learners to acquire knowledge and skills about these needs appraisal approaches are required. As well, further studies regarding the impact, feasibility, acceptability, cost-effectiveness, reliability, and validity of these tools in new care environments are required. Last, it is important that the results of CA and CSR studies require diffusion to those in CE worksites. In this way, such findings can be translated and imbedded into professional practice.

Jennett PA, Scott SM, Atkinson MA, et al. Patient charts and physician office management decisions: chart audit and chart stimulated recall. *J Contin Educ Health Prof.* 1995;15:31–39.

Abstract: Accurate assessment of clinical competence and performance in office practice is enhanced through a multi-tool approach. Two assessment tools that offer a complementary range of information, specific to the patient's chart, are chart audit (CA) and chart stimulated recall (CSR). This paper demonstrates how CA and CSR provide insights into the office management of osteoarthritis in the elderly. CA provides basic data for clinical choices when areas of problem identification, history, physical, investigations and treatments are examined. CSR illuminates the rationale behind decisions, as well as the choices considered and the options ruled out. Furthermore, CSR shows how individual patient and physician characteristics, practice and professional factors, and health care system and social factors, are influential variables on the physician's clinical management decisions. Supplementing the type of data extracted from the CA with those found through CSR allows for a broad range of information to be used in assessing a physician's ability to make clinical decisions. Physicians, educators, and assessors, will benefit from considering the value of using both of these patient chart approaches when reviewing clinical care.

Lewis CE. Continuing medical education: past, present, future. *West J Med.* 1998;168:334–340.

Abstract: Medical education can be divided into three segments: undergraduate, graduate, and continuing. Of these, continuing medical education (CME) clearly takes place for the longest time—if the practicing physician is to employ recent scientific developments that translate into optimal practice. Our assignment was to examine the past, present, and future of CME. We evaluated what forms it has taken and what forms it may take. We also include a review of the evidence of its impact.

Lomas J. Medicine in context: a neglected perspective in medical education. *Acad Med.* 1994;69:S95–S101.

Mann KV. Educating medical students: lessons from research in continuing education. *Acad Med.* 1994;69:41–47.

Abstract: Creating a true continuum of medical education from admission to medical school throughout a lifetime of professional learning is easier said than done. To do so, the various components on the continuum must be explored to determine where appropriate links might be made. The author considers selected concepts and evidence from the theory and practice underlying continuing medical education (CME) and continuing professional education (CPE) insofar as CME and CPE can inform undergraduate medical curricula, including its current innovations. Five conceptual and empirical approaches from CME and CPE are discussed in detail: social learning theory, how physicians learn and change, competence in business and the professions, how professionals learn in practice, and lifelong self-directed learning. Then the author describes the implications of these approaches for the ongoing development of undergraduate medical education. 1) The entire learning environment, and not merely discrete aspects such as curriculum content, must be examined and fully utilized to benefit learning. 2) The importance of the contexts in which learning occurs must be emphasized in several ways. 3) Learning should be centered around clinical problems. 4) The many benefits of small-group learning and other ways of learning from colleagues should be emphasized. 5) The undergraduate curriculum should emphasize the development of students' feelings of self-efficacy to ensure that students become physicians who are confident about their abilities. 6) CME research and CPE research reinforce the efforts in undergraduate medical education to emphasize the early development of students' process skills as well as content mastery.

Mazmanian PE, Daffron SR, Johnson RE, Davis DA, Kantrowitz MP. Information about barriers to planned change: a randomized controlled trial involving continuing medical education lectures and commitment to change. *Acad Med.* 1998;73:882–886.

Abstract: PURPOSE: To determine whether practicing physicians receiving only clinical information at a traditional continuing medical education (CME) lecture (control group) and physicians receiving clinical information plus information about barriers to behavioral change (study group) would alter their clinical behaviors at the same rate. METHOD: In a randomized controlled trial, the investigators matched 13 pairs of US and Canadian medical schools, assigning one school from each pair to study or control conditions. Following the commitment-to-change model, the investigators asked the primary care physicians attending control or study lectures on the management of cardiovascular risks whether they intended to make behavioral changes as a result of participating in the lectures and, if so, to indicate the specific changes. Thirty to 45 days later, the investigators surveyed the responding physicians to learn whether they had implemented those changes. RESULTS: Information about barriers to change did not increase the likelihood that physicians in the study group would report successful changes; they were no more likely to change than those in the control group. However, the physicians in both study and control groups were significantly more likely to change (47% vs 7%, p < .001) if they indicated an intent to change immediately following the lecture. CONCLUSIONS: Successful change in practice may depend less on clinical and barriers information than on other factors that influence physicians' performances. To further develop the commitment-to-change strategy in measuring the effects of planned change, it is important to isolate and learn the powers of individual components of the strategy as well as their collective influence on physicians' clinical behaviors. COMMENT: This study provides high quality evidence of the relationship between commitment to change and initiating change.

Mazmanian PE, Mazmanian PM, Waugh JL. Commitment to change: ideational roots, empirical evidence, and ethical implications. *J Contin Educ Health Prof.* 1997;17:133–140.

Abstract: Commitment to change may be applied as a tool for promulgating as well as evaluating behavioral change. Its ideational roots may be traced to communication, law, and philosophy. A commitment to change may be triggered by one's perception of uncertainty between himself or herself and the environment. Acquiring information may help to reduce uncertainty. Studies of planned change are reviewed in the present document. The reviews suggest that planners and learners experience higher rates of successful change when commitments to change are secured from learners than when they are not. As evidence for the success of planned change grows, the planners' armamentarium increases, and ethical questions regarding responsibility for controlling the behavior of others need to be resolved.

McClaran J, Snell L, Franco E. Type of clinical problem is a determinant of physicians' self-selected learning methods in their practice settings. *J Contin Educ Health Prof.* 1998;18:107–118.

Abstract: While much research has been written about physician-preferred learning methods and self-directed learning, no published study describes the physician's self-selected learning methods specific to problems arising in his practice. Study subjects were 366 primary care physicians asked to describe a recent clinical problem for which they needed more knowledge or skill to solve. For the specific problem of his/her own patient, each physician was asked how he/she gained the specific ability to solve the problem. Fifty-five learning methods were described by the study population and were categorized as three outcome variables: reading and related activity, 47.8% of study subject responses, formal and informal consultation and/or referral (33.3%), and formal continuing medical education (CME) (18.9%). Analysis for risk similarities led to progressive recombination of 64 problem categories to two predictive variables: clinical problems requiring more knowledge and clinical problems requiring more technical or communication skill to solve. Multiple logistic regression was carried out. The final predictive model revealed that of the factors studied, problem type was the major determinant of self-selected learning method in the practice setting. While reading is the most frequently selected method overall, physicians are more likely to select formal CME when the problem requires more technical expertise or communication ability to solve (odds ratio = 2.31, confidence interval = 1.25–4.25). Region and year of graduation added only slightly to the model. Gender, certification, and size of town did not add to the predictive model. CME providers must be aware of physicians' practice-based choices of learning method and incorporate this into their CME activities.

McDonald CJ. Medical heuristics: the silent adjudicators of clinical practice. *Ann Intern Med.* 1996;124:56–62.

Abstract: Robust scientific conclusions are too sparse to inform fully most of the choices that physicians must make about tests and treatments. Instead, ad hoc rules of thumb, or "heuristics," must guide them, and many of these are problematic. Physicians extrapolate from the small samples studied by clinical trials to general populations, but they do so inconsistently. Many physicians live by rules that dictate "not treating the numbers," correcting abnormalities slowly, achieving diagnostic certainty, and operating now to avoid "greater" risk in the future. Yet in each case, historical trends or statistical realities suggest either doing the opposite or investing in more discriminating heuristics. The heuristics of medicine should be discussed, criticized, refined, and then taught. More uniform use of explicit and better heuristics could lead to less practice variation and more efficient medical care.

Moore DE, Green JS, Jay SJ, Leist JC, Maitland FM. Creating a new paradigm for CME: seizing opportunities within the health care revolution. *J Contin Educ Health Prof.* 1994;14:4–31.

Abstract: Contents: Traditional CME Forces creating change in CME. Government and private efforts in health care reform. Increasing application of quality management in health care institutions. Expansion of biomedical information and technology. Advances in information and communications technology. A new paradigm for CME. Increasing emphasis on learning. Educational activities based on clinically-relevant data and collaborative planning. Continuous improvement of health care and its components using techniques that combine quality management and CME. Collaborative learning system that supports physician learners and CME providers. Emphasis on improving patient outcomes. CME as an integral part of the health care system. Factors that will facilitate the development of a new paradigm. Change in the culture of CME. Stable CME funding. Education of CME providers. CME research and development. CME involvement in health care policy making and discussion. Changes in accreditation and credit incentives. Enhanced status of the CME profession. CME leadership and management.

Moore DE. Moving CME closer to the clinical encounter: the promise of quality management and CME. *J Contin Educ Health Prof.* 1995;15:135–145.

Abstract: The purpose of this article is to set the context for the articles in this special edition on continuing medical education (CME) and quality management (QM). We provide a brief review of the evolution of the current forms of quality management and CME that will improve our understanding of each as we begin to examine how QM systems and CME can work together. This improved understanding about QM systems and how they work is an important prerequisite for developing working alliances between CME and QM systems.

Ockene JK, Lindsay EA, Hymowitz N, et al. Tobacco control activities of primary-care physicians in the Community Intervention Trial for Smoking Cessation. COMMIT Research Group. *Tob Control.* 1997;6 Suppl 2:S49–S56.

Abstract: OBJECTIVE: To compare tobacco control practices of physicians and their staff in Intervention communities with those in Comparison communities of the Community Intervention Trial for Smoking Cessation (COMMIT). DESIGN: COMMIT was a randomized trial testing community-based intervention for smoking cessation carried out over four years. SETTING: Eleven matched pairs of communities assigned randomly to Intervention and Comparison conditions. PARTICIPANTS AND INTERVENTIONS: Physicians in the Intervention communities participated in continuing medical education (CME). Training for office staff focused on tobacco control and office intervention "systems." OUTCOME MEASURES: Smoking control attitudes and practices reported by primary-care physicians in the 22 communities, smoking policies, and practices of 30 randomly selected medical offices in each community, and patient reports of physician intervention activities. RESULTS: Response rates to the physicians' mail survey were 45% and 42% in Intervention and Comparison communities, respectively. Telephone interviews of office staff had response rates of 84% in both conditions. Physicians in Intervention communities were more likely to attend training than those in Comparison communities (53% and 26%, respectively ($P < 0.0005$)). In both conditions, training attendees perceived themselves as being better prepared to counsel smokers than non-attendees ($P < $ or $= 0.01$) and reported more activity in smoking intervention. Intervention communities carried out more office-based tobacco control activities ($P = 0.002$). Smokers in Intervention communities were more likely to report receiving reading material about smoking from their physicians ($P = 0.026$). No other differences in physician intervention activities were reported by smokers between the Intervention and Comparison communities. CONCLUSIONS: The COMMIT intervention had a significant effect on some reported physician behaviors, office practices, and policies. However, most physicians still did not use state-of-the-art smoking intervention practices with their patients and there was little, or no, difference between patient reports of intervention activities of physicians in the Intervention and Comparison communities. Better systems and incentives are needed to attract physicians and their staff to CME and to encourage them to follow through on what they learn. The recently released Agency for Health Care Policy and Research clinical practice guideline for smoking cessation and other standards and policies outline these systems and offer suggestions for incentives to facilitate adoption of these practices by physicians.

Ockene JK, Wheeler EV, Adams A, Hurley TG, Hebert J. Provider training for patient-centered alcohol counseling in a primary care setting. *Arch Intern Med*. 1997;157:2334–2341.

Abstract: OBJECTIVE: To assess the impact of a brief training program on primary care providers' skills, attitudes, and knowledge regarding high-risk and problem drinking. DESIGN: Training plus pretesting and posttesting for program efficacy. SETTING: Ambulatory primary care clinic; academic medical center. PARTICIPANTS: Fourteen attending physicians, 12 residents, and 5 nurse practitioners were randomized by clinical team affiliation to a Special Intervention or usual care condition of a larger study. We report the results of the training program for the Special Intervention providers. INTERVENTION: Providers received a 2-hour group training session plus a 10- to 20-minute individual tutorial session 2 to 6 weeks after the group session. The training focused on teaching providers how to perform patient-centered counseling for high-risk and problem drinkers. MAIN OUTCOME MEASURES: Alcohol counseling skills; attitudes regarding preparedness to intervene and perceived importance and usefulness of intervening with high-risk and problem drinkers; and knowledge of the nature, prevalence, and appropriate treatment of alcohol abuse in primary care populations. RESULTS: After training, providers scored significantly higher on measures of counseling skills, preparedness to intervene, perceived usefulness and importance of intervening, and knowledge. CONCLUSION: A group training program plus brief individual feedback can significantly improve primary care providers' counseling skills, attitudes, and knowledge regarding high-risk and problem drinkers.

Oxman TE. Effective educational techniques for primary care providers: application to the management of psychiatric disorders. *Int J Psychiatry Med*. 1998;28:3–9.

Parboosingh J. Learning portfolios: potential to assist health professionals with self-directed learning [PC Diary/MOCOMP]. *J Contin Educ Health Prof*. 1996;16:75–81.

Abstract: While learning portfolios have been used by students enrolled in formal education courses for over 20 years, their potential to assist health professionals with their learning activities remains relatively unexplored. The increasing need for health professionals to manage change efficiently and the central role of practice-based self-directed learning provide the impetus for educators to find ways of assisting professionals to enhance the quality of their learning activities. This article explores the potential of the portfolio to enhance the quality of an individual's learning activities while respecting their desire for control of the education process. Physicians using a new computer software program called PCDiary report that it helps them to review and appraise their learning activities. It is predicted, based on these early experiences, that the integration of computer and telecommunications technology, and the traditional learning portfolio will produce a new generation of interactive learning tools. PCDiary, and future computer-based learning tools, will stand or fall on their ability to assist professionals to plan and appraise learning activities generated from their practice experiences. Computer "smart" portfolios will enhance learner interaction in ways that preserve the autonomy of independent learners. They will also be useful tools to research ways of helping professionals with their continuing learning.

Pathman DE, Konrad TR, Freed GL, Freeman VA, Koch GG. The awareness-to-adherence model of the steps to clinical guideline compliance: the case of pediatric vaccine recommendations. *Med Care.* 1996;34:873–889.

Abstract: OBJECTIVES: This article proposes, tests, and explores the potential applications of a model of the cognitive and behavioral steps physicians take when they comply with national clinical practice guidelines. The authors propose that when physicians comply with practice guidelines, they must first become aware of the guidelines, then intellectually agree with them, then decide to adopt them in the care they provide, then regularly adhere to them at appropriate times. METHODS: Data used to test this model address physicians' responses to national pediatric vaccine recommendations. Questionnaires were mailed to 3,014 family physicians and pediatricians who were working in communities of various sizes in nine states. RESULTS: The survey response rate was 66.2%. In the case of the recommendation to provide hepatitis B vaccine to all infants, guideline awareness among respondents was 98.4%, agreement 70.4%, adoption 77.7%, and adherence 30.1%. The data for 87.9% of physicians fit the model at every step. Significant deviation from the model occurred only for the 11% of all physicians who adopted the hepatitis B recommendation without agreeing with it. In the case of the recommendation to provide the acellular variety of the pertussis vaccine for children's fourth and fifth pertussis doses, guideline awareness among respondents was 89.8%, agreement 66.5%, adoption 46.3%, and adherence 35.2%. Data fit the model at every step for 90.6% of physicians. Greater likelihood of movement from each step to the next in the path to adherence was found for physicians with certain characteristics, information sources, and beliefs about the vaccines, and those in certain types of practice settings. Specific physician and practice characteristics typically predicted movement along only one or two of the steps to adherence to either the hepatitis B or acellular pertussis recommendations. CONCLUSIONS: These data on physicians' use of pediatric vaccine recommendations generally support the awareness-to-adherence model. This model may prove useful in identifying ways to improve physicians' adherence to a variety of guidelines by demonstrating where physicians fall off the path to adherence, which physicians are at greatest risk for not attaining each step in the path, and factors associated with a greater likelihood of attaining each step toward guideline adherence.

Premi JN, Shannon S, Hartwick K, Lamb S, Wakefield J, Williams J. Practice-based small group CME. *Acad Med.* 1994;69:800–802.

Pyatt RS. The role of CME and managed care. *N J Med.* 1997;94:55–56.

Richards BF, Rupp R, Zaccaro DJ, et al. Use of a standardized-patient-based clinical performance examination as an outcome measure to evaluate medical school curricula. *Acad Med.* 1996;71:S49–S51.

Schmidt HG, Norman GR, Boshuizen HP. A cognitive perspective on medical expertise: theory and implications. *Acad Med.* 1990;65:611–621.

> *Abstract:* A new theory of the development of expertise in medicine is outlined. Contrary to existing views, this theory assumes that expertise is not so much a matter of superior reasoning skills or in-depth knowledge of pathophysiological states as it is based on cognitive structures that describe the features of prototypical or even actual patients. These cognitive structures, referred to as "illness scripts," contain relatively little knowledge about pathophysiological causes of symptoms and complaints but a wealth of clinically relevant information about disease, its consequences, and the context under which illness develops. By contrast, intermediate-level students without clinical experience typically use pathophysiological, causal models of disease when solving problems. The authors review evidence supporting the theory and discuss its implications for the understanding of five phenomena extensively documented in the clinical-reasoning literature: (1) content specificity in diagnostic performance; (2) typical differences in data-gathering techniques between medical students and physicians; (3) difficulties involved in setting standards; (4) a decline in performance on certain measures of clinical reasoning with increasing expertise; and (5) a paradoxical association between errors and longer response times in visual diagnosis.

Schön DA. The new scholarship requires a new epistemology. *Change.* 1995;27:26–34.

> *Abstract:* This article argues that if higher education pursues the new norms of scholarship proposed by Ernest Boyer in "Scholarship Reconsidered," a new kind of action research is required that would conflict with the epistemology of the existing research university. An illustration of this kind of research is offered, and the epistemological, institutional, and political issues it would raise are discussed.

Slotnick HB. How doctors learn: the role of clinical problems across the medical school-to-practice continuum. *Acad Med.* 1996;71:28–34.

> *Abstract:* The author proposes a theory of how physicians learn that uses clinical problem-solving as its central feature. His theory, which integrates insights from Maslow, Schon, Norman, and others, claims that physicians-in-training and practicing physicians learn largely by deriving insights from clinical experience. These insights allow the learner to solve future problems and thereby address the learner's basic human needs for security, affiliation, and self-esteem. Ensuring that students gain such insights means that the proper roles of the teacher are (1) to select problems for students to solve and offer guidance on how to solve them, and (2) to serve as a role model of how to reflect on the problem, its solution, and the solution's effectiveness. Three principles guide instruction within its framework for learning: (1) learners, whether physicians-in-training or practicing physicians, seek to solve problems they recognize they have;

(2) learners want to be involved in their own learning; and (3) instruction must both be time-efficient and also demonstrate the range of ways in which students can apply what they learn. The author concludes by applying the theory to an aspect of undergraduate education and to the general process of continuing medical education.

Soumerai SB, Avorn J. Principles of educational outreach ("academic detailing") to improve clinical decision making. *JAMA*. 1990;263:549–556.

Abstract: Physicians' choices of drugs frequently fall short of the ideal of precise and cost-effective decision making. Evidence indicates that such decisions can be improved in a variety of ways. A number of theories and principles of communication and behavior change underlie the success of pharmaceutical manufacturers in influencing prescribing practices. Based on this behavioral science and several field trials, it is possible to define the theory and practice of methods to improve physicians' clinical decision making to enhance the quality and cost-effectiveness of care. Some of the most important techniques of such "academic detailing" include (1) conducting interviews to investigate baseline knowledge and motivations of current prescribing patterns; (2) focusing programs on specific categories of physicians as well as on their opinion leaders; (3) defining clear educational and behavioral objectives; (4) establishing credibility through a respected organizational identity, referencing authoritative and unbiased sources of information, and presenting both sides of controversial issues; (5) stimulating active physician participation in educational interactions; (6) using concise graphic educational materials; (7) highlighting and repeating the essential messages; and (8) providing positive reinforcement of improved practices in follow-up visits. The authors note the consistency of these principles with adult education theory. Use of these techniques by the nonprofit sector has been shown to reduce inappropriate prescribing as well as unnecessary health care expenditures.

Soumerai SB, McLaughlin TJ, Gurwitz JH, et al. Effect of local medical opinion leaders on quality of care for acute myocardial infarction; a randomized controlled trial. *JAMA*. 1998;279:1358–1363.

Abstract: CONTEXT: The effectiveness of recruiting local medical opinion leaders to improve quality of care is poorly understood. OBJECTIVE: To evaluate a guideline-implementation intervention of clinician education by local opinion leaders and performance feedback to 1) increase use of lifesaving drugs (aspirin and thrombolytics in eligible elderly patients, β-blockers in all eligible patients) for acute myocardial infarction (AMI), and 2) decrease use of a potentially harmful therapy (prophylactic lidocaine). DESIGN: Randomized controlled trial with hospital as the unit of randomization, intervention, and analysis. SETTING: Thirty-seven community hospitals in Minnesota. PATIENTS: All patients with AMI admitted to study hospitals over 10 months before (1992–1993, N = 2409) or after (1995–1996, N = 2938) the intervention. INTERVENTION: Using a validated survey, we identified opinion leaders at 20 experimental hospitals who influenced peers through small and large group discussions, informal consultations, and revisions of protocols and clinical pathways. They focused on 1) evidence (drug efficacy),

2) comparative performance, and 3) barriers to change. Control hospitals received mailed performance feedback. MAIN OUTCOME MEASURES: Hospital-specific changes before and after the intervention in the proportion of eligible patients receiving each study drug. RESULTS: Among experimental hospitals, the median change in the proportion of eligible elderly patients receiving aspirin was +0.13 (17% increase from 0.77 at baseline), compared with a change of −0.03 at control hospitals (P = 0.04). For β-blockers, the respective changes were +0.31 (63% increase from 0.49 at baseline) vs +0.18 (30% increase from baseline) for controls (P = 0.02). Lidocaine use declined by about 50% in both groups. The intervention did not increase thrombolysis in the elderly (from 0.73 at baseline), but nearly two thirds of eligible nonrecipients were older than 85 years, had severe comorbidities, or presented after at least 6 hours. CONCLUSIONS: Working with opinion leaders and providing performance feedback can accelerate adoption of some beneficial AMI therapies (eg, aspirin, β-blockers). Secular changes in knowledge and hospital protocols may extinguish outdated practices (eg, prophylactic lidocaine). However, it is more difficult to increase use of effective but riskier treatments (eg, thrombolysis) for frail elderly patients.

Tichy N. The teachable point of view: a primer. *Harvard Business Review*. 1999;77:82–83.

Abstract: Three things can be said about change in today's intense competitive environment: 1) It is hard; 2) It is necessary; 3) Most people are bound to resist it. The question for leaders, then is, what actually makes change happen? The answer is teaching. Or more specifically, teaching based on a mechanism that has been called the teachable point of view, which turns leaders into teachers and their students into teachers and leaders, and so on.

Weed LL. New connections between medical knowledge and patient care. *BMJ*. 1997;315:231–235.

COMMENT: This article highlights the directions we should be taking in learning outcomes. It outlines the downside of using knowledge tests to evaluate learning.